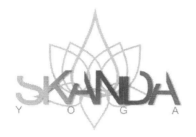

THE PRACTICE OF SKANDA YOGA
BY KENNETH F. VON ROENN III

Edited by Madison Moore & Dr. Lisa Paz

Published by ANAND

Photography by Nerissa Sparkman, Raquel Glottman, Gabriel Marquez, Wanderson M. Dos Santos, and Mauricio Velez.
Cover photo by Raquel Glottman.
Layout and cover design by Ferenc Rozumberski.

The purpose of this manual is to help students develop their yoga practice. It is not intended to supplement the guidance of a teacher. If you choose to practice any of the techniques or sequences in this manual, it is essential to have the guidance of a qualified teacher. Before beginning any physical practice of yoga, you must consult with your medical professional regarding any health issues, injuries, or physical limitations. It is recommended to read the book first before practicing any of the techniques or sequences.

www.skandayoga.com

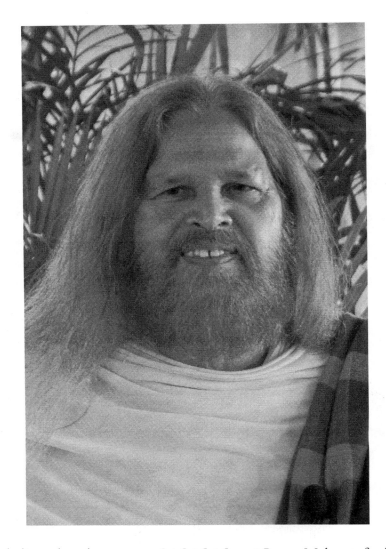

This text is dedicated to the satguru, Sri Sri Sri Svami Purna Maharaj, for his guidance, wisdom and supreme grace. May his blessings shift the awareness of humanity to the highest truth that dwells within all.

"If all the land were turned to paper,
And all the seas turned to ink,
And all the trees into pens to write with,
They would not suffice
To describe the greatness of the Guru."

Kabir

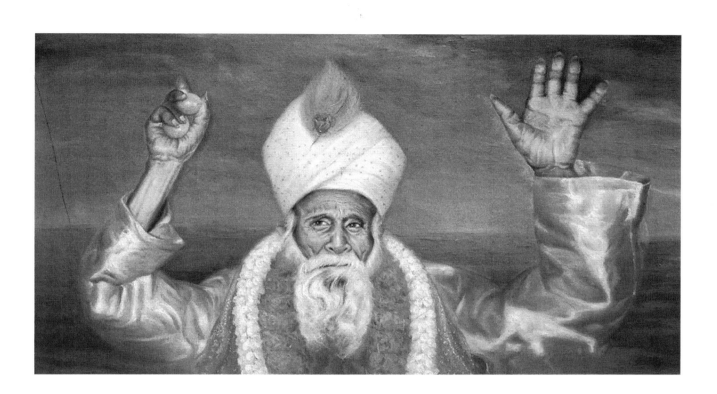

This text is also dedicated to
Sri Guru Maha Siddhar Kodi Thatha Svami
for his divine Grace and continuous work for humanity.

Guru Brahma, Guru Vishnu, Guru Devo Maheswarah
Guru Sakshaat Para-Brahma,
Tasmai Shri Guruve Namaha

The Guru is Brahma (Lord of Creation)
The Guru is Vishnu (Lord of Sustenance)
The Guru is Shiva (Lord of Deconstruction)

TABLE OF CONTENTS

PREFACE

It is with great honor and humility that I present this work on the practice of Skanda Yoga. This practice has changed my life in many ways and I hope it serves as inspiration for your own development through yoga. It was never my intention to create a yoga style or write a book, but these manifested out of necessity and the guidance of Grace.

I was a student at Arizona State University when my father suggested I take yoga to improve my flexibility for rock climbing. The first class I attended included a meditation practice and I was transfixed. I immediately knew that the trajectory of my life would somehow revolve around yoga. I began studying philosophy in school and practicing meditation and lucid dreaming.

I moved to Louisville, Kentucky to finish my degree in philosophy and to climb the high sandstone cliffs and rock walls of the Red River Gorge. By the time I finished school, I had torn rotator cuff muscles in both shoulders and impinged ligaments. I had torn hand tendons and developed scar tissue on a nerve in my foot. I was troubled by several other ailments as well and had been diagnosed with irritable bowel syndrome, acid-reflux disease and gastroparesis. I was a physical wreck. My injuries were a result of over-training and my dis-eases from physical and emotional stress. I seriously lacked balance in my life.

I enrolled in a yoga teacher-training program and had several reconstructive surgeries. My practice proved to be an invaluable tool in my rehabilitation and it eventually restored me to greater strength and flexibility than before my injuries. I decided to dedicate myself fully to all dimensions of yoga and travelled around the country to practice and study. I finally found my way to Miami, Florida and decided to settle there.

When I arrived in Miami, I was teaching Anusara® Yoga and so was Lina Vallejo, the talented teacher who would become my partner. Lina encouraged me to base my class themes on the cyclical patterns found in nature. She was convinced that this awareness would bring students into resonance with each other and with the larger flow of universal energy. She introduced me to the Dreamspell calendar and I began to integrate the teachings into my classes. I also began to include some of the scientific stretching techniques that I learned while practicing martial arts.

Skanda Yoga began to evolve from these beginnings and it grew along with the proficiencies and desires of the local yoga community. We were all developing in our practice and we needed something that could continue to challenge us and serve as a platform for higher spiritual aspirations. Lina and I formally established Skanda Yoga in 2008 and shortly afterward, we met the satguru Sri Sri Sri Svami Purna Maharaj – a siddha yoga master from the Himalayas and our guru. We feel blessed to be under his guidance and grace, and are humbled to share the sacred practice of yoga.

This manual was written for practitioners of all levels who wish to advance their yoga. It was also written for teachers who would like to introduce empowering techniques and new energies and sequences into their classes. Ultimately, it was written to align all who discover it with the guiding power of Grace and its manifestations of magic and synchronicity. We are the creators and architects of our lives and what we align with internally manifests as the world we experience externally. May this manual help you bring the two into harmonious attunement.

I am very grateful for all of the help and support I received to manifest this work. Deep gratitude to my partner in life, Lina Vallejo, for her patience, devotion, love, and divine light. Thanks to my father for directing me into yoga. Thanks to my mother for practicing with me. Thanks to my children, Adrian Wolfgang and Isabella Luna, for inspiring me. Thanks to Madison Moore for her stellar work initiating the editing process for this book. Thanks to Dr. Lisa Paz for helping finish up the editing. Thanks to Sarah Weeks and Amy Shelby for proofreading. Thanks to Nerissa Sparkman, Raquel Glottman, Garbriel "Archangel" Marquez, Wanderson M. Dos Santos, and Mauricio Velez for the great photography. Many thanks to all of my coaches and teachers over the years: Jim Kraeszig, J. Robinson, Tom Brands, Laura Spaulding, Amanda McMaine, Sianna Sherman, Mitchel Bleir, Darren Rhodes, Richard Freeman, Douglas Brooks, John Friend, and Sri Rudra Abhishek. Thanks to Cesar Lizarraga for believing in me and for all the laughs. Thanks to the Summit Series team at Powder Mountain for all the love. Thanks to Milijana at the Girl Skirt Mission for the beautiful pants. Thanks to Lama Glenn Mullin for the Dream Yoga initiation. Thanks to Sri Sri Sri Svami Purna for living and teaching the path to freedom. Thanks to the Skanda Yoga teachers for covering my classes so I could write: Kelly Gregorakis, Don Llopis, David Dorr, Gabriel Axel, and Zarid Urbina. A final thanks to all of my students and community for your great energy and open hearts. Much love to you all!!!

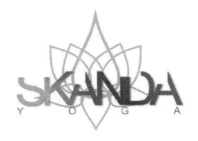

CHAPTER I

Introduction to Skanda Yoga and Origins of the Practice

Skanda Yoga is a new paradigm for the practice of *asana*[1]. It introduces alternate methods for achieving alignment, stretching and strengthening. It is a breath-inspired, alignment-based, power-style of practice. Skanda Yoga aims to develop the qualities of will, courage, and strength and, through them, prompt transformation on all levels of being. In this process, Skanda Yoga fits itself within the framework and energy of an ancient 13-moon, natural-time calendar to align with nature's cyclical patterns, and to create an almanac for revealing Grace and synchronicity. Skanda Yoga is derived from the traditional schools of Hatha Yoga and follows the path of *bhakti* or devotion. Before we delve deeper into the practice of Skanda Yoga, it is necessary to take a look at the origins and evolution of yoga as a science of spiritual alchemy and philosophy. This chapter will elucidate a historical account of how yoga developed into its modern expression.

Yoga as a spiritual discipline originated in India before 4,000 B.C.E., and existed as a meditative and ascetic practice to purify the body for higher states of consciousness. There have been artifacts discovered from the Indus Valley civilization (4000-2000 B.C.E.) that depict symbols associated with yoga and figures of cross-legged meditation postures. The Vedic period (2000-1000 B.C.E.) was inspired by the *rishis*, the sages of the forest, who were divine seers. The *rishis* heard the sacred Vedas while in deep states of meditation and trance. These revealed scriptures of divine origin are known as *agamas*, meaning "that which has come down." They are also known as *shruti*, "that which is heard," and are thus considered *apauruseya* (not of human agency).

The Vedas are a collection of the oldest spiritual books from India, and were written in the earliest form of Sanskrit. Veda means "wisdom," and comes from the root word *vid*, meaning "to know." The Vedas existed mostly through an oral tradition that was eventually compiled and then divided into four sections by the sage Vyasa (1800-1500 B.C.E.), but due to the fragile quality of the manuscripts, they would only survive for a few hundred years. The Vedas exist as an extensive collection of hymns, wisdom, stories, manuals, and discourses. They contain instruction in architecture, martial arts, and medicine.

---

1 *Asana* was originally defined as a sitting position but is now used to define any posture that promotes wellbeing.

The peak of the Vedas culminated in the advent of Vedantic philosophy (800 B.C.E.). Vedanta means "the end or the culmination of the Vedas," and refers to the philosophy of the Upanishads, which means "to sit near and listen," and is a collection of short stories of teachings from the gurus of antiquity. The teachings are to be transmitted by a guru to a disciple even in the modern age. Only then can a disciple receive the energy or *shaktipat* (divine energy transmitted from the guru to student).

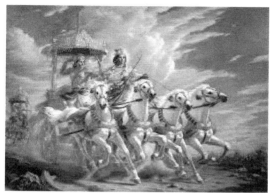

1.1 Arjuna and Krishna from Bhagavad Gita

The sacred texts of the Ramayana, Mahabharata, and the Puranas are all recognized as *smriti*, "that which is remembered," and are not divinely revealed as was the case with the Vedas. Instead they come from tradition, insight, and experience. The Mahabharata contains 10,000 verses and the Skanda Purana contains 84,000 verses. They are the two largest spiritual texts from India. The Bhagavad Gita ("Song of God") is the 18th chapter of the Mahabharata. It is an important scripture in Hinduism, composed between the 5th and 2nd century B.C.E., it consists of 700 verses. The work is culturally significant because it united the two streams of yoga: the *shramanic* ascetic path with the teachings of Vedas from the Brahmin caste. It made the spiritual path attainable for the householder, so anyone could practice the science of yoga regardless of their life circumstance.

The Bhagavad Gita is the story of the god-head incarnate, Krishna, who gives council to Arjuna, the warrior who is faced with great fear and indecisiveness. According to Krishna, the root of all suffering and discord is the agitation of the mind caused by selfish desire. The only way to douse the flame is by stilling the mind through self-discipline and a devoted spiritual practice. In the Bhagavad Gita, the aim of yoga is to attain self-realization and link action and perception in the moment while staying in remembrance of the Divine light in all beings. The words of Krishna made Arjuna see his actions in clear light. The battle on the plains of Kurukshetra was no ordinary war; it was a battle to relieve the earth goddess Bhoodevi from the burden of *adharma* (injustice).

Krishna counsels Arjuna on the greater idea of *dharma* as a universal law of harmony and duty. He begins with the tenet that the *jiva* (soul) is eternal and immortal. Any death on the battlefield would only involve the shedding of the physical form and the release of the soul. He teaches that Arjuna's hesitation comes from a lack of understanding of the nature of things. His fear has become an obstruction to the balance of universal order. Arjuna still wants to abandon action, and is warned that inaction would cause the cosmos to fall from order and truth.

Krishna then expounds the yoga paths of jnana yoga (yoga of knowledge), karma yoga (yoga of action), and bhakti yoga (yoga of devotion) to clarify his teachings. Fundamentally, the Bhagavad Gita teaches that true enlightenment comes from growing beyond identification of the ego and the ephemeral world, so that one identifies with the truth of the immortal self. Through detachment and the practices of yoga, it is possible to transcend the ego and identify with the supreme.

The myth is an allegory for experience, and is highly symbolic. The battlefield is the field of *dharma,* or the field of action. The war is the battle between good and evil. Arjuna represents the Lower Self that is filled with doubt, fear, and skepticism. Krishna represents the Higher Self that is all-knowing, and filled with trust and confidence. The chariot represents the body, and the horses represent the senses of the body, which pull the mind in every direction. The warrior who listens to the advice of the Divine from within will triumph in life and attain the highest good.

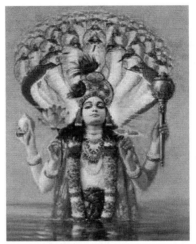

1.2 Vishnu with cosmic serpent

The Yoga Sutras were written by Patanjali around 200 C.E. He was the first to assemble and catalog the teachings of yoga that had been in circulation for some time. In Sanskrit, the name Patanjali means "a fallen prayer" or "the prayer of one who has fallen." It could also be interpreted as, "a prayer for those who have fallen from grace." The name 'Anjali' is in reference to *Adi Ananta Sesha (one-infinite-nothing),* the primordial serpent that supports the cosmos, which represents the three levels of consciousness (subconscious, conscious, and unconscious). *Vishnu* (the Sustainer of the cosmos) lies on the coiled serpent, and represents the *turiya,* the transcendental fourth state of super consciousness. Patanjali was the physical manifestation of this serpent. The serpent has an infinite number of heads with one tail, which shows that there are many teachings and many paths of yoga, but ultimately they all have the same root and will take you to the same place.

The Yoga Sutras exist as short aphorisms where the teachings were concise enough that a student could memorize all 195 sutras. These teachings had been around for centuries, and Patanjali organized them in their present form. Scholars have also theorized that there may have been interpolations throughout the Sutras' history. This is common for a great work that is practiced by so many. It is only natural that as the methods became more precise and refined, practitioners wanted to contribute to the text.

Patanjali organized the book into four chapters. Each one expands upon the former with more teachings and philosophy. The first is *samadhi pada*, which deals with the nature of *samadhi* (bliss). The second is *sadhana pada*, and deals with the practices to attain *samadhi*. It formalizes the practices of *Kriya* and *Ashtanga Yoga*. The third is *vibhuti pada* and outlines the attainment of super natural powers. The fourth chapter is *kaivalya pada*, literally meaning "aloneness," and deals with the state of liberation.

Patanjali starts with the highest teachings first and then expounds the philosophies of Kriya Yoga and Ashtanga Yoga for more support of the practice of *samadhi*.

Below are some of the key sutras that outline the philosophies:

Sutra 1.1 *atha yoganusasanam*

Now is the moment to embrace the practice of yoga. We offer our hearts and ask for blessings in return. No effort is lost on the path of self-awareness. Begin the practice again as if doing it for the first time every day.

Sutra 1.2 *yogah cittavritti nirodhah*

Yoga is attained when the fluctuations of the mind cease. *Niroddha* could also be translated as suppression, suspension, to still, or release. The seer stands still in its own form, and this is a state of enlightenment. Over-identification with *chitta vritti* causes suffering, and they must be controlled, or accepted for what they are without identifying with them. Absence of thought does not make yoga a non-intellectual practice. Yoga is the perfection of philosophy and the art of thinking. It is not just giving up, and deciding not to think. It is intelligently relating to the thoughts of oneself and others.

Sutra 1.3 *tada drastuh svarupe avasthanam*

Then, the seer dwells in his own splendor. The seer just sees, but is different from the seen. This only becomes apparent when the mind and senses are at rest, and only the seer remains. Union is the natural state of one's true Self, but we create a dualistic split by getting caught up in the mind. When we are wrestling with our mind, we feel separate from others and the source of creation. When we are at peace and rest, then we are returning to our natural state of being.

Sutra 2.1 *tapah svadhyaya Isvarapranidhanani kriyayogah*

Burning zeal in practice, self-study and study of scriptures, and surrender to God are the acts of yoga.

This outlines the three aspects of *Kriya Yoga*: tapas, swadhya, Isvara pranidhana. Entering the sacred space, and cultivating the center of being develops *tapas* (inner heat), which is necessary to burn off impurities to seek the path of enlightenment. *Swadhya* is self-reflection or self-study, a philosophical introspection to find the source of our suffering and our true self. Traditionally, this means the study of the Vedas, but in the modern world, it warrants a broader scope and application. *Isvara pranidhana* is the dedication of the fruits of one's efforts to the Supreme Being.

The purpose of kriya yoga is *samadhi*. The second purpose is to lessen the *kleshas* or the torments that block the experience of yoga.

Five *Kleshas*:

-*Avidya* (ignorance)

-*Asmita* (ego)

-*Raga* (passion)

-*Dvesha* (repulsion)

-*Abhinivesha* (fear of death)

The final *klesha* is *abhinivesha*, meaning "clinging to life," which is experienced as the fear of death. It is very intimately connected to the deeper aspects of yoga. The reaction to a personal loss is one of fear and panic, but this is the dawning of discriminative awareness, that everything is impermanent.

Kriya yoga removes *avidya*, ignorance, which is the cause of all torments. Until we have an experience of union, we aspire to repair the surface of things. It is like trying to decorate your prison cell without realizing you hold a key to get out. The practice of yoga is beneficial and successful when we are able to overcome the root of suffering. If we grasp for something, then we are clinging to something that is inseparable from the rest. When we grasp, then we also reach for its opposite, which is memory. Dissolution and pleasure are the natural state of mind. Once grounded in *samadhi*, it cannot be maintained due to an unconscious agitation. Patanjali prescribes the eight-limbs of yoga as a means to stay rooted in the practice in any situation.

The Yoga Sutras outline the philosophical system of yoga known as Raja Yoga (the kingly path) or Ashtanga Yoga (the eight limbed path). Ashtanga Yoga should not be confused with the Ashtanga vinyasa (*yoga chikitsa*) system of Krishnamcharya. The eight limbs of Yoga are: *yama* (self-restraints), *niyama* (self-observations), *asana* (posture), *pranayama* (breath liberation), *pratyahara* (sense withdrawal), *dharana* (one pointed focus), *dhyana* (meditation) and *samadhi* (bliss). The first four limbs are referred to as the external limbs, as they concern the body's appearance and attitude. The last four limbs are the inner limbs that are concerned with one's inner state of being. There are five *yamas* and five *niyamas*, each of which similar to the Ten Commandments to build an ethical and moral practice. However, one should not feel guilty if one of the *yamas* or *niyamas* is transgressed. The negative energy associated with the act will prevent one from practicing, and will lead to suffering. Maintain a steady practice and eventually the *yamas* and *niyamas* will come into alignment with your intentions to manifest the highest good.

Five *Yamas*:

-*Ahimsa*: non-violence, cause no harm, including to the Self. In yoga, it is important to be mindful of one's thoughts. It is easy to compare and judge one's performance negatively. This inner negativity is a form of violence because we are diminishing our self-worth. Also, if we avoid the poses that we aren't good at, or avoid a side because it is more difficult, then this creates a physical imbalance, which is another form of inflicting violence against oneself.

-*Satya*: truthfulness. Speak the truth and act in accordance. In yoga, be honest with one's level of practice. Don't push your body into a space it is not ready for.

-*Asteya*: non-stealing. Not to claim things for ourselves, but see all things as an interconnected whole. In yoga, remember that our power does not arise from within but is supplied by Grace.

-*Bramacharya*: celibacy. To act as a *Brahman* or to have an ethical sexual practice. A practice that follows *ahimsa*, *satya*, and *asteya*.

-*Aparigraha*: non-coveting. Yoga deals with love, and if the *yamas* are practiced, then love is allowed to flourish. Remain grateful for all that you have and you will attract more abundance in your life.

Five *Niyamas*:

-*Saucha*: cleanliness. Shower before a yoga practice to refresh the senses and not to offend others if attending a class.

-*Santosha*: contentment. Aligning as best we can, and being happy for no particular reason, but to suspend cares, worries, and desires. Contentment cultivates patience.

-*Tapas*: austerity, burning zeal, the heat generated from practice. We generate *tapas* through vigorous practices and long holds in *asana*.

-*Svadhya*: self-study. Study the Self through reading sacred texts, meditation, and *japa* (prayer repetition).

-*Isvara Pranidhana*: dedication to *Isvara*. Dedicate all our actions for the highest good.

Asana is described as that which enables meditation to arise spontaneously. There are only two verses in the entire Yoga Sutras on *asana,* which are listed for the purpose of meditation. The word *asana* comes from the verbal root *as*, meaning "to sit". The body is transformed into a good seat or platform. All *asanas* have two qualities: *sthira*, meaning "stable," and *sukham* meaning "happy" or "easy."

Pranayama is practiced after the poses are established in proficiency. It is traditionally said that *pranayama* is breath control, but the two root words are *prana* and *ayama*. *Prana* means "life force energy," and *ayama* means "to remove control or restrictions." *Pranayama* is thus a releasing or freeing of the *prana* by bringing structure to the breath.

Pratyahara is the withdrawal of the senses. Refraining from identifying with outer sensations. It is the turning of the senses within. To listen, feel, taste, and sense the inner space. The outer world we experience is a response to the inner world we cultivate. Take time each day to direct the senses within to contemplate the world you wish to create for yourself.

Dharana is a field of concentration. It requires an intention or desire to concentrate. It creates a wall from other sensory experiences so the mind can concentrate on a technique, *yantra* (geometric symbol), or *japa* (prayer repetition). *Dharana* progresses into meditation and a sense of ease in concentration.

Dhyana is uninterrupted absorption in meditation. The practitioner merges completely with the object of concentration. It is absorption into the field of concentration, so there are no longer internal or external pressures on *dharana*. There is a sense that the mind doesn't have to move for concentration to deepen.

Samadhi is the attainment of bliss. Ecstatic rapture, crying, or laughing can characterize it. There are many types and many levels to *samadhi*, which arises when there is no longer an observer who is observing. Through the practice of *samadhi,* the connection between body and soul can be suspended for as long as desired.

The eight limbs do not have to be practiced in progression. They are akin to branches of a tree, and all begin to flourish through the practice. Yoga is simply defined as paying close attention to what is presented in the moment, and through the practice, the three fundamental urges of the *gunas*[2] (qualities of nature) no longer have an object towards which they function.

Tantra Philosophy

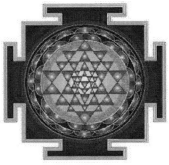

1.3 Sri Yantra

Tantra yoga developed around 600 C.E. and fully blossomed between the 9th and 13th century. The name tantra comes from the root word *tan*, meaning "to stretch." Tantra can be interpreted many ways, which has led to many definitions. Thus, it could mean: to warp reality, to loom, or to apply technique. In short, Tantra is the means by which knowledge is extended, and spread out. It is the continuity between the path of a worldly life, and that of liberation.

Tantric philosophy merged into the religious streams of Hinduism, Buddhism, and Jainism. It has been established in Southern Asia, China, Japan, Tibet, Korea, Cambodia, Burma, Indonesia, and Mongolia. Those who followed the philosophy were called *tantrikas*, and their teachers were called Siddhas. The Nath Siddhas are largely credited with the innovation of hatha yoga as a formal practice. Matsyendranath, Goraknath, and Jalendaranath were the greatest among them.

---

2 There are three *gunas*: *tamas* (low vibration, inert, dark, cool), *rajas* (high vibration, active, bright, hot), and *sattva* (balance, peace, pure).

Tantra does not affirm or deny other philosophies, but offers a dynamic synthesis and revision of elements from previous systems. The first revision was in relation to the concept of *prakriti* (matter). It had been previously viewed as a problematic element of nature, but in Tantra it no longer was an obstacle to overcome. *Prakriti* was now celebrated as a manifestation of the divine, and was known as *Shakti*, the feminine principle of creation.

In Tantra, there is an emphasis on absolute freedom (*svatatrya*), which is attained by the knowledge that matter cannot contaminate spirit, and that one has the ability to act perfectly in an imperfect world. This creative freedom in the domain of *Shakti* was known as the power of *Shiva*. To live with this awareness of liberation was the state of a *Jivamukti* (liberated soul).

The tantrikas taught that the Vedic teachings were too difficult to live during the Kali Yuga (iron age; the current world age of darkness and disillusionment), and that there was a simpler means that allowed access to the Divine. Tantra is not a single coherent system, but an accumulation of practices and ideas. The common characteristics are the use of the mundane to access the Divine, and the identification of the macrocosm within the mirocosm.

Tantra practitioners use many tools to cultivate the sacred space. Hatha yoga is practiced to increase awareness, strengthen the spirit, and purify the body. Mantras are used to evoke blessings, and yantras (geometric symbols) are used as visualization tools to strengthen *dharana* (concentration). Identification and internalization of the Divine is enacted through a complete association of one's Self with the deity of worship. This allows the attributes of mythical characters to be embodied within the individual.

Tantrism is the quest for spiritual perfection and supernatural power. The purpose is to achieve complete control over the forces of nature and oneself, and at the same time to release the desire to control, and accept all that is presented to the mind. The aim is to sublimate reality instead of negating it. The process of sublimation consists of three phases: purification, elevation, and the affirmation of pure consciousness as the central identity.

There are two approaches to the Tantric path. The right-handed path is *Dakshina Marga*, and is more conservative. *Kaula Marga* is the left-handed path, which employs radical techniques to attain realization. Left-handed *tantrikas* used ritual sexual intercourse, not for pleasure, but as a way of cultivating spiritual awareness and magical power. In the west, the name "Tantra" has become synonymous with "sex." This is a gross misunderstanding of the spiritual depth of the practice.

The Nath sect of *kanpatha* (split eared) yogins[3] formalized the practice of hatha yoga *asana* in the 8th century of our current era. It was developed as a reaction to the growing popularity of Buddhism in India. The yogins noticed that the long hours of meditation and study depleted the body of vital energy and created an imbalance between the physical and mental energies. The use of *asana* to strengthen the body for meditation and the inner practice was used before this time, but it had never been formalized into a practice unto itself. This has led to great confusion regarding the origins of the practice where Patanjali is often mistakenly attributed as the originator of yoga *asana*.

---

3 *Kanpatha* yogins were known as the 'split-eared' ones, because they would pierce their ears with heavy objects to stretch them out as a sign of knowledge and progress on the spiritual path.

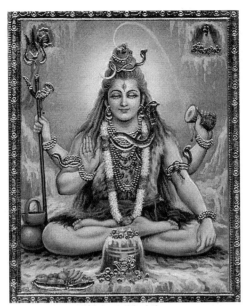

1.4 image of Lord Shiva

The origins of the Nath sect are enshrouded in myth. One day Shiva and Parvati were having a conversation about meditation near a body of water. A fish overheard the discourse and fell into a deep trance meditation. Shiva was very impressed by the fish and granted him a physical form. He became known as the sage Matsyendranath. His disciple was Goraknath, who founded the Nath sect, and is considered the father of modern hatha yoga.

The three main texts on hatha yoga are the Hatha Yoga Pradipika by Yogi Swatmarama (15th century), the Shiva Samhita (17th century), and the Gheranda Samhita by Yogi Gheranda (17th century). These texts helped to establish the development of several modern hatha yoga schools like the Bihar School of Yoga and the Himalayan Institute. Swami Sivananda (Sivananda Yoga) and Swami Satchidananda (Integral Yoga) have also contributed to the rise of yoga's popularity. There were several modern schools of hatha yoga that developed from the hatha yoga movement, but most have been influenced by Tirumalai Krishnamacharya, a yogi from Mysore, India (1888-1989).

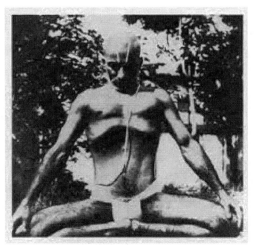

1.5 Krishnamacharya in mulabhandasana

Krishnamacharya traveled throughout India studying and debating philosophy. He realized he needed a true master, so he walked for two and a half months to reach the cave of Sri Brahmachari located in the mountains of Tibet. He lived there for eight years studying yoga, pranayama, and therapeutics. He returned to Mysore, and began teaching Ashtanga *vinyasa* yoga. His student Pattabhi Jois (1915-2009) founded the Ashtanga Yoga Research Institute, which is led today by his grandson Sharath Jois.

B.K.S. Iyengar was also a student of Krisnamacharya. He began studying Ashtanga *vinyasa*, but then began to teach the poses with the support of props and strict alignment. Poses were held for a longer duration to refine the form of each pose, as opposed to the Ashtanga *vinyasa* system, where each pose is held for a maximum of five breaths. The American yoga teacher John Friend was a student of Iyengar who developed Anusara® Yoga, an open-heart style that emphasized the Universal Principles of Alignment.

Skanda is the name of a character in Hindu mythology, a warrior and prince and an archetype of both attacking and uniting. The word *yoga* translates from Sanskrit as "union" or "to unite." *Hatha* is a word combined from two *beeja* or seed mantras[1]. *Ha* translates as "solar" and refers to *Prana* or life force, and *tha* to "lunar" and refers to mental energy or *manas*. The aim of hatha yoga is to unite the *Prana* or life-force energy with the *manas* or mental force. The two energies are also referred to as the god and goddess energies and in the Hindu pantheon of deities are represented by Lord Shiva and the Goddess Shakti. *Skanda* represents the union of these complementary opposites of *shiva* and *shakti* and symbolizes the energy of a spiritual warrior.

Skanda Yoga embodies the energies of the 13-Moon Dreamspell Calendar to align students and their practice with nature's cyclical patterns of time. While we may no longer be aware of these patterns, we tend to suffer when our actions fall out of sync with their energetic possibilities and thrive when we are attuned to them. Skanda Yoga utilizes many different techniques that allow *asana* to be practiced differently every day. There are four introductory sequences for beginners at level 0, and 20 unique sequences at levels I-III for beginners to advanced practitioners that are based upon the cyclical patterns found in nature.

Yoga is a physical, mental and spiritual practice that can become a way of life. In its demand for immediate focus and attention, it brings us into the moment; it centers our energy into presence. Every experience in life can either strengthen or diminish our energy. Yoga is a means of establishing and maintaining strength on all levels without letting doubt, skepticism, or negativity deter us from our dreams and goals. A commitment to our yoga practice helps us to stay committed to our beliefs and to the convictions of our heart. Ultimately, yoga is practiced to expand us by moving us beyond limiting concepts of the self and into a greater possibility of being in the world.

The aim of Skanda Yoga is to present a format for the practice that is engaging, fun, challenging, and transformative. Before we explore the practice, let's meet the character behind the name.

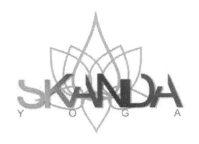

CHAPTER 2

Skanda in Hindu Mythology

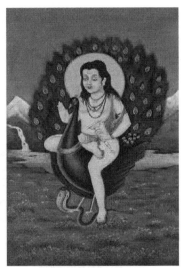

2.1 Skanda riding the peacock

Skanda Yoga takes its name from a warrior who appears in the early Hindu sacred texts[4]. His is the oldest historical myth of a son of god who is a hero and divine savior. Skanda's father is Shiva, the archetype of destructive forces. Shiva is a *mahadeva* – a great god – and he is one of the holy trinity or *trimurti* of gods in Hindu mythology. The other two are Brahma, the creator, and Vishnu, the sustainer and preserver of the universe. Vishnu incarnates ten times within human history, sending avatars to reestablish *dharma* – the way of virtuous action. His energy is regarded as that of the "higher self." Vishnu represents that aspect of god-within-human that is also referred to as the "son of Shiva." This makes Skanda, first-born of Shiva, an auspicious character who embodies the savior energy of Vishnu's avatars.

In the mythological stories of the sacred texts, Shiva noticed that there was great suffering in humanity. He approached Brahma to ask why. Brahma sprouted four heads to observe the four directions of his creation and became quite pleased with what he saw. After reflecting upon it, he sprouted a fifth head to hold his pride. This infuriated Shiva. He was disgusted with Brahma's pride and considered his response a lack of concern for the human condition. He chopped off Brahma's fifth head and retreated to the forest in anger.

---

4 The Hindu scriptures are comprised of the *Vedas, Upanishads, Puranas* and Sanskrit epics *Mahabharata* and *Ramayana*.

Shiva meditated in forests and in cremation grounds, embarked on austerities and engaged yogic practices. During this time, he encountered Sati, an avatar of the goddess Shakti, and Shiva's complementary opposite. Inevitably, They fell in love and married. Sati's family did not accept Shiva as a suitable mate for her. His skin and long dreadlocked hair were caked in cremation ash. He wore a necklace of skulls and was attended by fearsome ghosts and other unmentionables of society; he smoked ganja from a chillum. Sati's parents showed their disapproval of Shiva by omitting the couple from a guest list for a fire ceremony to which the family's close relatives had all been invited. Thinking the lack of invitation to be a mistake, Sati went anyway. When she learned that it was intentional, and that her father meant to publicly denounce Shiva, she walked into the fire and killed herself. Shiva arrived and exacted his revenge. His grief was unbearable and he again retreated to the places of shadows and death to become absorbed in meditation.

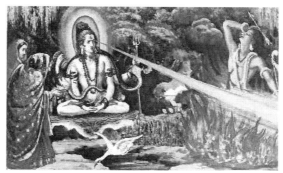
2.2 Shiva destroys the god of love

Shakti incarnated again; this time as Parvati, daughter of the mountain king Himalaya. She grew into womanhood and secluded herself on the mountain, pining for Shiva. Shiva was lost in meditation and disengaged from all else. Fearing that the two would never meet, the gods sent Kandarpa, a *kamadeva* or love god, to pierce Shiva with his arrow. Disturbed by the interruption, Shiva opened his third eye and burned Kandarpa to ashes. But the pair were destined to come together, as no position or thing can exist without its opposite. Shiva and Parvati married in a great ceremony at the home of her father.

At this time, demonic forces were at play in the world. Taraka, an asura[5], has been granted the boon of immortality by Brahma. Taraka's boon was conditional. He could only be defeated by the son of Shiva – a son who was yet to be born. Feeling invincible, Taraka and his demon cohorts, Surapadma and Simhamukha, terrorize the world with their awesome power.

There are several myths describing the birth of Shiva's first son. While they may differ in details, they all contain a symbolical birth sequence in which the life force is embodied into the five elements. The *tejas* represents the vital essence of life. In this myth, it is the semen of Shiva and was too potent and filled with heat for any to bear. It was carried by Vayu, the god of wind, and he offered it to the fire god Agni. Unable to sustain it, Agni gave it to the river Ganga, the goddess of water, who would *skandh* or spurt it up onto the shore. The seed came from *akasha* or space; it was carried by the wind, offered to the fire, given to the water, and finally, pushed onto the earth. The story of Skanda's birth represents the idea that the life force or spiritual essence of an individual is manifested through the five elements.

---

5 Asuras were described as dark and demonic. They are exactly opposite the devas who were thought of as the light and godly.

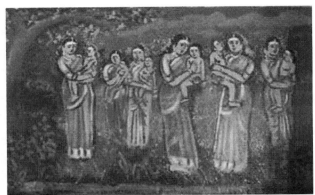

2.3 The Krittikas tend the babies

As it landed in a brilliant thicket of reeds, the seed produced a divine child, split into six beings. Indra, god of rain and thunderstorms, a principal deity and twin brother of Agni, brought the six Krittikas[6] to nurse the babies until Parvati arrived to take them. In Hindu mytho-astronomy, the Krittikas represent the six stars of the Pleiades constellation, which can be found exactly opposite the rotational center of the Milky Way galaxy. Like Shiva and Shakti, these opposing pairs represent duality and complementary yet opposite energies. The same model is found in the body where the galactic center is represented by the root or *mula chakra*[7], and the Pleiades the crown or *sahasrara*.

Parvati arrived to claim her offspring and assembled the six boys into one body with six faces and twelve arms. This act symbolically represents the six aspects of the higher self that combine at the *sahasrara*. They are *bala* (strength and valor), *jnana* (wisdom and knowledge), *vairagya* (detachment and dispassion), *keerti* (fame or recognition), *sri* (grace, beauty and prosperity), and *aishwarya* (affluence and divine powers). It is believed that the six qualities of the higher self develop naturally when one embraces the practice of yoga as the vehicle of transformation.

Skanda was born to defeat Taraka and his asura brothers Surapadma and Simhamukha. Together, the three represent the trinity of the ego mind – the dark forces of *karma* or accumulated actions, *kama* or pleasure, and *avidya* or ignorance. Skanda swiftly defeated them with his *vel*[8] and thus, the egoic energies were defeated by wisdom and one-pointed focus.

Skanda's mode of transportation or *vahana* was a peacock. When he was carried on its back, he had overcome the egoic energies of vanity and pride. When he dismounted, the peacock transforms back into the demon Surapadma. This is potent imagery that corresponds to our personal dedication to the practice of yoga. When we engage the practice fully we ride the peacock on a path of radiance. When we stop practicing, patterns, habits and negative tendencies are likely to return.

---

6 The Krittikas were sister-devas whose name translates to mean "the cutters." Since Skanda was raised by them, he is often referred to as Kārtikeya – him of the Krittika.

7 In Hindu metaphysical traditions, the *chakras* are energy centers located along the central axis of the body through which *prana* or vital life energy flows.

8 To defeat the asuras, Skanda's mother presents him with the *vel* – a divine javelin or spear. The gesture symbolizes the gift of the primordial cosmic energy or empowerment that is shakti.

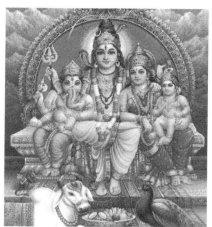

2.4 Skanda with his brother Ganesha and parents Shiva and Parvati

Although Skanda was the first-born son of Shiva and Parvati, he later lost his birthright in a competition with his brother Ganesha, who proved his cunning and wisdom. Their parents challenged the boys to race around the world three times for the pleasure of a beautiful golden mango. Skanda took flight on his peacock, but Ganesha had only a tiny bandicoot to ride. He departed quickly while Ganesha rested in contemplation. Ganesha realized that his parents contained all of creation within them. He circled them three times and they declared him the winner. Meanwhile, Skanda took his time to enjoy sacred sites as he circled the world. Upon his return, he was quite dismayed to find that his brother had outwitted him. To add insult to injury, Ganesha laughed at Skanda for his misplaced confidence. Skanda was outraged. He left their home in the Himalayas and travelled to south India.

Skanda is thought of as the lord of *lila* – the divine play and possibility. Skanda's *bhava* or attitude is broody, sometimes sweet and sometimes strong. Ganesha is the lord of *karma* and represents order and probability. His *bhava* is always happy and relaxed. Ganesha, as an elephant, is out in the open. He cannot hide and his next steps are always clearly visible. His actions are overt and his influence is always apparent. Ganesha represents the law of cause and effect and *karma*. Skanda is the unseen stalker of the moment, ready to pierce it with uncertainty and possibility. He hides in the forest of reeds and is hard to see. His actions are covert and his influence is always hidden. Skanda embraces and transforms energies that would otherwise be self-negating. He utilizes the energies of narcissism and nihilism to perfect the self and inspire others. Their stories represent aspects of our own consciousness as we play these opposing yet complementary roles in our lives. Ganesha represents the earth, order, stability and predictability, while Skanda represents play, magic and synchronicity. The two are ever present as *karma* (action) and *lila* (divine play).

The Skanda myth symbolizes the personal quest to become a warrior in the battle between *avidya* and *jnana* (ignorance and knowledge). The asura forces in the stories represent the lower, egoic nature, and the deva forces represent the higher energies of the divine. Helping us to find our way is the guru – the personification of the *skanda-shakti*. Skanda is the lord of the *shaktis* – the all-pervading, cosmic and spiritual powers. He marries Valli and Devayani, who represent *iccha* (intention and will power) and *kriya* (cleansing, purifying action); his *vel* represents *jnana* (spiritual knowledge). This places him as archetype of *iccha-jana-kriya shaktis*. It takes right intention and right knowledge to manifest a goal. To be successful in our attempts to overcome limiting patterns and the lower forces of our nature, we must first prove ourselves to be a dedicated aspirant or *adhikari*. Only then can we receive the *shaktipat* or *guru's* grace that fuels us on our path of transformation.

When the devas approached Vishnu and asked for a savior to defeat the marauding asuras, they had recognized that they couldn't do it themselves. Divine power was needed. This story suggests that we may need help in defeating the "asuric" forces that are within us. These forces are the patterns that keep us stuck in cycles of resistance and habits of reaction to situations, people and events that appear and arise in our lives. These patterns are the *samskaras* and their roots reach deep into our developmental conditioning. When we can begin to see our *samskaras* and recognize how they impact our mental and emotional well-being, we can develop an intention to work toward overcoming them. Skanda steps forth as the avatar of a higher power that has the grace to save us when we recognize that we can't do it ourselves.

The Skanda myth migrated to Persia and influenced Mithraism. Mitra was an Indian solar deity who became a benevolent Persian god. Over time, Mitra assumed attributes from Agni, Shiva and Skanda. Elements of the Skanda myth also influenced other savior myths like those of Adonis, Attis, Hercules, Krishna, Buddha, and Christ. They all represent the embodiment of the divine spirit and the godlike greatness that is latent in each and all. Their mythic tales represent the body as the temple and the mind as the battlefield. The prize of the war that is waged there is happiness and peace.

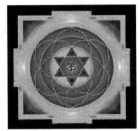

2.5 Skanda yantra

The *yantra* is a geometric symbol that is used as an instrument to balance the mind and focus it on spiritual concepts. The Skanda *yantra* has a six-pointed star in the center. This star is usually referred to as the Star of David but its use is ancient and far pre-dates the appearance of the symbol in Judaism. The star is comprised of intersecting ascending and descending triangles. The ascending triangle represents the upward-rising masculine energy that is characterized by Shiva. The descending triangle represents the manifesting, falling and coagulating energies of Shakti. The energies of god and goddess – *shiva-shakti* – are said to merge in the body at the heart space. Skanda represents the merger and union of the two energies.

In Skanda Yoga, the downward triangle is used to set daily intentions for physical action and the upward triangle for personal and spiritual aspiration. They each have a power, action, and essence (*iccha, jnana, kriya*) that are embodied through the practice to create the cellular memory, which leads to remembrance and embodiment.

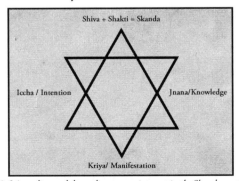

2.6 Ascending and descending powers intersect in the Skanda yantra

Now that we know a bit about the mythological Skanda and the powerful ideas he represents, we can be reminded of them as we engage the practical applications and expressions of *asana* in the body.

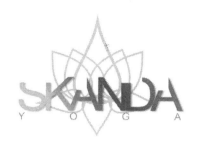

CHAPTER 3

The Foundations of Asana – Hands and Feet

The foundation in the yogic posture or *asana* provides and maintains alignment and integrity for the pose. More often than not, yoga practices focus on developing strength in all parts of the body except those that provide support. Since the possibilities in a pose match the energy and strength of the foundation, it is wise to develop the structures of the hands and feet. There are many foundation variations that can be practiced with sound technique. They can deepen an opening in the body and be utilized for the development of strength. The following positions in this chapter are presented as tools to enhance any hatha yoga practice.

The Hands

The hands are the foundation in *vinyasa,* which are the transition movements between poses that are matched to the initiation and length of the breath. It is necessary to set the foundation of the hands properly to prevent injury to the wrists. This is particularly important in arm-balance and inverted poses. When they provide all or part of the foundation for a pose, the hands are commonly positioned flat on the floor with fingers spreading out widely. It isn't possible to actually grip a flat surface unless the hands are active and, the more active they are, the more possible it is to grip and to maintain good form in the pose. If the weight of the body is borne by the outer edge of the hand, the result will be destabilization in the pose and strain in the connective tissue of the wrist. To begin to engage a strong foundation in the hands, the focus should be on rooting the index knuckle down. This keeps weight evenly distributed between the inner and outer edges of the wrist.

The most common positioning of the hands in a foundational application is with the outside edge of the wrist aligned with the outside edge of the shoulder (see figure 3.1). This placement automatically shifts more weight on the outer edge of the wrist. The hands then have to work harder to keep the index knuckle down. If the hands are wider and the midpoint of the hand—the space between the index and middle finger—is aligned with the outside edge of the shoulder, as shown in figure 3.2, then weight shifts to the center of the hands. This is of particular importance during *vinyasa* as it also initiates more external rotation in the top of the arm bones. This outer rotation reduces stress on the attachment tissues of the subscapularis muscle – one of the small, stabilizing muscles of the shoulder referred to collectively as the rotator cuff.

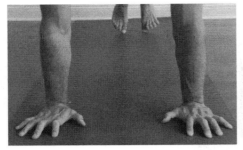 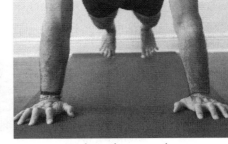

3.1 Hands in narrow position with active grip. *3.2 Hands in wide position with active grip*

In Skanda Yoga, the hands are placed in both the narrow and wide positions depending upon the *asana* and the practitioner. The hands are aligned with the outside edge of the shoulder when the arms are straight overhead. The hands are taken wider when the arms are bent and below the head. In both positions, the hands actively grip or claw the mat to protect the wrists and stimulate muscular engagement in the arms. The hands activate by pressing down through all corners and as a result, the palms of the hands lift up. This is known as *hasta bandha* or hand lock. When executed properly, the middle knuckle of the fingers also lifts off the mat. This places more power in the fingertips, and roots the base knuckle of each finger firmly down. These actions of rooting down lift more than the palm and center finger knuckles. They also draw the flexor retinaculum[9] up, which protects the connective tissue of the wrist. All of these actions strengthen the hands, fingers and wrists over time.

Establishing a Grip

When the hands are engaged as described above, the action of pulling the fingertips back toward the palms creates a strong grip. The middle knuckles will lift and the base knuckles—those closest to the hand—push down. At first, it may be difficult to engage all of the fingers in this way at once. If it is, start with the index finger and gradually engage the remaining fingers one by one. When the hand and fingers are fully engaged, they will resemble a tarantula.

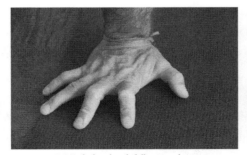 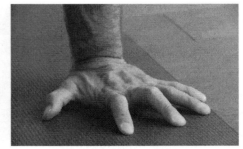

3.3 Right hand with fully engaged grip *3.4 Left hand with fully engaged grip*

---

9   The flexor retinaculum is a strong band of fibrous ligament that arches over the carpus and converts the deep groove on the front of the carpal bones into a tunnel – the carpal tunnel.

When the grip is executed improperly, or not at all, the index knuckle will lift. Weight will shift to the outside edge of the hand and can cause a strain in the wrist that can result in injury if performed habitually.

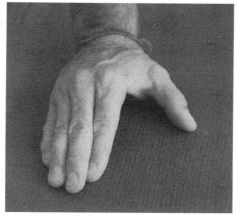

3.5 Unengaged hand

Engaging a Claw

Pressing the fingertips down strongly creates a claw-like appearance in the fingers and is another form of *hasta bandha*. This is done as an alternative to pulling the fingertips back toward the hand as described above. The fingers remain straight and the middle knuckle lifts while the base knuckle presses down. Depending on the practitioner, the claw may be easier to perform than the grip. In either case, the fingertips press down so strongly that they become whiter than the rest of the finger as the blood is dispersed away from the area by the pressure.

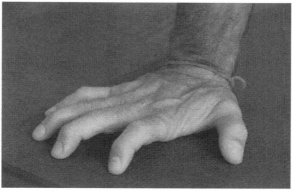

3.6 Fingers in a claw position

Hands Elevated to Ridgetops

Supporting the hand on the base knuckles of the fingers while lifting the palm of the hand off the floor is often referred to as a "ridgetop" position. The Sanskrit term is *utthita hasta,* or rising hand. This hand-placement variation is sometimes done to gain height and extension. It is also employed to produce strength in the hands. When used in a foundational position, the hands are not pointing straight ahead (see figure 3.7). When the fingers are pointing straight ahead and lifted to ridgetops, it is very difficult to grip with the fingertips. Turning them out makes the grip possible and ensures muscle energy in the hands. It strengthens the muscles between the metacarpal bones and those surrounding the wrists. The thumb is bent at the middle knuckle to increase strength and protect the joint. If the thumb is hyperextended or bent beyond its normal range of motion, it will become weak over time.

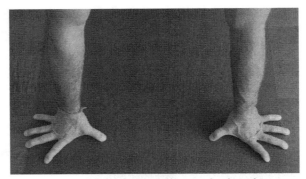

3.7 Front view of hands elevated to ridgetops in a foundational position

The outward turn of the hands in ridgetop position allows all four of the base knuckles of the fingers to root down evenly as the middle knuckles lift up. This stabilizes the hand. If the fingers point straight ahead, the weight borne by the hands will shift between the medial and lateral sides of the hand. Turning the hands out also allows more external rotation in the arm bones to stabilize the shoulder. Any time the wrists elevate, the sides of the body can lengthen more, increasing space between the vertebrae. This allows for safer and deeper back bending.

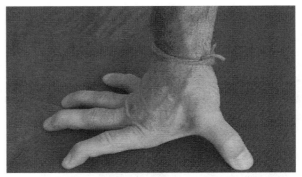

3.8 Detail of fingers and thumb with hand in elevated ridgetop position.

Hands in Reverse Ridgetop Position

Reversing the placement of the hands in ridgetop position allows for full external rotation of the arm bones. Reverse ridgetop placement of the hands initiates engagement in the back of the body. This helps to balance shoulder strength and can be used as a therapeutic technique for certain types of injuries. The thumbs point straight forward and the fingers back. The top knuckle of the thumb is bent so the tip of the thumb presses straight down. The Sanskrit term for this hand placement is *viparita utthita hasta* – reverse rising hand.

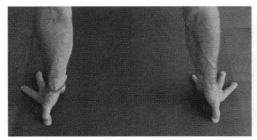

3.9 Hands in reverse ridgetop position

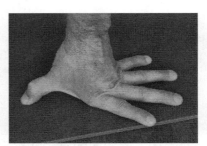

3.10 Detail of fingers and thumb with hand in reverse ridgetop position

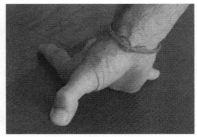

3.11 Detail of active thumb with hand in reverse ridgetop position

Hands Elevated on Fingertips or "Fiery Hands"

Elevating the hands onto the fingertips is referred to as "fiery hands;" in Sanskrit, this is *rajas utthita hasta*. To support weight in this position, the fingers hyperextend or move beyond their normal range of extension. This hand position should be used with caution and employed infrequently as a means to strengthen the tendons of the hand. If used too often, it will weaken the joints. It is recommended for use only in *vinyasas* or for support in standing poses. Arm-balance and inversion poses are unstable on fingertips. Most of the weight of the body would be borne by the thumb and little finger, and hyperextension under load can cause injury. When employing fiery hands, the thumbs point inward and the fingers flare out.

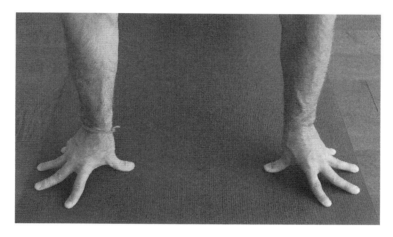

3.12 Fiery Hands

Hands in Jaguar Claws

Elevating the hands onto the thumbs and first two finger knuckles is referred to as "jaguar claws" or *pundarikam hasta*. The thumbs point toward each other. They are bent at a right angle and the thumb tips press down as they did in reverse ridgetop position (figure 3.11). The first two fingers are bent at the middle knuckles and, along with the thumb, create a tripod base. The ring finger and little fingers press in toward the palm of the hand. Elevating hands in the jaguar claw position creates superior hand strength and is recommended for use in *vinyasa* only.

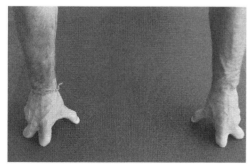

3.13 Hands elevated in jaguar claw position

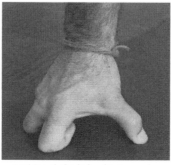

3.14 Detail of right hand in jaguar claw

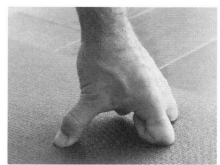

3.15 Detail of left hand in jaguar claw

Hands in Eagle Talons

In the eagle-talon or *garuda hasta* hand placement, the weight rests on the middle, ring and little fingers – on the part of those fingers between the first and middle knuckles. The index finger is folded in and locked off by the thumb. The eagle talon creates exceptional hand and finger strength.

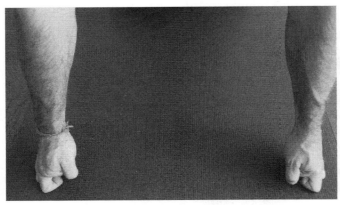
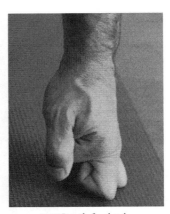

3.16 Hands in eagle talon position   *3.17 Detail of eagle talon*

Hands Supported on Fists

Folding all fingers into the palm of the hand creates a fist or *musti*. To elevate the hand and support weight in the fist position, the weight is placed on the outer three knuckles. The index knuckle hovers off of the floor a few millimeters (this keeps the back of the wrist straight and supported). The thumb can be used as an optional means of support and may be bent with the thumb tip pressed into the floor.

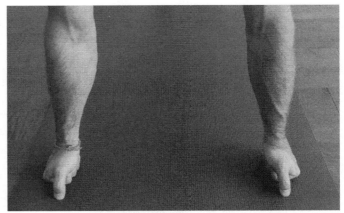

3.18 Hands in fist position with optional support from thumbs

Open-Handed Fists

With an open-handed fist (*amusti*), weight is supported on the tops of uncurled fingers. As the open fingers push down into the mat, the wrist lifts away from the floor and does not collapse. The thumbs are never used in this position, as they would compromise the strength being recruited into the hand.

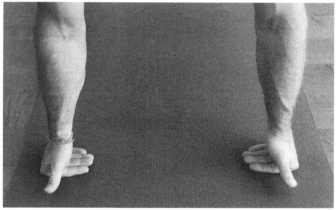

3.19 Open-handed fists

Bound Hands

The bound-hands (*baddha hasta*) foundation is created by interlacing the fingers with the palms of the hands pressing into the floor. With thumb tips touching, the index fingers press down into the mat. This hand position is good for strengthening the chest and the front of the shoulders, but is contraindicated if the shoulder girdle and stabilizing muscles of the rotator cuff are impaired or unbalanced.

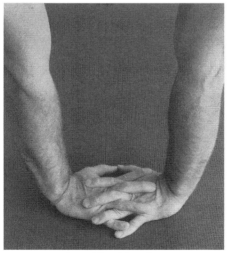

3.20 A bound-hand foundation

Revolved Bound Hands

To stimulate the creation of more strength and flexibility in the wrists, a revolved bound-hands foundation is practiced. Revolved bound-hands (*parivrtta baddha hasta*) places the backs of interlaced fingers on the floor. Practice on a thick mat or doubled mat to reduce compressive forces on the fingers and wrists.

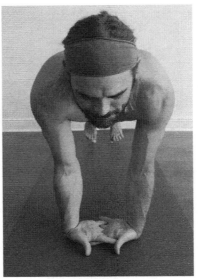

3.21 Revolved bound-hands

Diamond Hands

The diamond-hands or *vajra hasta* foundation is a good alternative to the bound-hands positions when shoulder instabilities are present. The palms of the hand press into the mat and are turned inward so the tips of thumbs and index fingers meet.

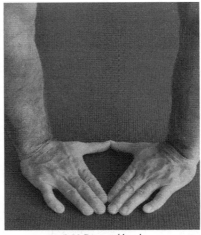

3.22 Diamond hands

Placement of Hands for Headstand

Three different hand positions can be used to create a foundation for headstand or *sirsasana* pose. The three positions correspond to the three qualities of matter: *tamas* (easy), *rajas* (active), *sattva* (balanced). *Tamasic* hands are fully open with fingers interlaced. The back of the head is held in the open palms. This position allows for more balance but less muscle energy. *Rajasic* hands are fully clasped and the head is placed between the forearms. This position increases muscle energy but decreases balance. *Sattvic* hands are tightly clasped, but with some space created for the head by the tips of the thumbs pressing together. This creates a balance between stability and strength.

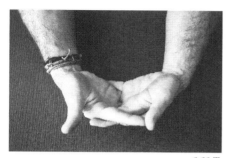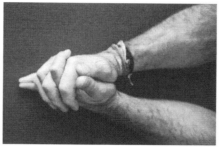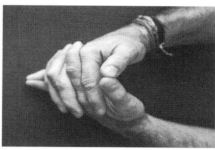

3.23 Tamasic, rajasic and sattvic hand positions create foundations for headstand

Placement of Hands for Forearm Balance

Like headstand, there are three main hand positions to work with in forearm balance, or *pincha mayurasana* pose. A palms-up hand position is *tamasic*. Muscle energy is decreased but balance is increased. *Rajasic* hands are placed palms down. They press into the floor with or without a block between the index fingers to maintain proper spacing. This hand position increases strength but decreases balance. *Sattvic* hands are very active and resemble the elevated ridgetop hand position. The base knuckles of the fingers press down and the wrists lift and push out to the sides. This creates a balance between stability and muscle energy.

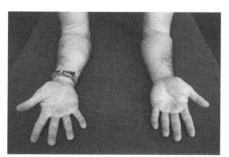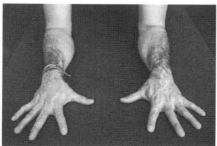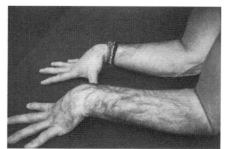

3.24 Tamasic, rajasic and sattvic hand positions create foundations for forearm balance

The Feet

The feet are the foundation for standing poses and, depending upon how they are placed, they can enhance or diminish alignment and action in *asana*. When standing in *tadasana* (mountain pose), the feet can be placed together or separated by the width of the hips. When the feet are together, the balance becomes challenged as the weight sways over the feet and around the central axis.

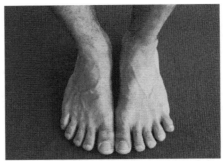
3.25 Standing with feet together

When feet are placed hip-distance apart, the body's weight is distributed evenly over the foundation of the feet and is centered at the midline or central axis of the body. This foot placement creates space for the thighbones to roll in and back, so the hamstring muscles can align and engage on the bone. This liberates the lower back and the backs of the legs in forward folds. The feet can be engaged in three positions: flexed, pointed or flointed. All three have different qualities of action in *asana*.

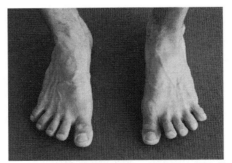
3.26 Standing with feet hip-distance apart and outer edges of heels aligned with the outer edges of the fourth toes

Feet Flexed

Flexing the feet brings the feet and lower leg into a right-angle position. This energetic action draws muscle energy in and up toward the core of the body. This decelerates actions and creates external rotation of the top of the thighbones or femur heads.

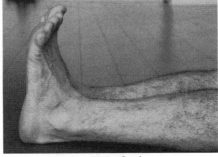
3.27 Feet flexed

Feet Pointed

Pointing the feet straightens the ankles and inclines the toes away from the shins. This action extends energy from the core of the body outward toward the periphery. It accelerates action in *asana* and creates more internal rotation of the femur heads. Depending on the *asana* and how it is performed, either flexing or pointing can be more advantageous.

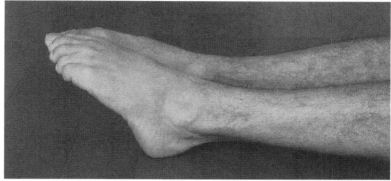

3.28 Feet in a pointed position

Feet Flointed

"Floint" is a hybrid word created by combining the words flex and point. Flointing of the foot blends both of those actions and results in energy extending out and drawing in at the same time. The big toes point away while the three middle toes flex back toward the body and the pinky toe extends out to the side. This creates extension from the four corners of the feet as the central pads lift. The common term for this action is *pada bandha,* or foot lock.

Flointed feet are often confused with "Barbie feet" where the toes are pulled back and the balls of the feet press strongly forward. This foot position serves no purpose to enhance any action in *asana.*

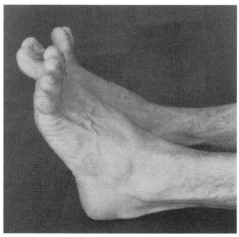

3.29 Flointed feet

Positioning the Feet with Legs Extended Behind the Body

When the legs are extended out behind the body in a prone or sitting position, as they are in cobra pose or *bhujangasana* (shown in figure 3.30), upward-facing dog or *urdhva mukha svanasana*, and pigeon (*eka pada rajakapotasana*), the feet should be actively drawing in towards the core. This drawing-in action has the effect of extending energy back out. When the toes root down and pull back, the heels lift and center themselves and energy extends back and out. If the toes don't press down and pull back towards the hips, the disengagement drops the heels out to the sides and this destabilizes the pose.

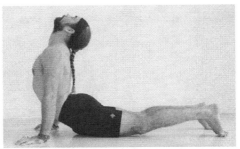

3.30 Cobra pose with feet engaged

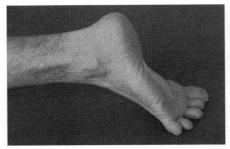

3.31 Toes pressing down and drawing back

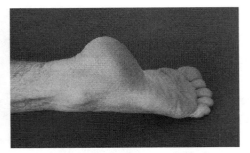

3.32 Foot disengaged and turning or "sickling" in

Foot Placement in Warrior I and Lunge Variations

In *virabhadrasana* I or Warrior I pose and lunge variations, there is a tendency to place too much weight into the foot of the trailing leg. This causes the knee of that leg to bend. Leaning forward onto the ball of the back foot allows the leg to straighten as the weight shifts forward. There should also be a few inches between the feet to increase balance and stability. To increase length in the stance, slide the rear foot back behind you a few inches. To increase the width, wiggle the forward foot out to the side. The outer edges of the feet are aligned with the outer edges of the thighs and hips in all standing poses that have a symmetric hip opening.

Warrior I is also performed with the back foot flat and the heels aligned. When the back heel turns down and in, then the hips are no longer symmetric and the backbend should be resisted by strength in the legs and core. The back heel pushes down and away while the ball of the foot pivots forward. This creates an inner rotation of the top of the thighbone that brings the back hip forward.

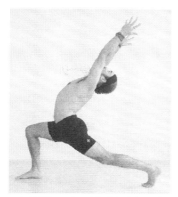

3.33 Warrior I with back heel elevated

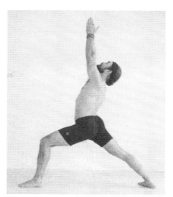

3.34 Warior I with back foot flat

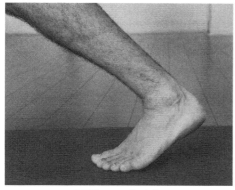

3.35 Inactive back foot

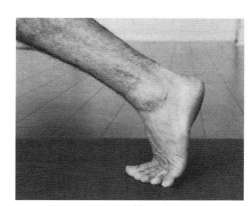

3.36 Activated foot and leg

Feet in Utthita Parsvakonasana and Utthita Trikonasana

The heels should be aligned with an asymmetric hip opening, or forward heel to the arch of the back foot for experienced practitioners. The foot of the trailing leg in *utthita parsvakonasana* (extended side angle pose) and *utthita trikonasana* (extended triangle pose) can be positioned with the toes pointing inward 30-60 degrees or with the outer edge of the foot parallel to the back edge of the mat. If the foot turns in, the thighbone rotates inward. This is advantageous for practitioners with less flexible hips. If the foot of the trailing leg is placed parallel with back edge of mat, the leg can strengthen more and be integrated more deeply into the hip socket.

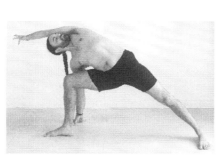

3.37 Utthita Parsvakonasana

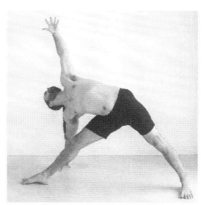

3.38 Utthita Trikonasana

A tendency in either alignment of the back foot in these standing poses is for the outer edge of the foot to lift off the mat. Focus on pressing down through the outer edge of the foot, and strive to create a *pada bandha* or foot lock by rooting through the big and little toe while lifting three middle toes off the mat.

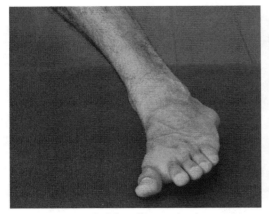

3.39 Back foot rolling onto the side

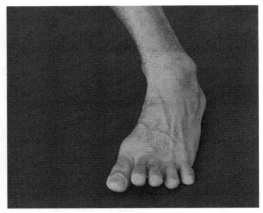

3.40 Pressing the big and little toes down to create a foot lock

Placement of the Feet in Parsvottanasana and Utthita Parivrtta Trikonasana

In *parsvottanasana* (side intense stretch pose) and *utthita parivrtta trikonasna* (revolved triangle pose), the feet can be positioned with front heel and back heel in alignment, or they can be placed with front and back heels hip-width apart. When the heels are aligned, the pelvis is narrowed and aligning the hips is more difficult. When the feet are placed hip-width apart, the thighs can press back and the hips can square to the front edge of the mat.

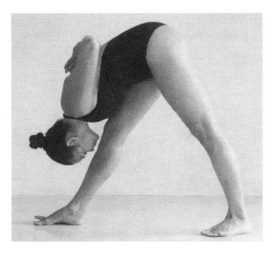

3.41 Parsvottanasana

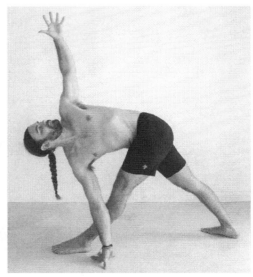

3.42 Utthita Parivrtta Trikonasana

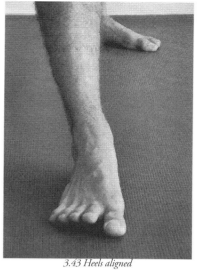

3.43 Heels aligned

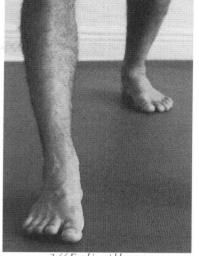

3.44 Feet hip-width apart

To deepen *parsvottanasana,* the back foot can be turned in. The foot flexes and the little-toe side of the foot presses down, lifting the heel. This is often referred to as "goofy foot" and it keeps the ankle, shin and knee in alignment. The hands must be used on the floor for support during this variation.

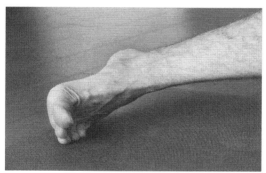

3.45 Goofy foot

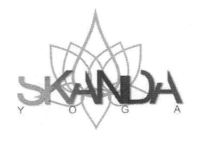

CHAPTER 4

Breath, Energy Locks, and Alignment and Action in Asana

Alignment of the inner and outer body is realized through the activation of three principal actions. *Ujjayi* or victorious breath is a type of deep and audible breathing. The *bandhas* are energy locks in the body. *Spanda* is the pulsation or motion of energy oscillating between opposite points. In this chapter, we will explore these alignment principles and the unique alignment actions of a variety of familiar poses.

Principles of Breath in *Asana*

Ujjayi breath creates an expansion of the inner body. The muscles of the lower abdomen draw in and the pelvis tilts forward. The ribs lift and expand. The glottis muscle at the back of the throat constricts and tones and the breath becomes slightly audible. The sound of the breath is smooth and resonant, as if it is swirling in the back of the throat.

- All actions are initiated with the breath.
- Inhalations decelerate actions as the inner body expands and the outer body contracts.
- Exhalations accelerate actions as the inner body contracts and the outer body expands.

Action-with-the-Breath Guidelines in *Asana*

- Standing poses with an asymmetric hip opening are entered on an exhalation and exited on an inhalation.
- Standing poses with a symmetrical hip opening are entered on an inhalation and exited on an exhalation.
- Twisting poses are entered with an exhalation and exited on an inhalation.
- Back-bending poses are entered on an inhalation and exited on an exhalation.
- Forward-bending poses are entered with an exhalation and exited on an inhalation.

Engaging Energy Locks and Aligning Internally

The Sanskrit word *"bandha"* is usually translated in the West as meaning "to lock" or "to bind." It also translates as "to join" and "to put together." Interestingly, engaging the energy locks in the body actually has the effect of unlocking the flow of energy.

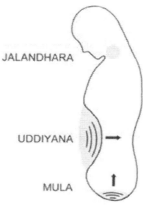

4.1 The three bandhas

The three *bandhas* are the *mula* (base or root lock), the *uddiyana* (upward-flying or abdominal lock), and *jalandhara* (flowing-like-water or chin lock). The engagement of the three *bandhas* draws energy into the *sushumna* – the central channel of the body. The breath becomes still (*kumbhaka*) with the cessation of exhalation (*rechhaka*). *Maha bandha* is the activation of all three *bandhas* at once and can only be performed at the end of an exhalation. It is generally only utilized during meditation and during the practice of *pranayama* – the consciously active control of the breath.

Mula Bandha

Mula bandha stimulates both the peripheral (sensory and motor) and autonomic nervous systems. It also minimally stimulates the parasympathetic[10] nervous system and the sympathetic system. Parasympathetic fibers exist in the cervical and sacral areas only, while sympathetic-nervous-system[11] fibers emerge from the thoracic and lumbar region of the spine. The performance of the *bandhas* has been shown to increase parasympathetic activity by decreasing heart rate, respiration, and blood pressure.

The aim of hatha yoga is to unite the two sides of the body – the masculine or right side, and the feminine, the left. Energetically, this is done by drawing the *ida* and *pingala nadis*[12] into a centralized flow up from the pelvic floor. *Mula bandha* is achieved by contracting or drawing the perineum up in men and the cervix up in women. This is generalized as lifting or toning of the pelvic floor. It activates the base of the central nervous system and the parasympathetic and sympathetic nervous fibers.

---

10 The parasympathetic nervous system is one of the main divisions of the autonomic nervous system (functioning below the level of consciousness). It affects heart and respiration rates, digestion, salivation, perspiration, sexual arousal, pupillary dilation and the ejection of urine from the bladder.

11 The sympathetic nervous system aids in control of most of the body's internal organs. It mobilizes the nervous system's flight-or-fight response.

12 *Nadis* are the channels through which the energies of the subtle body or *prana* flow, according to Indian medicine and spiritual science. Active energies (solar/masculine) are said to flow within the *pingala* channel and represent the right side of the body and passive through the *ida* (lunar/feminine), representing the left side. These two *nadis* interweave around the *sushumna* or central *nadi*.

The engagement of *mula bandha* in *asana* begins with relaxing the roof of the mouth, specifically the soft palate[13]. The dome of the mouth and the dome of the pelvic floor are intimately connected. When the palate lifts, the pelvic floor lifts. The energy raised from *mula bandha* becomes restricted in its flow if there is tension in the roof of the mouth. Therefore, to practice *mula bandha* efficiently, the palate must first release. The best way to free the soft palate is to smile inwardly, as if you were smiling from the inside of your mouth rather than from the outside. The relationship of the palate and pelvic floor can easily be felt by sucking strongly through a straw placed in a thick milkshake or smoothie. It can also be felt during a sneeze or a cough. You'll notice that the pelvic floor lifts every time the roof of the mouth lifts. Kegel[14] exercises can strengthen the control of the pelvic floor. The muscles used in the Kegel exercises both hold and release the flow of urine. The action of *mula bandha* is maintained throughout the entire *asana* practice.

Uddiyana Bandha

Uddiyana bandha is performed by drawing the lower abdominal muscles in or back toward the spine while the internal organs are sucked in and lifted after exhalation. *Uddiyana bandha* compresses the internal organs and tones the sympathetic nervous system. It physiologically stimulates the sympathetic nervous system and energetically heats the *prana* (upward-flowing energy) while channeling the *apana* (downward flowing energy) upwards. The practice of *uddiyana* is different from *uddiyana bandha*. It is simply a toning of the lower abdominals while not lifting the internal organs. It can be held on inhalation and exhalation. During *pranayama*, *uddiyana bandha* is only held after exhalation. *Uddiyana* should be held throughout the entire *asana* practice to maintain core alignment and *ujjayi* breath.

Jalandhara Bandha

Jalandhara bandha is performed on exhalation by drawing the muscles of the throat in and resting the chin to the chest while the chest lifts towards the chin. This seals energy within the body to nourish all the vital organs and activates both the parasympathetic and sympathetic nervous systems. *Jalandhara bandha* stimulates the upper endocrine glands, the pineal, pituitary, thyroid, parathyroid, and thymus. It also tones the parasympathetic nervous fibers at the base of the medulla oblongata[15].

Jalandhara bandha is most commonly utilized during *mudras* and *pranayama* and can be held after inhalation or exhalation. Like *uddiyana bandha*, *jalandhara bandha* can be practiced without the lock of holding the breath. The muscles of the throat are slightly toned consistently with the breath. It is possible to activate *jalandhara* without the *bandha* of holding the breath in poses that bring the chest and chin together (e.g., plow pose or *halasana*, ear-pressure pose or *karnapidasana*, and shoulder stand or *sarvangasana)*.

The actions of *mula bandha, uddiyana* and *jalandhara* are always utilized during *asana* practice. *Mula bandha* balances the pelvic floor as the tailbone and pubic bone reach towards each other. *Uddiyana* widens the kidneys as the navel draws in. *Jalandhara* strengthens *pratyahara* and *dharana*.

---

13 The soft tissue at the back of the roof of the mouth.
14 Exercises that repeatedly contract and relax the muscles of the pelvic floor were devised by gynecologist Arnold Kegel and came to be known as Kegel exercises.
15 The medulla oblongata is the lower half of the brainstem that contains the cardiac, respiratory, vomiting and vasomotor centers and deals with autonomic involuntary functions such as breathing, heart rate and blood pressure.

Spanda Action in Asana

The Sanskrit word *spanda* translates to a vibrating, pulsing activity, beat or motion. It describes the incessant throb of contraction and expansion seen in all beings and things in the natural world. In *asana*, pulsating with the breath, undulating the spine, or linking actions with the breath, embodies the *spanda* principle. It is utilized by the engagement and lengthening of the muscles through concentric and eccentric actions. On inhalation, the muscles hug into the bone and draw in from the periphery to the core. On exhalation, the muscles and bones extend out from the core to the periphery. There are many subtleties of the *spanda* principle that take one deeper into experience every time it is utilized.

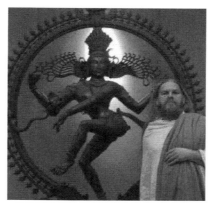

4.2 Sri Svami Purna standing before a Chola bronze of Shiva in the ecstatic dance of Nataraj

During *asana* practice, when we try to hold a pose too statically, the full flow of breath and energy are denied. When all poses are performed with the pulsing undulation of *spanda,* the *prana* or life force energy can be utilized. In reality, there are two poses within every posture – the inhale pose and the exhale pose. It is the point of transition between the two that distinguishes them as separate and complementary opposites (*shiva-shakti*). This transition point allows the dance of *spanda* to occur. This is the dance of energy and matter described in modern physics and it is the dance of *Shiva Nataraja*[16]. T.S. Eliot[17] wrote of it in one of his poems from the *Four Quartets*: "At the still point of the turning world…there the dance is. Except for the point, the still point, there would be no dance, and there is only the dance."

This distinguishing pause between inhalation and exhalation is an *anusvara* point. It is thought to contain both everything and nothing, a finite space with the power of the infinite. Like dusk and dawn, when light gives way to darkness and darkness to light, it is neither ascent nor decline. When this transition point is consciously lengthened in *asana*, it allows the two energies to meet and converge in a harmonic resonance. This space between the breaths is a midpoint of *spanda.* These midpoints are thought to be opportunities for our thoughts to suspend and for an experience of union with opposite states and with all that seems separate or other. *Skanda* attacks to unite and this point of neither-this-nor-that is the manifestation of his energy and the merger of *Shiva* and *Shakti* into a singularity. This point between the breaths should be extended but not held.

---

16 The image of Lord Shiva in an ecstatic dance was depicted in the famous Chola bronzes carved between 850-1250 C.E. Shiva's form portrays the concept of dualities engaged in the vibrating motion or frictive pulsation from one state to the other. This rhythmic dance is the source of all movement in the universe.
17 Thomas Stearns Eliot was a Nobel-Prize-winning poet, publisher, playwright and literary and social critic.

Alignment Options in Basic Poses

Practicing proper alignment in *asana* is relating muscles to bones in optimal ways. It is important for creating good body mechanics in poses and transitions, which results in ideal postural alignment when the body is at rest. All of this helps to prevent injuries. Proper alignment in the physical body also aligns us energetically with the inner or spiritual reality as well.

Yoga poses can be performed with two different types of alignment. The word "alignment" is defined as an arrangement in a straight line and as the positioning of components for coordinated functioning. Many yoga *asanas* can be practiced with these two types of alignment. In Skanda Yoga, we refer to the first as "type A" or "standard alignment," where *asana* is practiced in alignment with straight lines and geometric angles. This type of alignment requires the aid of observer, mirror, photograph or video to see and acquire an ideal form. It builds strength and requires more concentration, body awareness and effort than the second type of alignment. What we refer to as "type B" or "dynamic alignment" is based on spirals, curves, and arches. This type of alignment is found in much of the natural world, where forms appear in curvilinear arrangements. Our DNA spirals, our bones curve and our muscles curl as they wrap over the bones. Dynamic alignment is performed from the perspective of the internal observer. It positions the components of the body for ideal form and enhanced performance. It requires less strength and enhances flexibility by creating greater openings in the body. Depending on the pose, dynamic alignment can be used as a preparation for standard alignment.

Standard and dynamic alignments both have benefits and neither is more right or proper than the other. The type of alignment practiced should always seek to relate the inner body with the outer body. The inner body is often imagined as an etheric or substance-less double of our internal organs and deep muscles, and it is believed that it can become misaligned with the outer form of the body. This can easily happen when muscles and bones are out of alignment and muscular holding patterns are formed. In practicing *asana*, the energetic body should be aligned before the outer form of the physical body.

The body will naturally exaggerate certain actions and holding patterns in *asanas*. When practitioners become aware of this tendency, it is possible to make corrections to maintain balanced actions in the body. For example, the foundation (trailing and stabilizing) leg of a standing pose will naturally rotate externally. This action is always counterbalanced by internally rotating the leg. The expanding (forward) leg creates an opening and will naturally rotate inward. It is counterbalanced by externally rotating the leg. Whether the legs are lifted or extended, depending upon the *asana,* the counterbalancing actions should never override the integrity of the pose.

Following is an exploration of alignment options, *spanda* actions and the alignment focus of a variety of basic and well-known poses. As you come to understand the differences in the alignment shapes of the poses, and how the breath and the body pulsate from drawing in to expanding out, you can come to apply the same principles to any pose. A photo of the *asana* in standard alignment follows the pose name. Additional images illustrate dynamic alignment and important actions.

Tadasana (mountain pose)

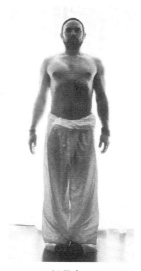

4.3 Tadasana

Standard Alignment: The feet are together. This decreases stability but provides the benefit of challenging the balance to hold to the midline.

Dynamic Alignment: The feet are hip-distance apart; the second outer toe is aligned with the outer edge of the heel. This increases stability and allows more space for the thighbones to root back with greater ease.

***Spanda* Action:** On inhalation, the leg muscles draw in from the periphery to the core and squeeze in to the midline. On the exhalation, they push out from the core to the periphery. On inhalation, the shoulder blades widen apart; on exhalation, they curl in to the heart. The spine moves in a subtle wave like motion from base of the pelvis at the beginning of the inhalation and reaches the crown of the head at the end of the breath. The spine is still and neutral on exhalation.

Alignment Focus: The thighbones stay rooting back and don't pop forward or turn out. The soft palate is aligned over the central axis.

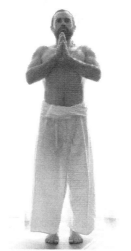

4.4 Tadasana in dynamic alignment

Uttanasana (intense stretching or forward-bending pose)

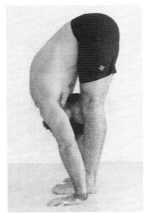

4.5 Uttanasana in standard alignment

Standard Alignment: The feet are together and the upper back is rounded. The upper body is completely folded over from the hips.

Dynamic Alignment: The feet are hip-distance apart and the shoulder blades engage to lift up towards the hips. The upper body does not completely fold. There remains a small gap between the lower floating ribs and the top of the thighs. This increases muscular engagement and protects the hamstrings from becoming over-stretched.

***Spanda* Action:** The legs squeeze towards each other as the leg muscles engage and draw up. On the exhalation, the thighs widen apart and the shins continue to squeeze in toward each other. On inhalation, more weight is placed on the big toe and outer edge of the heel. On exhalation, weight is shifted to the inner edge of heel and outer edge of the top of the foot. This creates a reverberation of energy that spirals up the legs and enhances the muscular engagements. The spine undulates with the inhalation and exhalation. On inhalation, arch the lower back slightly to extend the spine and generate a wave that travels to the crown of the head. On exhalation, release the head and bring the spine into flexion.

Alignment Focus: The hips are centered over the ankles; they do not push back. The shins squeeze in and the thigh muscles lift up. The inner thighs are engaged to push the thighbones apart.

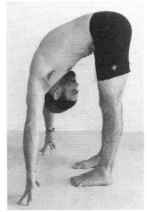

4.6 Uttanasana in dynamic alignment

Chaturanga Dandasana (four limbed staff pose)

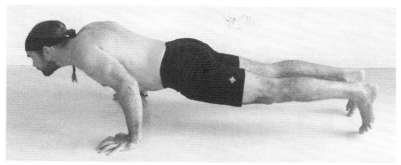

4.7 Chaturanga Dandasana

Standard Alignment: The outside edges of the hands are aligned with the outside edge of the shoulders and the fingers point straight ahead. The tops of the shoulders are aligned with the elbows.

Dynamic Alignment: The mid-point of the hand is aligned with the outside edge of the shoulder, and the index finger points straight ahead. Spreading the fingers and measuring one-third of the space between the index and the middle finger determines the midpoint. This wider hand placement protects the wrists and allows for an engagement in the back body that is stronger than that in the front body.

***Spanda* Action:** At the last moment of descent, when the upper arm bones become parallel with the elbows, the sitting bones lift and widen (see figure 4.8). The tailbone scoops into this space as the hips push down. This creates momentum to rise up into *bhujangasana* (cobra pose) or *udrhva mukha svanasana* (upward-facing dog pose) and relieves stress from the front of the shoulders. There is no undulation of the spine in *chaturanga dandasana*.

Alignment Focus: The shoulder blades are engaged on the back rather than winging off to the sides. The tops of the shoulders are at the same height as the elbows.

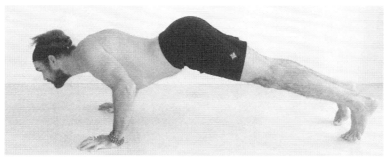

4.8 Chaturanga Dandasana with spanda action at the moment of descent

Urdhva Mukha Svanasana (upward facing dog pose)

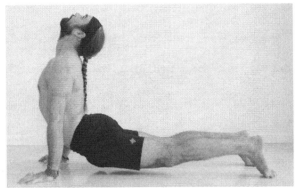

4.9 Urdhva Mukha Svanasana

Standard Alignment: The arms are straight and strong and the shoulders are aligned over the wrists. The thighs, knees and hips are lifting away from the floor. When the bones are completely straight, there is a decrease in muscular energy and the effects of the backbend will be felt in the lower back.

Dynamic Alignment: The mid-point of the hand is aligned with outside edge of shoulder. The arms are micro-bent a few millimeters. The upper arm bones and shoulders angle back. This allows for a stronger muscular engagement and for more external rotation of the arm bones. It takes the engagement into the back body and relieves the front of the shoulder. When performed correctly, the collarbones are invisible.

***Spanda* Action:** On the inhalation, the hands and feet pull in towards the core of the pelvis. On the exhalation, the pelvis pushes down, and the energy disperses from the core out to the periphery. The arms create more external rotation as they slowly begin to straighten.

Alignment Focus: The pad of the index knuckle stays weighted, as the collarbones pull back. The collarbones should be invisible. The "eyes" of the elbow are in line with the thumbs, or they point straight ahead if working an alternate hand position with wrists lifted. The forearms always roll in while upper arms roll out.

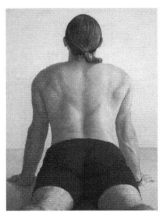
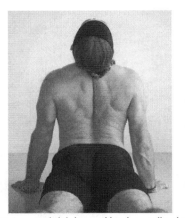
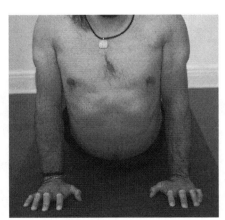

4.10 Arms straight with hands pushing down.	*4.11 Arms are slightly bent and hands are pulling back toward the hips.*	*4.12 The collarbones are not visible*

Adho Mukha Svanasana (downward facing dog pose)

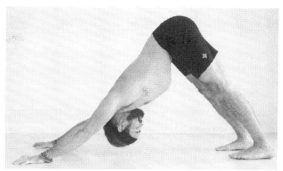

4.13 Adho Mukha Svanasana

Standard Alignment: The outer edge of the hand is aligned with the outer edge of the shoulder. The feet are parallel and placed hip-width apart. The arms actively lift away from the floor as the chest descends. The lower abdomen is firm and the neck releases. The thighbones are pushing back into the hamstrings.

Dynamic Alignment: The hands are placed in the same way as in the standard alignment, with the outer edge of the wrists aligned with the outer edge of the shoulders. This allows for greater extension of the arm bones out of the shoulder sockets. If a practitioner has difficulty keeping the arm bones straight with the index knuckles pressing down, the hands can be taken wider and rotated out to the sides. The tops of the shoulders are always rotating out and the collarbones are widening apart. To accentuate the curve in the spine and take some weight off of the arms, the knees can be bent.

***Spanda* Action:** On the inhalation, the armpits lift as the hands push down and pull back. The feet push down and draw in towards the hands. The legs squeeze into the midline as the core lifts. On the exhalation, the upper back curls and energy is pushed down from the shoulders through the hands as it is simultaneously pushed back out through the feet. The legs widen and root back. When these actions are maintained, they generate the undulation on inhalation and exhalation. Each pulsation should take you deeper into the pose.

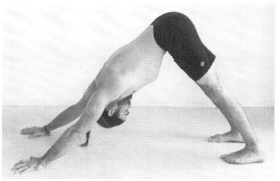

4.14 Adho Mukha Svanasana in dynamic alignment

Alignment Focus: The inner creases or "eyes" of the elbows face towards each other. The creases of the wrists and the shoulders are aligned parallel to the front edge of the mat.

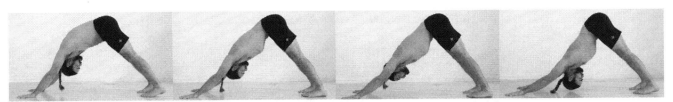

4.15 Detail of how the form of the pose changes through two series of inhalations and exhalations

Utthita Parsvakonasana (extended side angle pose)

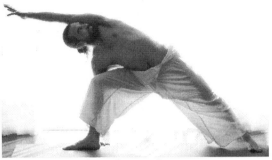

4.16 Utthita Parsvakonasana

Standard Alignment: The leading leg is bent at a 90-degree angle so the thigh is parallel to the floor. The trailing leg is straight. The grounding hand is placed beside the foot as the expanding arm reaches overhead with the palm pointing face-down.

Dynamic Alignment: The grounding hand and arm rotate outward; the hand is placed five to six inches away from the foot. The arm bone angles in so that there is always contact between the bicep and the outer knee. The extending arm rotates outward and curls back. It is nearly parallel with the floor and twists as the head pushes the arm bone back (see figure 4.17).

***Spanda* Action:** On the inhalation, the legs and arms draw in towards the core of the body. The thigh of the grounding leg roots back. On the exhalation, the leg and arm bones push out from the core to the periphery, as the tailbone scoops forward. The spine undulates rising from the pelvis through the crown to take the pose more toward a backbend with each breath.

Alignment Focus: The back leg is straight, and the core is held strong.

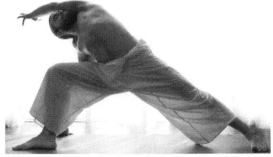

4.17 Dynamic alignment of Utthita Parsvakonasana

Utthita Trikonasana (extended triangle pose)

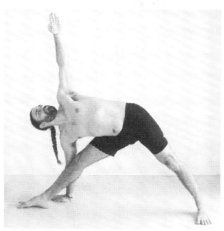

4.18 Utthita Trikonasana

Standard Alignment: The arms are aligned perpendicular with the floor. The grounding arm bone rotates inward and the wrist joint is under and in alignment with the shoulder. The heads turns and the eyes look up at the extended hand.

Dynamic Alignment: The grounding arm rotates outward and the hand is placed five to six inches away from the leg (see figure 4.19). The shoulder blades are engaged and drawn together on the back. The head curls back to open the throat and chest.

***Spanda* Action:** On the inhalation, the legs and arms draw in towards the core of the body. The thighbones root back into the hamstrings. On the exhalation, the leg and arm bones push out from the core to the periphery. On inhalation, the head moves back. On exhalation, the twist is deepened. These actions are maintained with the breath while the spine undulates.

Alignment Focus: Both legs are straight and the torso is aligned over the midline of the leading leg.

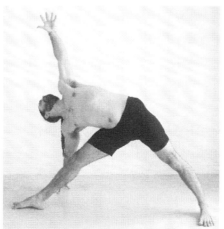

4.19 Utthita Trikonasana in dynamic alignment

Virabhadrasana I (warrior I pose)

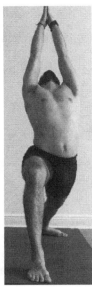

4.20 Virabhadrasana I with standard alignment

Standard Alignment: The heel of the trailing foot is on the floor and arms are straight overhead. The core and legs are strongly engaged to resist the backbend. The hands are placed together with the arms squeezing into the center.

Dynamic Alignment: The heel of the trailing foot is lifted and the hips are squared to the front edge of the mat. In this shape, the backbend can be deepened. The hands are apart to allow more curvature in the upper back.

***Spanda* Action:** On the inhalation, the legs draw together while a lift of the hips is resisted. On the exhalation, the legs are pushed apart and the hips are moved down. There is no pulsation in standard alignment.

Alignment Focus: With the core engaged and strong, the lower abdomen and rib cage squeeze in. The tailbone scoops without gripping the outer gluteal muscles. The trailing leg is straight and the knee of the leading leg is in line with the outer edge of the foot and the hip.

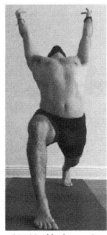

4.21 Virabhadrasana I in dynamic alignment

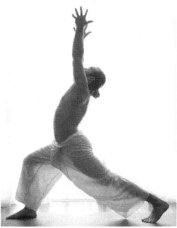

4.22 Form of the pose on inhalation

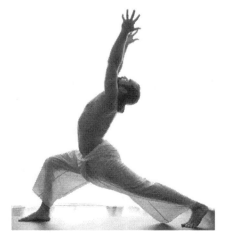

4.23 Form of the pose on exhalation

Vasisthasana (sage Vasisthasa's pose)

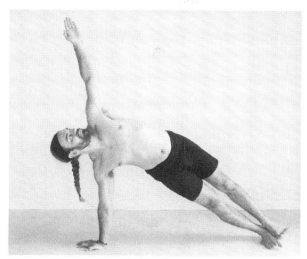

4.24 Vasisthasana

Standard Alignment: The supporting hand is placed directly under the shoulder with the fingers pointing straight ahead; the other arm reaches straight up. The foot of the top leg is stacked directly on top of the foot of the bottom leg.

Dynamic Alignment: The supporting hand is placed four to five inches in front of the shoulder and the arm and fingers are turned outward. The rising arm reaches back. The hips lift. The soles of both feet are on the floor. The torso twists and arches back as the head moves back and the chest lifts (see figure 4.25).

***Spanda* Action:** On the inhalation, the hips lift. On the exhalation, the torso twists and curls toward a backbend. There is no pulsation in standard alignment.

Alignment Focus: The shoulder heads move to the back of the body. The shoulder blades are engaged on the back.

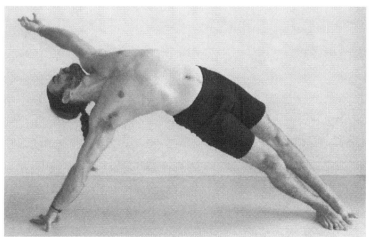

4.25 Vasisthasana in dynamic alignment

Bakasana (crane pose, also known as crow pose)

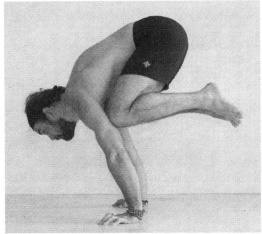

4.26 Bakasana

Standard Alignment: The knees are balanced on the backs of the upper arms and the hips are lifted. The feet are pointed and the inside edges are drawn together. The outside edges of the wrists are aligned with the outer edges of the shoulders. Arms are straightened.

Dynamic Alignment: Knees are wider than the arms and the feet are flointed. The midpoint of the hand is aligned with the outside edge of the shoulder. Alternatively, the pose can be performed on fists or ridgetops; this improves balance and increases the ability to lift the back higher.

***Spanda* Action:** On the inhalation, the legs are squeezed toward the midline. On the exhalation, the arms are straightened as the lower back rounds and the kidneys lift up. There is no pulsation in standard alignment.

Alignment Focus: Maintaining a strong grip or claw with the hands.

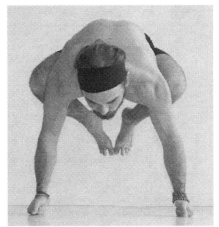

4.27 Bakasana in dynamic alignment, front view

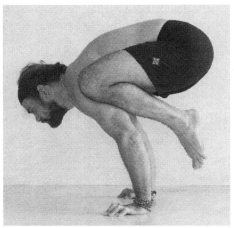

4.28 Bakasana in dynamic alignment, side view

Adho Mukha Vrksasana (downward facing tree or handstand)

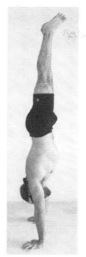

4.29 Adho Mukha Vrksasana

Standard Alignment: The outside edges of the hands are in line with the outer edges of the shoulders. The feet, hips, shoulders and wrists are aligned.

Dynamic Alignment: The spine is curved, allowing the chest to descend towards the floor. To avoid low back compression, the chest spreads open and the tailbone tucks strongly in. The increased arch improves stability.

***Spanda* Action:** On the inhalation, the body's weight descends and the arm bones sink into the shoulder sockets. On the exhalation, energy is pushed from the top of the shoulders down through the hands as the arm bones rotate outward. On inhalation, the legs are pressed together in the midline. On exhalation, energy is extended from the tailbone up through the heels. There is no pulsation in standard alignment.

Alignment Focus: The tailbone is strongly tucked and the legs squeeze into the midline. The heels are slightly separated so the thighs can rotate inward and the tailbone has space to extend energy up through the heels. The collarbones and shoulder blades are widening apart. The retinaculum of the wrists lifts up as a result of *hasta bandha* engagement (see Chapter Three).

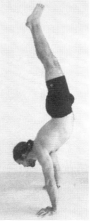

4.30 Adho Mukha Vrksasana in dynamic alignment

Eka Pada Rajakapotasana (one foot king pigeon pose or pigeon prep pose)

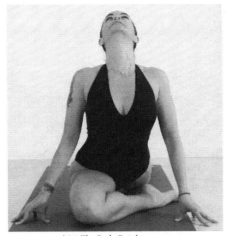

4.31 Eka Pada Rajakapotasana

Standard Alignment: The thigh of the leading leg is parallel to the outer edge of the mat. The knee is closed and pointing forward and the heel of the foot is close to the opposite hip.

Dynamic Alignment: The thigh of the leading leg moves away from the body at an angle that places the knee toward the edge of the mat. The shin slides up toward the front of the mat but is not parallel with the front edge. Placing the forward leg at a 90-degree angle creates a torque in the knee and strains connective tissue. Instead, the ankle should be just a few inches in front of the opposite hip.

***Spanda* Action:** On the inhalation, the legs draw together to initiate muscle energy. On the exhalation, the hips push down while the legs remain engaged. There is no pulsation in standard alignment.

Alignment Focus: The legs are active. The forward leg is pushing down and pulling back simultaneously. The shoulder blades are integrated on the back. The trailing leg pushes down and presses in toward the midline.

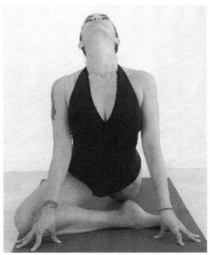

4.32 Eka Pada Rajakapotasana in dynamic alignment

Upavishta Konasana (seated wide angle pose)

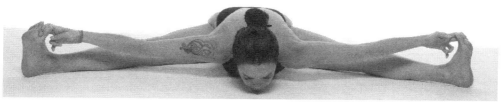

4.33 Upavishta Konasana

Standard Alignment: The legs are spread widely out to the sides and are engaged. The toes and kneecaps point up to the ceiling. The index and middle fingers grasp the big toes. The upper back is rounded as the torso and chin descend toward the floor.

Dynamic Alignment: The hands are placed on the mat in front of the thighs to support the forward extension. The arms lift to squeeze the shoulder blades together on the back. The spine is both arched and extended in the forward fold.

***Spanda* Action:** On the inhalation, the tops of the thighs are rotated inward and the leg bones are drawn back into the hip sockets. On the exhalation, the thighs are rotated outward and the leg bones are pushed away from the hips. These actions evenly lengthen the three muscles that make up the hamstring group on the back of the leg. On the inhalation, the hands are pulled back to tilt the pelvis and the lower back is arched. On exhalation, the lower abdomen is engaged and the torso is pulled forward. The big toes point toward the midline on inhalation and the little toes pull back on exhalation.

Alignment Focus: The thighbones are rooting down and the leg muscles are engaged. The lower back is arching to keep the top of the pelvis moving forward. The arms lift away from the floor and the feet are flexed or in *pada bandha*.

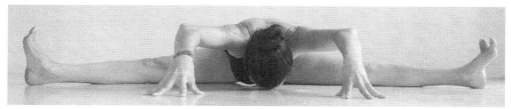

4.34 Upavishta Konasana in dynamic alignment

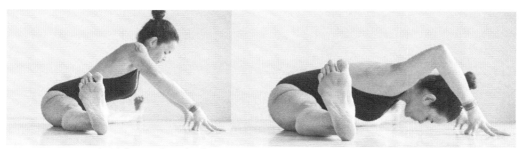

4.35 Side views of upavihsta konasana in dynamic alignment on inhalation and exhalation.

Urdhva Dhanurasana (upward bow pose)

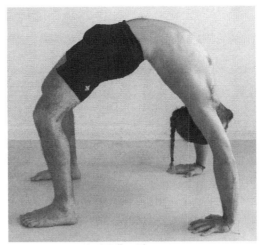

4.36 Urdhva Dhanurasana

Standard Alignment: The outer edges of the hands are aligned with the outer edges of the shoulders. The feet are flat and press down for strength; the toes are pointing forward.

Dynamic Alignment: The hands are placed wider than in standard alignment and can be rotated outward. This helps to open the chest and shoulders and takes stress off of the wrists. The heels lift to create a greater opening in the hips and greater extension of the spine.

***Spanda* Action:** On the inhalation, the tops of the thighs are rolled in and the hips are lowered a few inches. On the exhalation, the legs are pressed toward the midline as the tailbone is scooped under and the chest is pushed forward. On the inhalation, the legs push down and back. On exhalation, the legs are straightened and the chest is pushed forward.

Alignment Focus: The legs hug the midline as *uddiyana* and *mula bandha* are engaged. The big toes squeeze in as the heels push apart. The tops of the arm bones rotate outward.

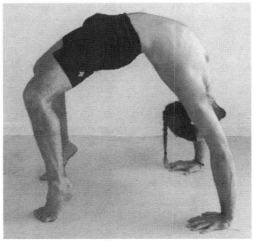

4.37 Urdhva Dhanurasana in dynamic alignment with heels lifted

Ardha Matsyendrasana (half sage Matsyendra pose - lord of the fish pose)

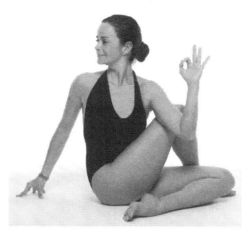

4.38 Ardha Matsyendrasana

Standard Alignment: Both sitting bones are rooted into the floor evenly. The lower back is arched. The lower abdomen is drawn in and back as the chest lifts up.

Dynamic Alignment: The pose is performed in standard alignment and becomes dynamic when practiced with *spanda*.

***Spanda* Action:** On the inhalation, the twist is released slightly while the lungs are expanded fully. On the exhalation, the twist is deepened by pushing the back of the lifted arm against the thigh of the elevated leg. The spine undulates from the pelvis through the crown on inhalation.

Alignment Focus: Both sitting bones are grounded evenly while the lower back arches. The hand on the floor behind the hips is elevated to ridgetop or fingertips.

Bharadvajasana II (sage Bharadva's pose)

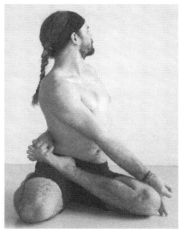
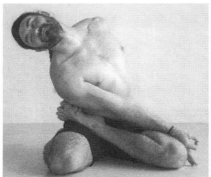

4.39 Bharadvajasana II   *4.40 Bharadvajasana II in dynamic alignment*

Standard Alignment: The entire torso is twisting in one direction as the sitting bones root into the floor.

Dynamic Alignment: The twist moves in two directions. The leading arm and shoulder pull back while the trailing arm and shoulder twist in the opposite direction. This creates two separate spirals of energy that travel up the spine and move away from the center (see figure 4.40).

***Spanda* Action:** On the inhalation, the twist is released slightly while the lungs are expanded fully. On the exhalation, the twist is deepened by pushing the back of the trailing hand against the thigh of the leading knee. The spine undulates from the pelvis through the crown on inhalation.

Alignment Focus: The lower back arches and *uddiyana* remains engaged.

Supta Padagusthasana I (reclined big toe pose or single leg stretch)

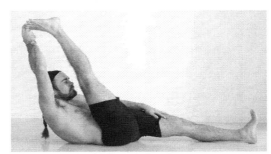

4.41 Supta Padagusthasana

Standard Alignment: The lower back is flat and the upper back is rounded. The big toe is taken by the index and middle fingers. The head and shoulders lift up towards the knee of the elevated leg. The leg resists the stretch by pushing the thighbone away.

Dynamic Alignment: The lower back arches and the shoulder blades are flat on the floor. The head lightly pushes back down. The arch in the low back is maintained as the leg comes closer to the chest. The hands are clasped behind the hamstrings or take a strap placed behind the hamstrings.

***Spanda* Action:** On the inhalation, the stretch is resisted by pressing the leg away from the pull of the hands with approximately ten percent of your strength. On the exhalation, the straight leg is slowly brought towards the chest as a bend in the knee is resisted. There is no undulation of the spine in supine poses and there is no pulsation in standard alignment.

Alignment Focus: Both legs are kept straight and the muscles of the legs are engaged. Both feet are held in *pada bandha*.

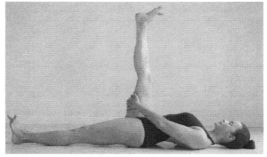

4.42 Supta Padagusthasana in dynamic alignment

Supta Virasana (supine hero's pose)

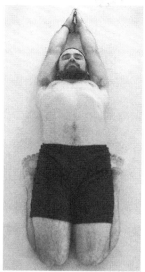

4.43 Supta Virasana

Standard Alignment: The ankles are placed outside the hips and the calf muscles spread out evenly to accommodate the thighs. The knees stay together and the shoulders rest on the floor.

Dynamic Alignment: The ankles are placed outside the hips and the knees are spread hip-width as the upper body rests back onto the mat. This alleviates pressure in the knees and should only be performed if the feet can stay active in alignment.

***Spanda* Action:** As a restorative pose, *supta virasana* would not engage *spanda* action.

Alignment Focus: The toes are spread wide with the fourth and fifth toes pushing down into the floor. The ankles squeeze in toward the hips. The tailbone scoops but does not override the descent of the pubic bone.

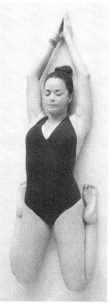

4.44 Supta Virasana in dynamic alignment

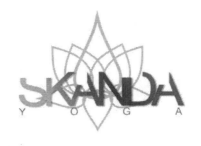

CHAPTER 5

Scientific Stretching Techniques

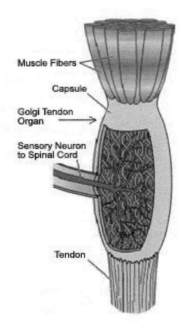

5.1 The musculotendinous junction

We often think of stretching as the act of lengthening tendons and muscles by placing parts of the anatomy in a greater-than-usual range of flexion or extension. Runners and other athletes can be seen manipulating arms and legs into these types of positions as a preparation for engaging their sport. A close look at the anatomy of our tendons reveals that, at best, this type of stretching doesn't actually produce greater tendon or muscle length and, at worst, can cause injury.

The contractility of skeletal muscle cells allows them to shorten significantly in order to pull on bones and other tissues to create movement in the body. Their extensibility can elongate them up to three times their contracted length and their elasticity returns them to their normal length when not in use. To maintain tendon and, thus, joint stability, the range of extensibility must be monitored and protected. This is the job of the golgi tendon organ (GTO), an innervated spindle structure found at the musculotendinous junction. The GTO senses changes in tension that can result in a stretch reflex – the initiation of a contractile force within the muscle that opposes and prevents elongation. Even with this monitoring system in place at the origin and insertion points of our muscles, it is possible to push the tissues into an overstretched position. The result is a strain or pulled muscle – a tearing of muscle or tendon fibers. This is the most common injury in many athletic activities, including yoga.

You may be wondering how it is possible to achieve greater ranges of motion with this guardian system in place. The answer lies in working with the system rather than against it. The stretch reflex and injury are likely to occur when we attempt to lengthen muscles that are not contracted or engaged, and when we ask for too much length too quickly. In examining the physiology of muscular lengthening, we can see that when the muscles are stretched, the GTO-containing spindles are stretched as well. To passively override the stretch reflex initiated within the spindle, we can apply greater and greater lengthening slowly over time; this gradually habituates the system to assuming increased length. To actively override the stretch reflex, the spindles can be shortened while the muscles and tendons are lengthened. This is accomplished by contracting or engaging the muscles that are to be stretched. Let's look at these two methods in greater detail.

Advanced Stretching Techniques

There are many different ways to engage a muscle to create greater length. The Skanda Yoga system employs a system that we refer to as "active dynamic stretching." The muscles that are to be lengthened are consciously engaged and the engagement is linked with the breath. On the inhalation, the muscles and limbs are drawn in towards the core of the body in a concentric action. On the exhalation, the muscles and bones are extended away from the core in an eccentric action. The engagement is never released, and should be of the same intensity between the agonist and antagonist muscles. These actions are maintained by the *spanda* or pulsation of the breath. The pulsation takes us deeper into the experience and meditative qualities of the pose, while cooperating with the central nervous system to safely strengthen and create more muscular length. By maintaining the muscular engagement of 10-15% of possible tensile strength recruitment during concentric and eccentric actions, we keep the stretch reflex from triggering and progressively retrain the nervous system to increase the range of motion and opening.

Proprioceptive Neuromuscular Facilitation (PNF) and Reciprocal Inhibition

PNF is an active method of achieving safe musculotendenous lengthening[18]. It is applied by strongly contracting the muscle that is to be stretched. The agonist muscles resist the stretch, offset the stretch reflex, and cause the GTO to release. The muscular engagement should be between 25% and 50% of

---

18 Proprioceptive neuromuscular – The GTO is a proprioceptor or sensory receptor that makes a connection between the muscular and neurological systems.

maximum strength and should be held for a minimum of six seconds and maximum of 30. Within this period of time, the GTO reads the tension in the engaged muscles as a signal that lengthening can be done safely. To illustrate, let's examine how this technique can be used to gain greater muscular length in a split-leg pose (*Hanumansana*). If the knee of the leading leg is bent and the heel is pushed into the floor, the muscles on the front of the leg engage. When the leg is pulled down and back toward the hip, the muscles on the back of the leg engage. These muscular engagements are held between six to 30 seconds. The muscles are then released, the leg straightens, and the pose is deepened. In this position of a greater "facilitated" stretch, engagement of opposing muscles will support the muscles being stretched. This is known as "reciprocal inhibition" and in *Hanumanasana*, the engagement of the quadriceps muscles on the front of the leg will support a lengthening of the hamstring muscles at the back of the leg. This method produces fast, effective results that retrain the nervous system and allows for increases of flexibility as well as strength.

After performing PNF, the muscles are released, the pose is deepened, and then PNF can be repeated or followed up by active dynamic stretching or reciprocal inhibition, which is a form of active-static stretching. As mentioned earlier, passive-static stretching involves a surrender and relaxation of the muscles that are targeted for lengthening. In yoga, this is found primarily in restorative poses where props are used for support. Keeping the muscles disengaged while challenging their length in a pose is unsafe when sustained for longer than 30 seconds at a time. Athletes who engage in passive stretching before a run or other strenuous activity should also engage in active, facilitated stretching afterward. As a general rule, it is unwise to vigorously stretch before strenuous exercise, as this can increase susceptibility to injury.

Pneumo-Muscular Flexibility Training (PFT)

PFT is a facilitated stretching technique that is performed in conjunction with PNF. Strength has been shown to increase when intra-abdominal pressure increases; this is known as the "pneumo-muscular reflex." One method of creating intra-abdominal pressure is by holding the breath in while every muscle in the body is engaged and pulled strongly toward the core at the same time. This is held for as long as possible. As the breath flows out and the muscles relax, the energy moves from the core out to the periphery and this outward release of strength makes it possible to move more deeply into a pose. Active dynamic stretching or active static stretching can now be used to make even greater increases in flexibility.

Shutdown Threshold Isometrics (STI)

STI is a facilitated stretching technique. It is performed by first creating the strongest engagement possible of the muscle that is to be stretched. The engagement is held until the GTO "collapse" and the muscle reaches contractile failure. The pose is subsequently deepened through gravity. This is an extremely advanced technique that should only be performed by an experienced practitioner who has the help of a spotter who can assist in safely exiting the pose.

Applying These Techniques in Asana

Let's examine how these techniques are applied in a variety of basic poses with which we are probably all familiar. You'll recognize some of the same poses used to establish alignment principles in the previous chapter. As you develop an understanding of how these advanced techniques are applied in these forms, it becomes easier to apply them in other poses as well.

Utthita Trikonasana (extended triangle pose)

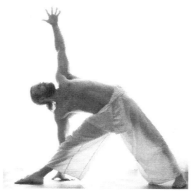

5.2 Utthita Trikonasana

PNF Technique: Lift the ball of the foot of the leading leg and push the heel down and back. The knee is slightly bent for a stronger engagement and a block can be used for support (see figure 5.3). Pulling the whole leg back engages the hamstring muscles on the back of the leg. Hold this for between six and 30 seconds, then release the muscular engagement as you lower the sole of the foot to the mat and stretch deeply into the pose. When you feel that you have reached the outer edge of your lengthening capacity, re-engage the legs and perform active-static or active-dynamic-stretching techniques.

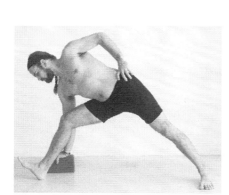

5.3 Muscles engaged and energy drawing up

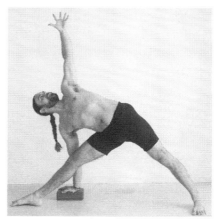

5.4 Energy moves out as musclar engagement is released for lengthening

Active Static Stretching: Hold the pose in a static position with the leg muscles fully engaged and the energy lifting up from the foot toward the hips. Focus on recruiting more strength in the quadriceps.

Active Dynamic Stretching (spanda technique): On an inhalation, squeeze the legs towards each other, engaging the adductor muscles[19]. Keeping the muscles engaged, widen the thighbones apart and exhale. This action continues with the breath and becomes more refined with practice. The big toe and outer heel will press down more during an inhalation and the little toe and inner heel will press down more on exhalation.

Parsvottanasana (intense side stretch)

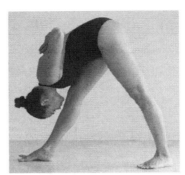

5.5 Parsvottanasana

PNF Technique: The same actions engaged in *utthita trikonasana* are applied to the leading leg in this pose. The muscular engagement is held for between six and 30 seconds and then released as the leg straightens. Then, the torso is moved toward the leading thigh. Place the hands on the floor a few inches behind the leading foot or bring them into reverse prayer position as shown above.

Active Static Stretching: Engage the quadriceps strongly. The hamstrings will lengthen as the thigh bones are pushed back behind you. More strength can be recruited in this pose by clasping the hands around the back of the trailing thigh. The arms pull forward on the thigh as the thigh pushes back into the hands.

Active Dynamic Stretching (*spanda* technique): On an inhalation, pull the thighbone of the leading leg firmly back into the hip joint. The leg will rotate outward as the opposite hip rolls forward. On exhalation, the thighbones continue to pull back firmly into the hip sockets; this keeps the hamstring muscles engaged. From the hips, the legs are pushed out in opposite directions.

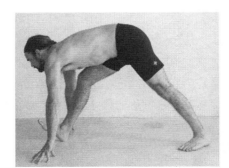

5.6 Muscles engaged and energy drawing up toward the hip

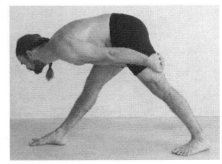

5.7 Recruting more strength for a greater opening

---

19 Adductor muscles bring a part of the anatomy closer to the midline of the body. In the legs, the adductor muscles are located in the upper, inner thigh.

Utthita Hasta Padangusthasana (standing hand to big toe posture)

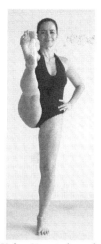

5.8 Utthita Hasta Padangusthasana

PNF Technique: Place the leading leg on a stable, elevated platform such as a bookshelf, windowsill, desk or kitchen counter, or work with a partner who can provide the support and assistance. Press your heel down with 25-50% of maximum strength of the hamstring muscles. Hold for six to 30 seconds then release and raise the leg higher to gain more length in the stretch. The torso can remain upright or bow over the lifted leg. Repeat the exercise one to three times.

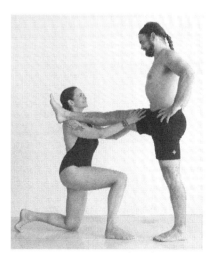

5.9 Partner-assisted stretch

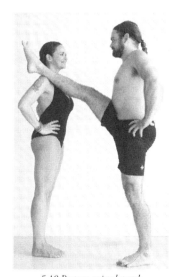

5.10 Partner-assisted stretch

Active Static Stretching: Draw the kneecap up to engage the quadriceps muscles and take the leg higher. This should be done following the PNF technique, but may also be performed on its own.

Active Dynamic Stretching (*spanda* technique): On an inhalation, engage the quadriceps and the hamstring muscles by pressing the lifted heel down while holding the big toe. Keep that muscular engagement as you raise the leg higher on exhalation. As you breathe, alternate between the two actions. On inhalations, press the heel down to resist upward movement and on exhalations, lengthen the back of the leg.

Prasarita Padottanasana (wide-legged standing forward bend)

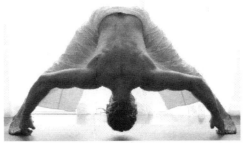

5.11 Prasarita Padottanasana

Active Static Stretching: The hands are on the floor under the shoulders for support. Bend the knees, arch your lower back and push your head up to create a strong inner rotation of the upper thighs. Squeeze the inner thighs toward each other and then slowly straighten the legs. Draw the navel in and scoop the tailbone, while holding a strong engagement in the quadriceps. Engage the muscles of the legs strongly and hold this strong contraction in the legs as you bow forward. Either take the big toes, or bring fingertips or forearms to the floor as the head moves to or toward the floor.

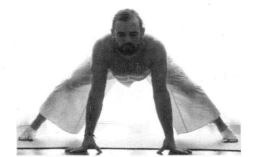

5.12 Engaging the adductor muscles in preparation for active static stretching

Active Dynamic Stretching (*spanda* technique): Place the hands on the floor under the shoulders for support. Engage the quadriceps and the hamstrings while linking inner and outer rotation of the thighs with the breath. On the inhalation, draw the legs in towards the midline and rotate the thighs inward. On the exhalation, push the legs apart and rotate the thighs outward.

Vira Prasarita Padottanasana (powerful wide-legged standing forward bend)

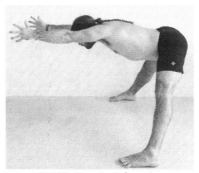

5.13 Vira Prasarita Padottanasana

PNF Technique: Create a strong inner rotation in the top of the thighs. Draw the navel in and scoop the tailbone then lean the hips back. Reach both arms straight ahead. Hold for ten seconds then relax the legs and place the hands on the floor; move the feet wider apart. Lift the torso parallel to the floor again; reach with the arms and create a full engagement in the leg muscles. Repeat the exercise one to three times.

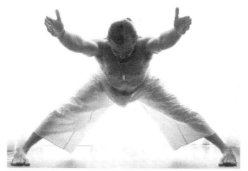

5.14 Using PNF to create greater length in the hamstring muscles

PFT Technique: Repeat the PNF instructions given above. When the arms lift, hold the breath in and engage every muscle in the body. Pull the muscular energy strongly into the midline to create as much internal pressure as possible. Release the muscle engagement and the breath at the same time and then, with the head, arms and/or chest on the floor, stretch the adductor muscles on the inside of the thighs as deeply as possible. Hold the release at the edge of your ability to lengthen and then re-engage the leg muscles to hold the pose longer; otherwise, exit the pose.

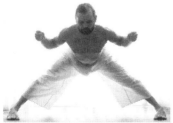

5.15 Using PFT to create internal pressure for greater strength and opening.

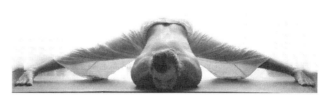

5.16 A deep stretch will take the inner thighs closer to the floor.

Samakonasana (same angle pose)

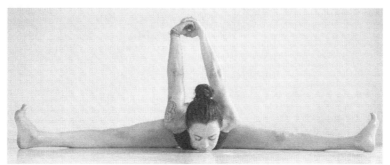

5.17 Samokonasana

When taken to a deeper level of opening, with the thighs rotated outward, feet pointing up, and the legs open at a 180-degree angle, *Vira Prasarita Padottanasana* becomes *Samakonasana* (with torso on the floor) or *Rajasamakonasana* (with torso elevated).

STI Technique: To engage the shutdown-threshold isometrics technique, place blocks under the heels with the legs open to a 180-degree angle. Place fingertips on the mat, or on a chair in front of you, and press the legs down into the blocks. Then, lean the upper back against a wall, push down through the legs and lift the arms overhead. Hold the engagement until the muscles of the legs reach a state of exhaustion. Release and move more deeply into the stretch. Hold for just a few breaths and then exit with the help of a spotter.

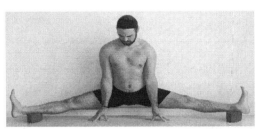

5.18 Moving into samakonasana with heels on blocks.

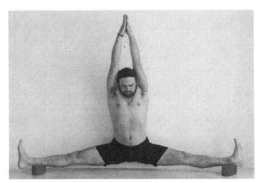

5.19 Descending into a deep stretch after releasing the engagement of the leg muscles

Eka Pada Rajakapotasana I (one foot king pigeon pose preparation)

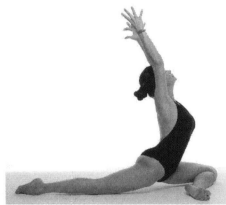

5.20 Eka Pada Rajakapotasana

PNF Technique: Pull the leading leg back toward the body as you pull the trailing leg forward. Hold a strong muscular engagement in the legs for six to 30 seconds, then push the legs apart and release the hips down.

Active Static Stretching: Bow the torso forward over the leading leg. Bring the forehead to the floor. Lift the elbows up and draw the shoulder blades together on the back. Push the leading leg down and pull it back toward the body. The sitting bones will move down toward the floor. Push the trailing leg down and rotate the thigh inward.

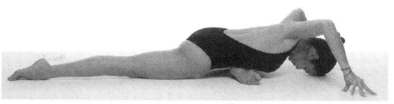

5.21 Active static stretching

Active Dynamic Stretching (*spanda* technique): Draw the legs toward each other on an inhalation and push them away from each other on an exhalation. The leading leg will rotate inward as you inhale and outward as you exhale. The trailing leg will rotate inward on inhalation and this must be held during exhalation.

Baddha Konasana (bound angle pose)

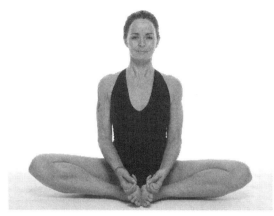

5.22 Baddha Konasana

PNF Technique: For the first stage of this technique, cross the forearms and bring the hands to the biceps. Place the crossed arms on the inside of the bent legs. Squeeze the legs into the arms strongly for six to 30 seconds. This will engage the muscles that adduct the legs into the midline of the body. For the second stage, bring the legs together and tightly wrap the arms around the outside of the legs. Attempt to force your arms apart by strongly pushing the legs outward. Hold for six to 30 seconds to engage the muscles that abduct the legs away from the midline of the body. Release and enter *badha konasana* fully, as shown in figure 5.25.

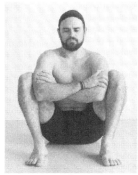

5.23 Pressing legs in to engage adductor muscles

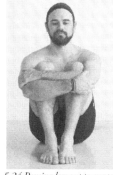

5.24 Pressing legs out to engage abductor muscles

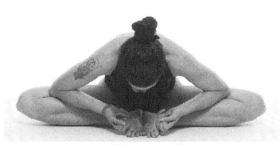

5.25 Forward folding into Baddha Konasana

Janu Sirsasana (head to knee pose)

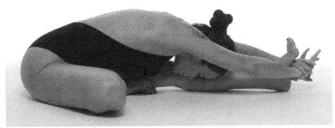

5.26 Janu Sirsasana

PNF Technique: Bend the leading leg and pull the heel back toward the hip to engage the hamstring muscles. Hold this engagement for six to 30 seconds then straighten the leg and release the hamstrings. Bow forward and reach for the foot. Re-engage the leg muscles to deepen the stretch using active static or active dynamic stretching.

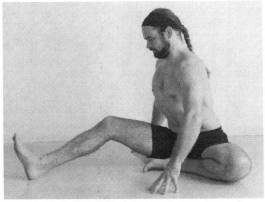

5.27 The heel is pulled back to engage the hamstring muscles

Active Static Stretching: Engage the quadriceps by pulling the kneecap up and pushing the thighbone down toward the floor while the hamstrings lengthen.

Active Dynamic Stretching: Engage the quadriceps and the hamstrings evenly, contracting them strongly onto the bones. On the inhalation, draw the leg back into the hip and flex the foot. On the exhalation, push the leg out away from the hip and point or floint the foot. These actions link the inner and outer rotations of the thigh with the breath.

Upavishta Konasana (seated wide angle pose):

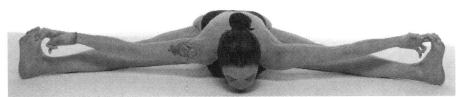

5.28 Upavishta Konasana

PNF Technique: Bring the arms beside the chest or raise them straight overhead; arch the lower back and bow halfway forward. Hold the muscular engagement in the legs for six to 30 seconds. Release the engagement and open the legs wider, then bow forward with the hands on the floor or clasp the big toes as shown above.

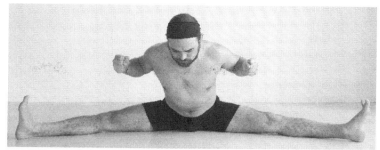

5.29 Engaging the leg muscles muscles prior to releasing into the stretch using the PNF technique

PFT Technique: Repeat the PNF technique as described above and at the same time, hold an inhalation and engage every muscle in the body. The arms are held off the floor as the whole body contracts. On the exhalation, release the muscles and stretch deeply into the pose.

Active Static Stretching: Engage the quadriceps by pulling the kneecaps up and pushing the thighbones down toward the floor while the hamstrings lengthen.

Active Dynamic Stretching (*spanda* technique): Engage the quadriceps and the hamstrings while linking inner and outer rotations of the thighs with the breath. On an inhalation, draw the thighbones into the hips, arch the lower back more and push the head up. This causes inner rotation of the thighbones, aligning the hamstring muscles on the bones. On the exhalation, bow forward, releasing the head down, then push the legs out from the hips with actively engaged feet; this results in outer rotation of the thighs.

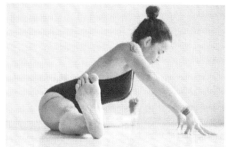

5.30 Active dynamic stretching on inhalation

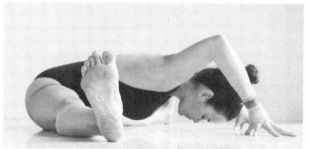

5.31 Active dynamic stretching on exhalation

Hanumanasana (Hanuman's pose)

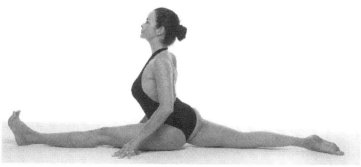

5.32 Hanumanasana

PNF Technique: Bend both legs and isometrically draw them toward the body for six to 30 seconds. The leading heel pushes down and pulls back to engage the hamstrings. The trailing knee pushes down and pulls forward to engage the quadriceps. Release the muscular engagement and push the legs away from each other to deepen the stretch in the pose.

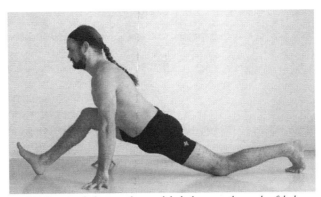

5.33 Drawing the legs strongly toward the body engages the muscles of the legs

STI Technique: Engage the shutdown-threshold isometrics technique by drawing the legs strongly toward the body as you reach the arms overhead. Hold the muscular engagement until you feel as though you are reaching a state of exhaustion. Release the engagement and stretch more deeply into the pose. For a more advanced technique, place blocks under the ankles. Push down into the blocks and draw the legs toward the body. This will elevate the hips. When you feel that the muscles have reached a state of exhaustion, push the legs in opposite directions to stretch deeply into the pose. Release the engagement as you bring your hands to the floor for support and stretch more deeply into the pose.

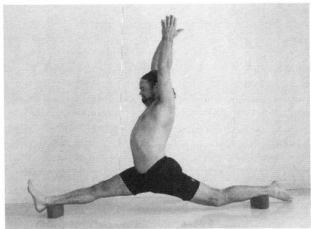

5.34 Pressing down and drawing in to engage the muscles of the legs to a point of exhaustion

Active Static Stretching: Activate the quadriceps and the hamstrings by pushing down through the legs and the feet. Hold the engagement as you lengthen the muscles into the stretch.

Active Dynamic Stretching: On an inhalation, draw the legs toward the body and toward the midline. On an exhalation, push the legs away from each other while maintaining the pull toward the midline of the body. The leading leg will rotate inward on an inhalation and outward on an exhalation. The trailing leg will rotate inward on the inhalation and this inner rotation must be maintained on exhalation as the leg pushes down and back.

Gomukhasana (cow face pose)

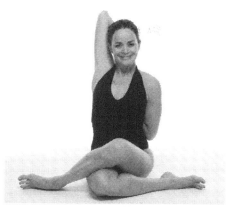

5.35 Gomukhasana

PNF Technique for arms: Place one hand at the level of the sacrum and one behind the head with each hand clasping a strap or belt. Pull the strap apart strongly for five to ten seconds. Release and bring the hands closer together. Repeat two to three more times until the hands reach each other enough for the fingers to clasp.

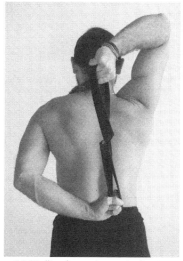

5.36 Pulling the strap in opposite directions

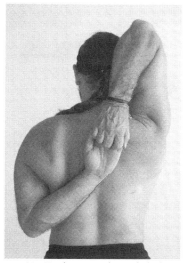

5.37 Hands come together on the back

Supta Agnistambhasana (reclined fire log pose)

This pose and the one that follows it are executed with the help of an assistant, and the instructions that are given have been written from the assistant's perspective. Passive stretching should only be done in restorative yoga with the support of props or with the assistance of a partner who can monitor proper alignment and breath. These poses create a deep opening for the hips and should only be held for up to three minutes. They do not occur in the Dreamspell class sequences but can be performed in private sessions, workshops, or as an alternative on Red days after *agnistambhasana* if the class is small.

Passive Static Stretching: With the practitioner in a reclined *agnistambhasana*, place one hand on the ankle and the other on the knee of the top leg. As the practitioner exhales, gently push the knee down toward the floor until they report that they have reached their maximum opening or until the top shin is lying on top of the bottom shin. Hold the pose at their edge and let them release the mental tension associated with the physical holding pattern.

PNF Technique: With the practitioner in a reclined *agnistambhasana,* place one hand on the heel and the other hand on the knee of the top leg. Ask them to push the top knee up into your hand for six to 30 seconds. As they release the pressure with an exhalation, gently push the knee down. This can be repeated if necessary. When the top shin is making contact with the bottom shin, passive static stretching can be performed.

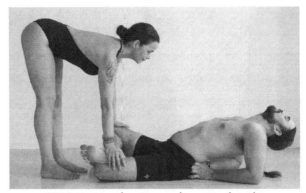

5.37 Assistant provides resistance and pressure on the top knee

Adho Mukha Agnistambhasana (downward facing fire log pose)

Passive Static Stretching: Press down slowly on the elevated ankle, as shown in figure 5.38. The practitioner's top knee may slide off of the bottom ankle and out to the side. If this occurs, hold the top knee in position by the placing your foot or knee against it. With the top knee stabilized, place one hand on it and the other hand on the ankle and gently begin to press the ankle down toward the knee of the bottom leg. Eventually, the shin of the top leg will stack on the shin of bottom leg.

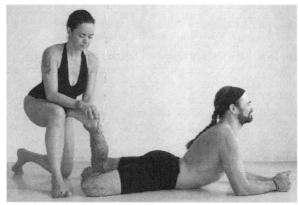

5.38 Assistant provides pressure to top ankle

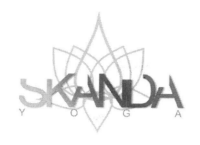

CHAPTER 6

The Energy Body

The philosophies of yoga hold that all living beings are infused with a life-force or enlivening energy. The Sanskrit word for this is *prana*. It circulates around and through the physical body, creating a "form" of its own – a *pranic* body. Within the *pranic* body are vortex centers where the energy cyclones in and out, and these areas of concentrated movement stimulate the endocrine system. They relate to specific locations in the physical body and are known as *chakras*, which translate from Sanskrit to "wheels." The *chakras* also relate to facets of our personality. When they are fully opened and balanced through yoga practice, we function at our optimal radiant health.

We can increase our awareness and sensitivity in the practice of yoga with knowledge of the *pranic* body and its influence upon the physical body. If the *pranic* "winds" become disturbed, they can be rebalanced through the practice of *asana, pranayama, mudra* and *bandha*.

Body of Light

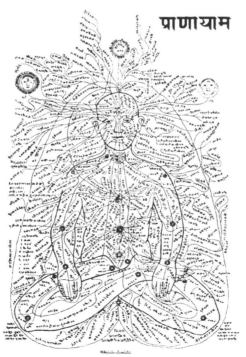

6.1 A traditional India- medicine and spiritual- science depiction of the nadis or energy channels

The *pranic* body is also referred to as a "light" or "aura body" because its energy has been observed as light. It is the vitalistic energy called "qi" that is the focus of the Chinese discipline Qigong. Its existence has been recognized by cultures all over the world and there are nearly 100 different names for the phenomenon. Individuals who have developed sensitivity to energy emanations have reportedly seen the light body. This was a skill that the spiritual masters or *rishis* engaged through what has been referred to as an opening of the spiritual or third eye. Coronal electrical emanations are believed to be captured using a technique known as Kirlian photography, which portrays the discharges on photographic film[20]. They have also been recorded in a number of well-designed scientific experiments.

Soviet Scientists from the Bioinformation Institute determined that organisms emit energy vibrations at a frequency between 300 and 2,000 nanometers. In her book *Hands of Light*, Barbra Ann Brennan explains that these findings have been confirmed at the Medical Sciences Academy in Moscow and are supported by researchers in Great Britain, the Netherlands, Germany and Poland. Dr. Valerie Hunt, from The University of California, Los Angeles, recorded low-millivoltage-frequency signals emanating from the body. Her information was analyzed and the wave patterns were translated by Fourier and sonogram frequency analysis[21]. This was the first electronic evidence of frequency, amplitude, and time of the body's energy emanations and, amazingly, they correspond to the colors the ancient spiritual seers perceived of the *charkas*.

Dr. Zheng Rongliang, of Lanzhou University[22] has made measurements of *prana* using a photo-quantum device and Dr. Hiroshi Motoyama, President of the International Association for Religion and Parapsychology, has created two different machines for detecting the energy emitted by the body. The first of Dr. Motoyama's machines that measures acupuncture meridians is the "Apparatus for Measuring the Function of Meridians and Corresponding Internal Organs" (AMI). The second is the *Chakra* Machine. It can measure the entirety of energy emissions without the use of attached electrodes.

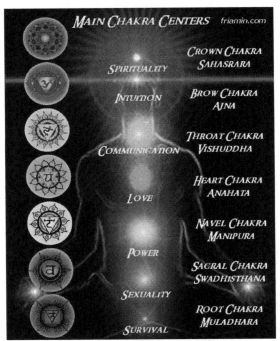

6.2 The chakra system

---

20 Named for its founder Semyon Kirlian, Kirlian photography is thought to produce images of the energy field or aura that surrounds living things.
21 Named for Joseph Fourier, Fourier analysis is the study of the way general functions can be represented or approximated by sums of simpler trigonometric functions. A sonogram analysis, also called a spectrogram, analyses the frequency modulations of sounds.
22 Lanzhou is a major research University located in Gansu Province, China.

The *Chakra* System

As mentioned earlier, *chakras* (pronounced cha-kra*)*, are vortices of energy that travel through the body. There are seven main *chakras* found along the body's central axis or spinal column. There are also several minor *chakras*, which are located in the ears, palms, elbows, knees and feet. *Chakras* transform non-physical energies into energies that can be utilized by the physical entity. The energy comes into the body through a *nadi* or energy channel and enlivens the nervous, circulatory and endocrine systems. Traditional Indian medicine and spiritual science establishes the existence of approximately 72,000 *nadis*.

Vital energy is supplied to the body's systems through each *chakra* and those systems are balanced and governed by them. Before disease or an imbalance develops in the physical body, it first manifests as a disturbance in the flow of *prana* through the *chakras*. Traditionally, *chakras* are described as flowers with each petal corresponding to the number of energies entering the body. The Sanskrit alphabet corresponds to the petals of the *chakra* system. The energies of each *chakra* encode specific sounds and they form the basic sounds found in the Sanskrit language. The ancients believed that every word, sound, syllable or group of words has causal energies. They arranged and repeated words into sacred prayers or *mantras,* which they believed had the ability to manipulate energy through the *chakras* and even to prompt a spiritual transformation. Certain *mantras* activate certain energy centers and the sound *aum* (most often spelled and sounded as "om") activates them all.

One of the aims of yoga is to open and balance each *chakra* so that *prana* can flow into and through the body without impediment. To work with the energy of the *chakras* directly, the most logical place to start is at the bottom, with progression upward – from the root or *muladhara chakra* to the crown or *sahasrara*. It is possible, however, to start anywhere in the system and to work on one or several areas simultaneously. Classes that include *asanas* from each of the main groups of movements are often organized around this principle and might effectively achieve this goal within the timeframe of the class. For example, standing poses will activate the root *chakra* as they create stability. Hip openers activate the second *chakra*, which leads to increased fluidity. Twists and poses that place pressure on the abdomen activate the third *chakra* by increasing digestive fire and will power. Backbends activate the heart *chakra* by opening the thoracic spine and stimulating the thymus. Inversions activate the throat *chakra* by directing *prana* into the thyroid. The brow and crown *chakras* are opened with seated mediation and breathing practices.

The *chakras* can be opened and activated during meditation and by visualizing or focusing on specific symbols, such as *yantras*[23]. *Mantras* are used in the same way and *pranayama,* or directed control of the breath, can manipulate the flow of energy through the *chakra* centers. Learning about the *chakras* and the dynamics of the energy body can help us pinpoint imbalances of energy, which are believed to be the result of our misinterpretation of past events and of holding onto strong emotions, fears or attachments.

There are guiding energies and emotional states associated with each *chakra* – from the drive to survive and assert one's will, to the impulse to communicate, know and love. When there are imbalances of energy in one center, others are affected. When too much energy exists in one or more *chakras*, certain mental and emotional states will predominate and when they are absent, those states will diminish. The hormones

---

23 Yantras are geometric figures or symbol patterns that are used to balance the mind and focus it on particular ideas. They represent the sacred architecture of the multidimensional reality. The translations of this Sanskrit word include "machine," "instrument," "engine" and "motor."

excreted by the endocrine system have a direct effect on our moods, and yoga's action on the various glands in the endocrine system results in a reciprocal response in the nervous system. Each *chakra* center can be balanced through yoga postures that stimulate the gland associated with it. For example, hip-opening postures stimulate the reproductive glands and belly-down backbends stimulate the glands associated with digestion and the assimilation of nutrients. When the nerve plexus and endocrine system function properly, energy is unfettered, the mind is balanced and the body feels better.

CHAKRA CHART				
	Location	Sanskrit Name	Color	Endocrine Gland
7	Crown	Sahasrara	Violet / White	Pineal
6	Brow	Ajna	Indigo	Pituitary
5	Throat	Vishuddhi	Blue	Thyroid
4	Heart	Anahata	Green	Thymus
3	Solar Plexus	Manipura	Yellow	Pancreas
2	Sacral	Swadhisthana	Orange	Gonads / Ovaries
1	Base	Muladhara	Red	Adrenals

Muladhara Chakra

The base of the *chakra* system is located at the perineum and represents grounding, as well as all the basic human needs associated with survival. *Muladhara* means "root place." It is the center of our sexual energy, desire for material needs, and security. These must be satisfied for the *chakra* to be open. When this *chakra* is balanced, we have a sense of being grounded in life. The base *chakra* has the densest energy and the slowest vibration. It connects us to the earth element by being dense, inert, heavy and rooting. It is the origin of sexual energy and, if imbalanced, we may experience fatigue, anemia, lower back pain, sciatica or depression. This *chakra* can be stimulated by physical exercise, standing yoga *asanas*, restful sleep, gardening and using the color red.

Svadhistana Chakra

The sacral *chakra* is associated with procreative instincts and sexual relationships. It is where we store our emotions and *samskaras* – the energetic conditioning and habits that we develop through experience. *Svadhistana* means "one's own dwelling place." It connects to the water element and is the center of all our emotions. Our desire to have relationships comes from this center and it gives us our sense of self. If this *chakra* is open, we will flow in life with creativity. If this center is blocked, it will lead to negative self-approval and anti-social behavior and can lead to eating disorders, drug abuse, and depression. The *chakra* is stimulated by hot aromatic baths, massage, swimming and hip-opening yoga *asanas*. Using the color orange or essential oils also stimulate this center.

Manipura Chakra

The *chakra* at the solar plexus embodies the energies of personal will and power. It balances the energies of the intellect, self-confidence and ego. *Manipura* means "city of jewels." It is the seat of our personal power and is associated with the fire element. When this center is open and balanced, we will excel at our talents and gifts. We will work not for self-serving gratification, but as an offering for the greater good. If this center is imbalanced, it can lead to digestive problems, ulcers, diabetes, toxicity and nervousness. To stimulate this center, engage in twisting yoga *asanas*, read books, sun bathe and detox the body. Using yellow colors and lemon or rosemary essential oils also stimulates this center.

Anahata Chakra

The heart center is the merging point of the ascending and descending energies. It is where the body and mind interconnect. *Anahata* translates to mean "unstruck" and "vibration that emanates independently." Love centers the energies of the heart and generates self-acceptance, approval, compassion and balance. Imbalances in this *chakra* will manifest as heart conditions, breathing disorders, breast cancer, high blood pressure and immune-system dysfunction. The heart center is activated by time spent in nature, and with family and friends. Green juices, clothing, and gemstones also stimulate this center, along with the essential oils eucalyptus or pine. This *chakra* is associated with the air element.

Vishudda Chakra

The energy center of the throat governs our power of speech and communication. *Vishuddha* translates to "pure" and is associated with the element of ether. This center clarifies energy to awaken the higher centers. When it is open, we express ourselves freely in alignment with our truth. When it is blocked or imbalanced, we may experience thyroid problems, swollen glands, fevers, flu, infections and mood swings. This center is stimulated by chanting, pranayama, and lucid dreaming. This *chakra* is stimulated by the use of the color blue in gemstones or clothing and essential oils such as jasmine, ginger, geranium and sandalwood.

Ajna Chakra

The energy center of the brow or the "third eye" is our power to see through illusions and perceive the ultimate reality. *Ajna* translates to mean "perceive" and "command" and, as the energy of soul, spirit and subconscious, it is beyond elemental reality. *Ajna* is the center of discriminative awareness and allows us to perceive the meta-pattern that unites all. When the center is open, our intuition and psychic abilities become more refined. When the center is imbalanced, we can have learning challenges, coordination problems and sleep disorders. The brow center is stimulated by meditation, star gazing, and using the color indigo and with the use of essential oils such as patchouli and frankincense.

Sahasrara Chakra

The *chakra* at the crown of the head embodies spiritual transformation and the energies of universal consciousness. *Sahasara* means "thousand-petaled lotus." Its opening or unfoldment represents the state of enlightenment. The crown *chakra* is where we integrate consciousness and the subconscious into the super-consciousness. Our views of God or a higher intelligence can affect this energy center. If it is imbalanced, we may experience headaches, mental illness, blood vessel problems and skin rashes. It is stimulated by focusing on dreaming, journaling, using the color violet, and the essential oils lavender or jasmine.

According to some yoga philosophies and traditions, *prana*, the great, potential energy and life force that invigorates all, is thought to lie like the coil of a rope–*kundala*–at the base of the spine or *muladhara chakra*. Through meditative and yogic practices, it is awakened and aroused to higher and more refined energetic frequencies. This liberates the dormant spiritual energy and allows it to ascend though the *chakras* above. This coiled energy is often envisioned as the goddess *Shakti*[24], who represents the primordial, creative power and dynamic force that moves through the entire universe and, as such, it is known as the *kundalini Shakti*. Just as it is possible to split atoms and release their potential energy, yogis seek to liberate the dormant potential of energy that lies within the bodily form. Yogic practices like *asana* and *pranayama* can manipulate, store and expand the life force and thus awaken greater and greater spiritual energies. When we know how the *prana* flows through the body, we can increase our sensitivity to it and even influence it. This is *prana vidya*, the knowledge of *prana*, and how to direct it with the mind into specific areas of the body.

The Energy Sheaths or *Koshas*

As a partial expression of universal consciousness, individual consciousness forms the illusion of separation. According to Vedantic yoga philosophy, consciousness is the ultimate reality out of which matter and mind arise; all beings and things are not only infused with it - they *are* it. From a single blade of grass to the highly evolved organization of a human being, consciousness exists in a broad spectrum of levels. As perhaps the most complex, human consciousness is believed to spread out in layers that are organized around the seed or kernel of an unmoving, infinite and eternal center. That center is described as the truth of the self and its state as pure bliss. It does not exist to be experienced; it is simply the organizing principle of the whole. It is referred to as the *Atman*, a Sanskrit word that means "soul" or "spirit." It is equivalent in meaning with the term "self." It is unchanging and untouched by the events of a life and those events are experienced and known by the first layer that covers it – the ego.

In the same way that yoga acts upon and organizes the energies that flow through the body, it acts upon the layers of consciousness that express the human being. By first recognizing the ego's concepts and judgments and its role in the formation of a life, it can be distinguished from the *Atman*, which can then be glimpsed or experienced. This can make way for the utilization of mind in its purposeful union with breath and body to achieve yoga. The early philosophers believed this refinement of the organization of human consciousness to be the ultimate and true aim of yoga.

The *Anandamaya Kosha* is the truth of the self. It is the sheer bliss of consciousness that exists beyond multiplicity and differentiation. The *Vignanamaya Kosha* represents the ego and learned concepts. It governs the function of thinking, reasoning, and discrimination. The *Manamaya Kosha* is the mind. It affects the function of awareness as well as passions and emotions. *Pranamaya Kosha* is the breath – the vital air that constitutes the five *pranas*. The *Annamaya Kosha* is the body – the physical system and the organs of perception and action.

---

24 *Shakti* is thought of as the manifesting and feminine force that is name and form and the manifested world. *Shakti* is one and same with its complementary opposite, *Shiva* – the masculine force and the ground of all - the latent potentiality. The universal goal of spiritual life is the experience of collapsing the apparent duality of *shakti* and *shiva* to experience creation and its potential, feminine and masculine, as one indivisible unchanging substratum of reality.

Five Primary *Pranas*

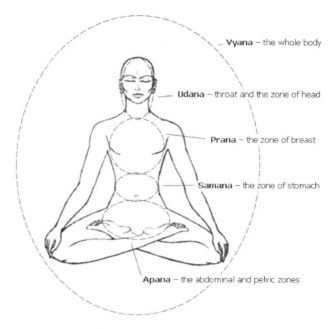

6.4 The five primary pranas

Prana, the life-force energy that supports all of life, is generated, stored, and expanded through yogic practices. Although there is one *Prana,* also known as the *Mahaprana* or "great *prana,*" it has distinct functions in the body. These different functions are known as *vayus* or "winds" and they influence the regulation of digestion, respiration, nerve impulses, circulation and conscious activity. The five vayus are: *prana, apana, samana, udana,* and *vyana.* Each of the *prana vayus* can be activated through *asana* to enhance their flow and influence on the body's vital functions. They can also be stimulated through the use of conscious or *ujjayi* breath. Knowing the flow of the vital winds and their function is important for yoga practitioners who wish to enhance their influence and increase vitality.

Prana vayu

An upward-moving energy from the bottom of the heart to the throat that regulates the heart and inhalation, *prana vayu* is the energy that receives air, food, liquids and perceptions into the body. In *asana*, it is experienced when we rise up out of the hips and create an inner expansion of the torso. *Prana vayu* literally means "forward moving air." As it moves inward toward the center of the body, it creates a feeling of openness and expansion and allows us to experience open-hearted joy. The standing warrior poses can be used to experience and build *prana vayu.* They cultivate an awareness of lengthening and maintaining length in the sides of the bodies as the inner body expands with *prana vayu.* This experience can eventually be replicated in all *asanas.*

Apana vayu

A downward-flowing energy from the navel to the legs, *apana vayu* controls exhalation, childbirth and the elimination of bodily fluids. Translated to mean "the air that moves away," *apana vayu* balances the incoming energies of *prana vayu.* When it is not functioning properly, toxins and detrimental thought patters can build up in the body and repeat in the mind and energetically and mentally deplete us. It is activated in *asana* by rooting down through the legs and pelvis in standing or seated postures. *Apana vayu* is associated with the earth element and the *muladhara chakra*, cultivating grounding and stability.

Udana vayu

An upward-moving energy from the throat to the head, *udana vayu* carries energy upward. It regulates breath and voice, muscle function and strength in the extremities and function of the sense organs. It seats the head high on the spinal foundation and prevents it from tipping forward and dropping down with age. In yoga asana, it is stimulated by inversions and by extension of the spine. It is associated with the element of space or ether, as it is within the region of the head that we gain awareness of the absolute.

Samana vayu

A downward-flowing energy from the bottom of the heart to the navel, *samana vayu* regulates digestion, vitality and balances every level of being. As the "balancing air," it pulsates in and out of the *kanda*, which is the origin of all nadis, and the source of the beat or vibratory pulse of being (*spanda* in Sanskrit). In *asana*, *samana vayu* governs the contraction and expansion of life force energy with muscle energy. It is the controlling power of the metabolism and assimilation of the oxygen from the air we breathe. It is associated with the element of fire, creating "digestive fire" physically and *tapas* or "inner heat" spiritually.

Vyana vayu

This energy pervades the whole body, governing coordination and balance of the nervous system. It translates to mean "outward moving air" and coordinates all the powers of the body as it runs through the entire energetic system of the 72,000 *nadis*. It regulates the circulatory system, and coordinates all the powers of the sensory system, as well as joint and muscle functions. In *asana*, it is activated by linking inner and outer rotations with the pulsation of breath and *spanda*.

In the practice of yoga *asana*, we strive to convert *apana* or downward-flowing energy into *prana* or upward-moving energy. One way that this is accomplished is by engaging the lock or seal at the root *chakra* – the *mula bandha* throughout the *asana* practice. This is believed to revert the aging process and direct the spiritual energy upward to awaken the higher *chakras*.

Ujjayi breath and *pranayama* techniques can also influence the *prana vayus*. Inhalation activates *prana* and exhalation activates a*pana* energy. *Udana* is activated in the space between the breaths. When the pause between the breaths is lengthened, *samana* is activated. *Vyana* is activated by the entire conscious breath. Overall, the practice of yoga keeps these winds of the life force flowing smoothly and this prevents imbalance and disease. If the flow of *prana* is not balanced and regulated through regular practice, the body will feel disturbed, restless, depressed and imbalanced.

Five Secondary *Pranas*

The five secondary *pranas* govern other functions within the body, which can be manipulated and regulated with the breath and awareness.

Naga is located in the abdomen and relieves stomach pressure by belching. *Kurma* is located in the head and controls the movement of the eyelids. *Krkara* is located in the throat and causes sneezing or coughing. *Devadatta* is located in the solar plexus and causes yawning. *Dhananjaya* is found throughout the whole body where it remains after death, causing the body to swell.

Exercises to Feel *Prana* and the *Pranic* Body

The concept of *prana* in Indian traditions is the same as the Japanese concept of *Ki* and the Chinese concept of *Chi*. Eastern traditions hold that *chi* follows *yi* and *yi* is mind or attention. When we place our attention somewhere in the body, energy is affected or activated there. It is possible to feel, see and dowse *prana* by concentrating our attention in certain exercises. As with any other activity, our skills will sharpen with practice. By practicing exercises to feel, see and measure the flow of *prana,* we are able to increase our sensitivity to its presence. We become more aware of its influence physically as well as spiritually, and learn to channel and control it as we practice yoga *asana.*

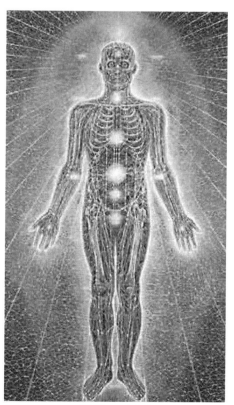

6.5 The pranic body

83

- Begin by rubbing your hands vigorously together until a good degree of heat has been created. Separate the hands about twelve inches apart and turn the palms facing toward each other. Gently move the hands a little closer and then apart. Concentrate on the space between your hands. Consciously direct the energies of your breath into that space while you focus on the sensations in the palms of the hands. You may be able to feel a gentle wind between the hands that pulsates with the movement of your own breath.

- Find a partner to work with and stand about ten feet across from and facing them. Rub your hands together strongly. Hold your hands up in front of you with your palms facing outward. Slowly begin to walk towards your friend. Pay close attention to the sensations in the palms of your hands. You may be able to feel a distinct pressure in your hands as you near the edge of your partner's energy field. Try this exercise with your eyes closed to decrease distraction and increase sensitivity.

- Stand behind a partner who is seated and in silent meditation with their eyes closed. Rub your hands together to create heat in the palms then hold both hands about three feet over the crown *chakra* point at the top of their head. Become sensitive to the feelings on the palms of the hands as you gently move them closer to the head and then further away. You may be able to feel a slight change in sensation as your hands approach the outer edge of your partner's *pranic* body.

Exercises to See Prana

- Begin by establishing *ujjayi* breathing. Adopt and hold *khecari* mudra by moving the tip of your tongue as far back toward the soft palate as possible without straining. Concentrate on and direct the energies of the breath toward your brow or *ajna chakra*. Do this for two to three minutes then hold your hands out in front of you and spread your fingers. You may be able to see streams of energy flowing between the fingers.

- Ask your partner to stand with their back against a bare, white wall. Begin *ujjayi* breath and adopt and hold *kechari* mudra. Look at the wall space that surrounds your friend. Allow your eyes to go out of focus and your gaze to become relaxed. It is easiest to see the crown *chakra* and the outer sheaths or layers of energy. Bring your gaze to the space above their head. You may be able to see what looks like a swirling cyclone or tornado of energy. You may be able to see what looks like vapor rising out of their head, like heat on a hot road during summer.

- Practice seeing the auras of trees and birds against a clear, blue sky, and of other plants and animals.

Detecting the Flow of Prana through the Chakras by Pendulum Dowsing

- Begin by focusing your attention on the movements of your breath. Become aware of the invigorating energy that courses in and around your body. Set an intention that you will become aware of yourself as an open channel for this divine energy.

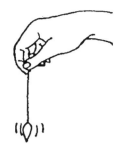

6.6 Holding a pendulum

• Hold the pendulum cord with the thumb and first three fingers, as shown in figure 6.6. Allow the pendulum to dangle a few inches down from your hand. With your partner standing in front of you, hold one hand a few inches away from a particular *chakra*. With the subject lying down, hold the pendulum a few inches above the *chakra*.

• Observe the movement of the pendulum as it comes under the influence of the *pranic* energy. Its motions can be used to diagnose the *chakra's* conductivity, as follows.

– An open circle moving clockwise indicates that the *chakra* is balanced and energy is flowing through it freely. The size of the circle relates to the conductive strength of the *chakra*.

– An open circle that moves in a counter-clockwise direction indicates that the *chakra* is impeding energy. This can be caused by repeating thoughts and persistent beliefs that are negative in nature. If a person is fearful of being able to meet their basic needs of food and shelter, for example, the root *chakra* may be blocked. If they believe they are not loved or not worthy of love, the heart *chakra* may be impeded.

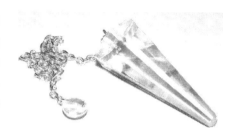

6.7 A crystal pendulum

– When the pendulum moves to the right in an ovoid circle or elliptical shape, it indicates an inclination toward active (masculine) rather than passive or receptive energies (feminine).

– When it moves in an oval shape to the left, it is an indication that receptive energies are more developed than active inclinations.

– When the pendulum moves in a vertical line, it is indicating that energy is moving upward. This can be due to changes or difficult situations.

– When it moves in a horizontal line, the energy is impeded. Movement to the right is an indication of aggressive energies, and to the left of passive energies.

– When there is a lack of movement, the *chakra* is closed and no energy moves through it.

– When the pendulum moves in a chaotic manner, the energies are moving in the same way. The individual may be going through extreme changes or experiencing difficulties; they may be filled with inner turmoil. This type of chaotic energy presentation is best cleared, as it will often lead to illness or disease.

Restorative and *Chakra*-Balancing Sequence

The following sequence is for activating each *chakra* from root to crown. When each *asana* is combined with mantra and visualization, the energy flow is strengthened and awareness becomes more sensitive. This routine can be practiced daily or on rest days when needed.

Muladhara – Base, 1st *chakra*

Visualize the color red and draw energy up from the pelvic floor.
Activation Mantra: *Om Bhur*
Asana: Sphinx pose and supported Sphinx pose

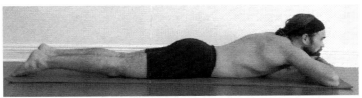

6.8 Downward corpse pose

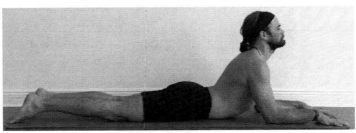

6.9 Sphinx pose

Lie flat on the belly and bring elbows under the shoulders. Gently pull the arms back, so the lower back muscles tone. Hold Sphinx pose for one minute then rest the head down on stacked fists in *apanavasana* or downward corpse pose.

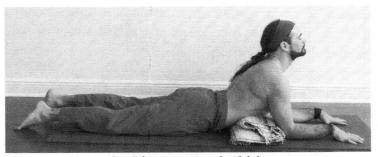

6.10 Sphinx pose supported with bolster

A bolster or blankets may be placed under the lower ribs, raising the top of the pelvis off the floor.

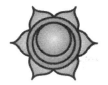

Swadhistana – Sacral, 2nd *chakra*

Visualize the color orange and breathe into the lower abdomen and sacral region.

Activation Mantra: *Om Bhuva*

Asana: *Paschimottanasana* (west side stretch, seated forward bend)
and *Salambha Paschimottanasana* (supported)

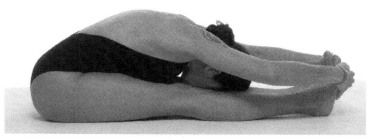

6.11 Paschimottanasa

Create strength in the legs by pushing them down as you fold forward. Keep the shoulders lifting above the ears and pulling down the back. Extend the heart forward. Use a strap around the feet and blankets under the hips to maintain spinal extension if necessary. Hold the forward fold for at least two minutes. Exit on an inhalation. Place the fingertips or hands on the floor behind the hips to reengage the lower back and lift the spine, stretching the neck. Repeat and go deeper, or perform a supported west side stretch. To support the seated forward bend, place a rolled blanket or bolster underneath the knees. Arch the lower back on inhalation, then fold forward and take the feet or a strap around the feet. Alternatively, place a bolster can be laid across the top of the thighs to support the torso as it folds toward the legs.

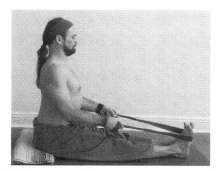

6.12 Paschimottanasa with a strap to maintain extension of spine

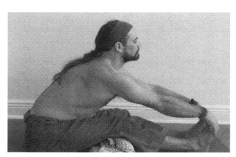

6.12b Supported Paschimottanasa

Manipurna – Solar Plexus, 3rd *chakra*

Visualize the color yellow in the upper abdomen.
Activating Mantra: *Om Swaha*
Asana: *Ardha Matsyendrasana* (half Lord of the Fishes pose)

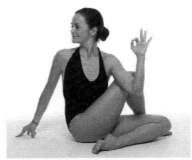

6.13 Ardha Matsyendrasana

On an inhalation, lift the spine and twist the torso in the direction of bent leg and bring the back of the elbow or arm to the outside of the bent knee. On an exhalation, deepen the twist. Hold the pose for two to five minutes and switch sides.

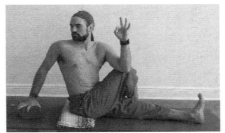

6.14 Using props in Ardha Matsyendrasana

By placing a blanket under the hips, the pelvis can achieve a forward tilt and the spine can lengthen from the natural inward or lordotic curve of the lumbar or low back. Use a block under the supporting hand to maintain length in the side body.

Alternatively, or in addition to using the supports shown above, the twist can be done lying down on a bolster or blanket. Look toward the knees for an easy twist, and look away from them to deepen the twist in the upper vertebrae.

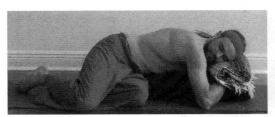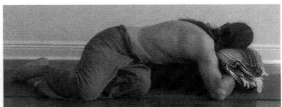

6.15 Ardha Matsyendrasana reclined over a bolster and blanket

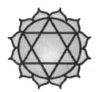

Anahata – Heart, 4th *chakra*

Visualize the color green in the heart center.
Activating Mantra: *Om Maha*
Asana: *Ustrasana* (camel pose) and *Salamba Supta Virasana* (supported reclined hero's pose)

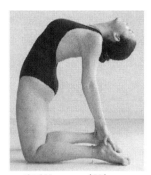

6.16 Unsupported Ushtrasana

This *asana* can be performed unsupported, as shown above or by pushing the hips into a wall as in image 6.17. Hold for up to five minutes and rest as needed in *vajrasana* or *virasana*.

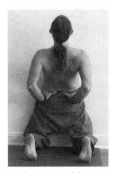

6.17 Ushtrasana with hips to a wall

To provide support for *supta virasana*, sit on the edge of a bolster then lie back over another bolster or blanket; this supports the spine. If any strain is felt in the knees, place a rolled towel behind the knee and between the upper and lower legs and adjust the supporting props higher.

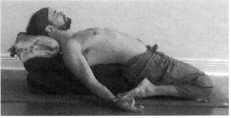

6.18 Salamba Supta Virasana (supported supine hero pose)

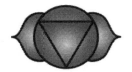

Vishuddhi – Throat, 5th *chakra*

Visualize the color blue at the throat center.
Activating Mantra: *Om Janah*
Asana: *Salamba Sarvangasana* (supported shoulder stand)

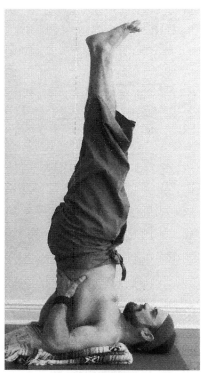

6.19 Supported Shoulder Stand

Place one or two folded blankets under the tops of the shoulders, as shown. The head will rest on the mat just beyond the blankets and this will preserve the curve of the cervical spine. Hold the post for five to 20 minutes. Alternatively, bring the hips to a wall and lift the legs up vertically in the resting pose *viparita karani*.

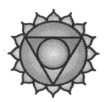

Ajna – Third Eye, 6th *chakra*

Visualize the color violet at the center of the forehead.
Activating Mantra: *Om Tapah*
Asana: *Salamba Upavishta Konasana* (supported seated wide angle posture)

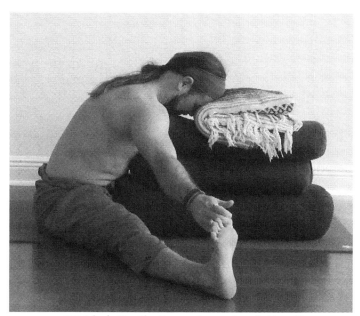

6.20 Salamba Upavishta Konasana (supported seated wide angle)

Sit with legs extended out to the sides and rest forward on a foundation of bolsters and/or blankets.
A light pressure at the brow will support the head and stimulate the third eye *chakra*.

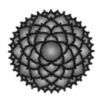

Sahasrara – Crown, 7th *chakra*

Visualize the color white at the top of the head.
Activating Mantra: *Om Satyam Purnam*
Asana: *Sirsasana I* (headstand I), *Supta Baddha Konasana* (supine bound angle pose),
Salamba Shavasana (supported corpse pose)

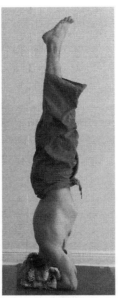

6.21 Sirsasana I with the support of a blanket

The pose can be done with or without support. If props are needed to support the neck or pad the head, use a blanket over the forearms and under the head. If avoiding inversions, perform a plank pose on forearms.

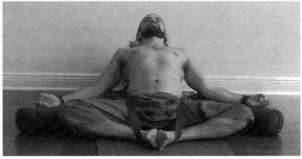

6.22 Salamba Supta Baddha Konasana (supported supine bound angle)

Supta Baddha Konasana (supine bound angle pose) is practiced at the end of the routine as a final relaxation pose or is followed by a supported corpse pose. It balances brain hemispheres and opens all *chakras*. Lie back on two or three bolsters that are stagger-stepped so there is no empty space behind the back. A blanket may be used as a pillow. Place blocks under the knees and a belt can be placed over the feet and around the lower back, as shown. Place any additional props under the forearms for support and greater relaxation.

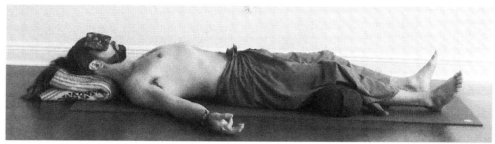

6.23 Salamba Shavasana (supported corpse pose)

For *Salamba Shavasana*, place a bolster under the knees to release tension from the lower back. Place a blanket under the head for support and a pillow over the eyes to increase relaxation.

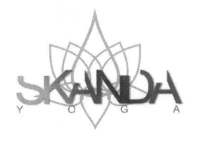

CHAPTER 7

Mudra and Pranayama

Mudras are used during the centering meditation in the beginning of a Skanda Yoga class to reaffirm the energy and intention of the day. The *mudras* that correspond to each practice can be found with the appropriate class sequence in chapter 16. Repetition of practice creates cellular memory and so the *mudras* are learned and integrated to be practiced anywhere at anytime. *Mudras* serve as tools to stay in remembrance of the higher aims of the practice while engaging the mind in subtle energies. This creates a refined awareness of one's being and of the *prana,* or life force energy.

Mudra

Like many Sanskrit words, the word "*mudra*" has numerous and varied translations. The word has its root in *mud,* meaning joy and bliss. It is most often used to describe the symbolic hand gestures or arm, leg and foot movements commonly portrayed in depictions of Hindu worship and dance. However, the word's most significant translation is that of sealing, stamping, imprinting, closing or locking. This would indicate that the physical gestures are the means of "officially" imprinting and locking certain concepts, ideas or energies upon and into a body, a ceremony, a community, etc.

Beyond the particular placement or movement of fingers and hands in ritual or prayer, the entire body can express *mudras.* The gestures we make with arms and hands as we speak are thought of as *mudras* and so are *asanas* themselves. These physical movements can alter mood, attitude and perception, expand awareness and deepen concentration. Therefore, *mudras* are emotional, devotional, psychic and aesthetic expressions.

In all of their tiny and large expressions, *mudras* can be performed in combination with the *bandhas, pranayama* and with visualization techniques. The *Hatha Yoga Pradipika* and other yogic texts consider *mudra* to be an independent branch (*yoganga*) of yoga practice because it requires awareness of the subtleties of energy that is gained with practice and proficiency in *asana, bandha* and *pranayama.*

The positions assumed with a *mudra* practice establish links between *annamaya kosha* (the physical body), *manomaya kosha* (the mental body) and *pranamayama kosha* (the *pranic* or energetic body). They redirect energy that would otherwise emanate from the body back within and act as barriers that seal energy inside the body. This creates balance in the *koshas* and enables the practitioner to channel energy to the upper *chakras*.

For example, when we perform *bhairava* or *bhairavi mudra*—with the hands resting palms-up in the lap during meditation or *pranayama*—we are establishing an intention to balance energies and connect to the highest. This requires using the physical form of the hands to activate *annamaya kosha*, the mental intention *manomaya kosha*, and the balancing of energies is *pranamayama kosha*.

Mudras also activate the primary elements of the body and move energy through the *chakras*. For example, *vayu mudra* balances the air element, which is associated with the heart *chakra*. Practicing *vayu mudra* creates an expansion of heart energy. *Shunya mudra* activates the element of ether that corresponds to the throat *chakra*. Practicing *shunya mudra* directs *prana* to this center to enhance communication. The practice of *mudra* can have an overall affect on your general health and emotional wellbeing.

Through the practice of *mudra* in *dharana*[25]-concentration - and *dhyana*[26]-meditation - the practice of turning the focus of the mind inward is strengthened as it is drawn away from outer forms. This is the practice of *pratyahara*, or sense withdrawal.

Mudras are tools to support and deepen meditation by engaging the mind and energizing the *chakras*. Their use allows us to access and influence the unconscious instinctive habits and patterns that originate in the primitive areas of the brain around the brainstem. The practice of *mudra* strengthens dendrites and creates new neural pathways in the brain, which can lead to new patterns of behavior. This affirmation of positive energy can have healing effects for the physical body and for specific organs, particularly when the *mudra* is aligned with an intention.

Each area of the hand corresponds to a specific area of the body. Most of the body's *nadis* or energy channels end in the hands and feet and energy flows through them from the periphery into the core. Manipulation and intentional direction of energy into and through the body influences the elements, *vayus*, and *chakras*. The body's systems and organs become stimulated through *mudra* in ways similar to the stimulation achieved with reflexology, acupressure and acupuncture

There are five general categories or groups of *mudra*, each having its own specific purpose and effect.

---

25   *Dharana* is the sixth of Patanjali's eight limbs of yoga. It is the ability to practice concentration and is made possible through the practice *pratyahara,* which is made possible by the four limbs that precede it.
26   *Dhyana* is the seventh limb of yoga. It is the state of being keenly aware that is achieved through meditative practice. More on Patanjali and the eight limbs of yoga can be found in chapter one.

Hasta Mudras – **Hand Energy Seals**

Hasta Mudras are meditative gestures that seal into the body the energy that would otherwise emanate from the hands. They are also seen in Indian classical dance where they are used to express the meaning of songs and the flavor, feelings and moods they evoke. Those used during the centering meditation at the beginning of Skanda Yoga classes follow.

Anjali Mudra (prayer and reverence)

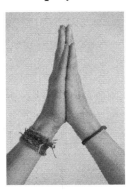

The palms are placed together with the the fingers straight, and the thumbs touch the chest. The fingers can be together or spread apart. The former position accelerates the *prana* and the latter decelerates it.

Chin Mudra (psychic gesture of knowledge)

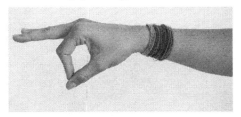

The tip of the index finger is placed on the inside edge of the thumb while the remaining three fingers extend straight. In a meditative posture, the hands rest on the knees with palms facing down.

Jnana Mudra (psychic gesture of consciousness)

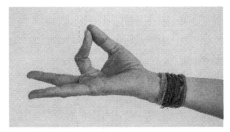

The tip of the index finger is brought to the inside edge of the thumb with the remaining fingers extended, as in *chin mudra*. In a meditative posture, the hands would rest on the knees and the palms would face upward. Both *jnana* and *chin mudras* are believed to strengthen meditation.

Hridaya Mudra (heart gesture)

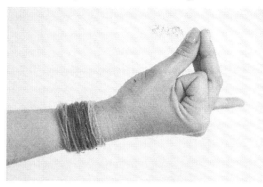

The tip of the index finger is placed at the root of the thumb and the tips of the middle and ring fingers are placed on the tip of the thumb while the little finger extends straight. This *mudra* is thought to improve the vitality of the heart and stimulate a connection with the true or divine wisdom at the core or center of everything.

Vayu Mudra (air or wind gesture)

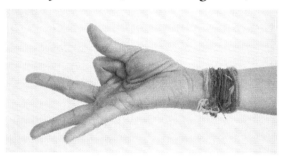

The index finger is folded into the base of thumb and presses down while the remaining fingers extend straight. This *mudra* balances the air element within the body and this, in turn, balances the *Anahata* or heart *chakra*.

Shunya Mudra (heaven gesture)

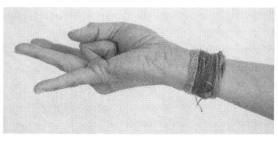

The middle finger is folded into the base of the thumb and lightly pressed down while the remaining fingers extend straight. This *mudra* balances the ether element within the body and thereby stimulates the throat *chakra*.

Prithivi Mudra (earth gesture)

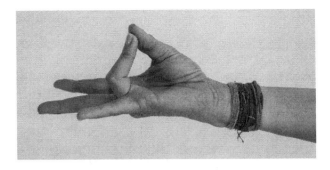

The tip of the ring finger is placed against the tip of the thumb while the remaining fingers extend straight. This *mudra* stimulates the earth element, which is associated with the *muladhara* or root *chakra*.

Varuna Mudra (water or god of water gesture)

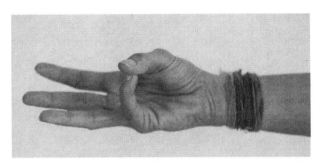

The tip of the little finger is placed against the tip of the thumb while the remaining three fingers extend straight. This *mudra* stimulates the *svadhistana chakra,* which is associated with the water element in the body.

Rudra Mudra (ruler of the solar plexus gesture)

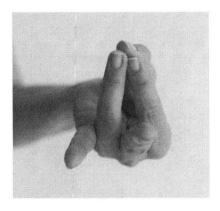

The tips of the thumb, index, and ring fingers are joined together while the middle and little fingers extend straight. This *mudra* is used to stimulate the *manipura* or solar plexus *chakra,* and is associated with the fire element.

Hakini Mudra (ruler of the third eye)

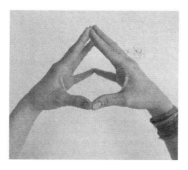

The tips of all four fingers join the tip of the thumb and the palms of two hands face each other at a distance of four to five inches. This *mudra* stimulates the *ajna chakra* at the center of the brow and balances the two hemispheres of the brain.

Makula Mudra (bud seal)

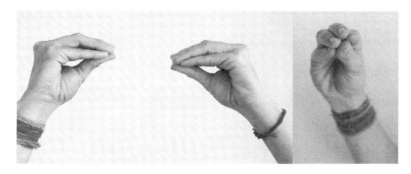

The tips of all four fingers and the thumbs are joined together. This *mudra* concentrates and directs the energy into the *chakras* or areas in need of healing. It is used for rejuvenation and balance.

Kali mudra (goddess seal)

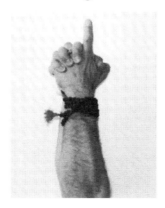

The outer three fingers and thumbs cross. The index fingers are pointing straight up. This *mudra* can be used during meditation or *asana* practice. It develops strength of spirit and determination in action. The left thumb is on top for females, and the right is on top for males.

Bhairava Mudra (gesture of a fierce or formidable attitude)

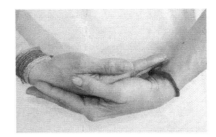

The back of the right hand is placed on top of the upward-facing palm of the left hand, the two hands are rested in the lap. When the left hand is placed on top of the right, the *mudra* is *Bhairavi*. This *mudra* balances the *sahasrara* or crown *chakra* and stimulates divine consciousness.

Vishnu Mudra (seal of Vishnu)

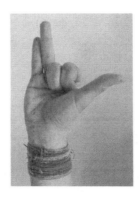

The index and middle fingers are folded in to touch the palm. The thumb, ring and little fingers extend up. It is used to alternate the breath through the nostrils during a form of *pranayama* called *nadi shodana* (see *pranayama*). This *mudra* balances opposing the energies of *anuloma,* or going with the grain, and *viloma,* going against. It is thought to stimulate the development of psychic abilities. The right hand should always be used, unless it is physically impossible.

Ganesha Mudra (seal of Ganesha)

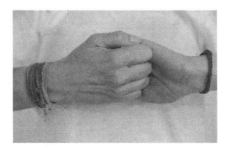

The fingers of the hands are clasped in front of the heart with the left hand turned down. The hands are lightly pulled apart so that the arms are engaged. This *mudra* supports the overcoming of obstacles.

Skanda Mudra (seal of Skanda)

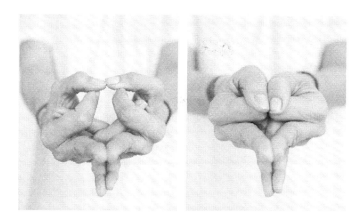

The ring fingers cross and the middle and little fingertips touch as the fingers extend straight up. The index fingers bend and curl around the tops of the crossed ring fingers and the thumbs press into the middle knuckles of the index fingers. The hands point straight up. This *mudra* is believed to build one-pointed focus and enhance *jnana shakti* – the power or energy of knowledge.

Sankalpa Mudra (seal of intention)

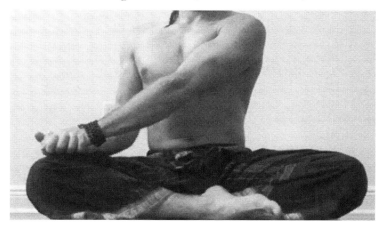

Place the right-hand palm face-up on top of the thigh. Reach the left arm across the heart and place it on top of the right palm face-down. Formulate an intention for the practice and seal it within the heart space.

Mana Mudras - (head energy seals)

This group of *mudras* utilizes the sense organs of eyes, ears, nose, tongue and lips and involves the engagement of subtle muscles.

Shambhavi Mudra (eyebrow center gazing)

Attempt to gaze at the center of the eyebrows without straining. Move the eyes toward each other and upward. This *mudra* is thought to strengthen concentration and mental stability and stimulate the pineal gland.

Nasikaga Drishti Mudra (tip of the nose gazing)

Focus the eyes on the tip of the nose by moving them toward each other and down. This *mudra* is thought to strengthen concentration and stimulate the root *chakra, muladhara.*

Khechari Mudra (to move the sky seal)

Place the tip of the tongue on the soft palate at the roof of the mouth. This *mudra* is believed to increase concentration and lower heart and respiratory rates. It activates the parasympathetic and sympathetic nervous systems and stimulates energy to rise up the central channel through the *chakras.* It increases *dharana* and deepens *ujjayi* breath. *Khechari* mudra can be practiced during meditation, *pranayama* and *asana.*

Shanmukhi Mudra (closing the six gates)

Close the ears with the thumbs, the eyes with the index fingers, the nostrils with the middle fingers, and the mouth by placing the ring and little fingers above and below the lips. As breathing is stopped, this *mudra* is usually performed with lungs full of air and the breath is held or locked inside – a *pranayama* called *antara kumbhaka.* This *mudra* strengthens *pratyahara,* relaxes the muscles of the face, and is reported to relieve stress.

Kaya Mudras – Postural Energy Seals

This group of *mudras* utilizes the whole body in combination with breath and concentration.

Viparita Karani Mudra (inverted psychic attitude)

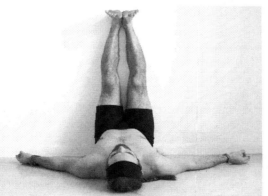 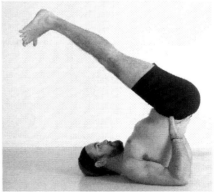

Lie with the hips placed against the wall and the leg extended up the wall, as shown in the first image, above. Alternatively, come into a supported shoulder-stand posture and reach the legs and feet over the head, as shown in the second photo. This *mudra* is believed to improve circulation, relieve stress and balance thyroid function. Practitioners with high blood pressure or heart conditions should consult their physician before practicing it.

Pashinee Mudra (folded psychic attitude)

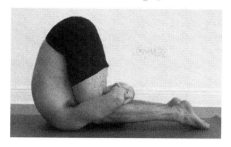

Assume *Karnapidasana or* ear-pressing *asana*. Balance on the back of the shoulders, draw the knees next to the ears and press them inward, then clasp the hands behind the knees as shown above. This *mudra* is believed to stimulate the parasympathetic nervous system. It should be avoided by practitioners with neck and cervical spine issues.

Tadagi Mudra (barreled abdomen technique)

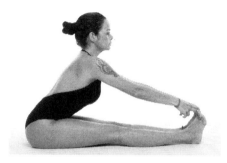

Sit with both legs together and extended straight ahead. Place the hands on the knees then take a deep breath in, hold the breath and allow the abdomen to protrude. Keep the spine long as you slide your hands toward your feet to clasp the big toes. Gaze straight ahead. This *mudra* is thought to improve circulation of blood to the internal organs and release tension in the diaphragm and the pelvic floor after the pose is exited. Practitioners who are pregnant or who have a hernia may choose not to practice it.

Maha Bheda Mudra (the great separating attitude)

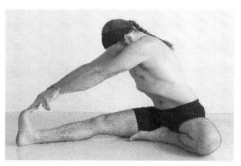 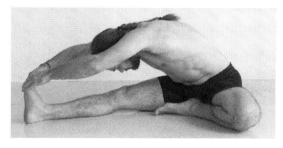

Assume *janu sirsasana*. From a seated position, bend one knee and move it out to the side, bringing the heel of the sole of the foot to the upper, inner thigh of the opposite leg with heel of the foot at the groin. Lengthen the spine, exhale fully, initiate *khechari mudra*, and engage the three *bandhas*. Hold the breath out, release, and then fold forward, as shown above. This *mudra* is believed to stimulate the parasympathetic and sympathetic nervous systems.

Maha Vedha Mudra (the great piercing attitude)

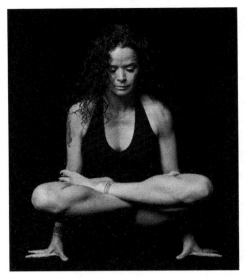

Sit in *padmasana* or lotus pose. Place the hands on the floor beside the hips. Lift the body off the floor then lower it back down with no resistance. This is usually repeated three times at first and, with practice, increased to a maximum of 11 repetitions. This *mudra* is believed to stimulate the *muladhara chakra* and draw energy from the root up the central channel of the spine. Practitioners with inflammatory, hip or pelvic ailments may wish to forego this *mudra*.

Pranayama –Breath Expansion Techniques

Pranayama is the science of utilizing and working with the breath in yoga. The word is derived from the root words *pran* (life force) and *ayam* (to extend); thus, the meaning of *pranayama* is to bring extension to the life force. It is often referred to as "breath control" because techniques are used to govern the breath, which liberates and expands its energy. Through *pranayama* techniques, the breath brings control to the fluctuations of the mind or *chitta vritti*. Most schools of yoga avoid teaching *pranayama* to a student until they are proficient in *asana* or have been practicing for a minimum of two years. This is recommended before doing a practice only of *pranayama* that consists of 20-60 minute sessions.

Before beginning a *pranayama* practice, it is recommended to perform the yogic cleansing techniques. The original aim of yoga was to eliminate toxins of the body through *shatkarmas* (cleansing techniques). *Shatkarma* is composed of two words: *shat* meaning 'six' and *karma* meaning 'art' or 'process'. The word *kriya* or *krama* is used in hatha yoga in a technical sense regarding a technique of cleansing or positive action. It is not necessary to perform all of them everyday, but it is important to know when and how to practice if needed. The six practices are:

– *Neti* (nasal cleansing)
– *Basti* (colon cleansing)
– *Kapalbhati* (purification of frontal lobes)
– *Dhauti* (cleansing the digestive tract)
– *Trataka* (candle gazing)
– *Nauli* (abdominal massage)

Mixing a non-iodized salt with water to create a saline solution in a neti pot performs **neti**. It is then poured up one nostril and drains out the other. The angle of the head is slightly tilted; if it is extreme, then water will flow into the ear canal. It takes practice to find the right angle. The water should always be boiled first to purify, and then left to cool until slightly warm.

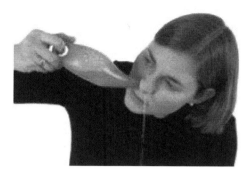

Basti is the cleansing of the colon. It used to be performed using archaic techniques, which are now rudimentary. It is more efficient to have a hydro-colonic periodically with the seasons to keep the colon and intestines clean, and/or to perform a regular enema with saline water.

Kapalabhati is a traditional *pranayama* technique where *prana* is channeled into the upper *chakras* by emphasizing a strong exhalation and a quick inhalation. Engage the lower abdominals strongly on exhalation. The exhalation is made forceful and quick, while the inhalation is passive. This *pranayama* clears mucous disorders, decompresses cerebral spinal fluid, and increases *prana* in the upper *chakras*.

Swallowing a saline solution and then vomiting performs **dhauti**. Swallowing a gauze roll and pulling it back up also performs *dhauti*. This is recommended only once a week.

Trataka is a meditation that is performed by gazing at the tip of a candle to increase *ekagrata* (one pointed concentration) by focusing the mind on a single point. On inhalation, breathe the light from the candle to your brow *chakra*. On exhalation, extend light from the brow *chakra* to the candle.

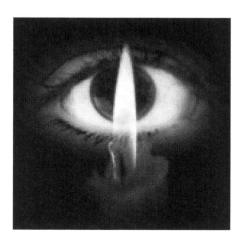

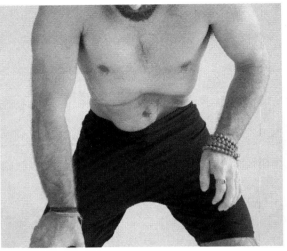 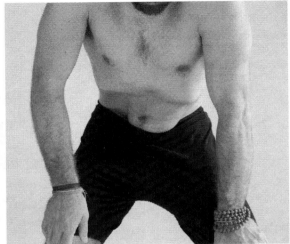

Nauli is performed to break up stagnation in the digestive system. Lean forward and place the hands on the knees. Pull the lower abdomen in and back to engage *uddiyana bandha*. Lift one hand and press down with the opposite hand. As you engage that side of the rectus abdominis muscles, the opposite side lifts. Repeat the exercise on the opposite side. Continue until the abdominal muscles churn in a waving motion from side to side.

Abdominal massaging exercises are believed to ignite the digestive fire, remove indigestion and clear constipation. Other forms include:

Dakshina Nauli is performed by rotating the abdomen from left to right or counter-clockwise.

Vama Nauli is performed by rotating the abdomen from right to left in a clockwise motion.

Madhyama Nauli is performed by engaging the abdominal muscles and protruding them while *uddiyana bandha* is held.

Agni Sara is performed with *uddiyana bandha* engaged and the abdomen is pumped in and out like *bhastrika*, but with no breath.

Pranayama Technique

Suryabheda (vitality stimulating breath)

Close the left nostril with the thumb with *Vishnu mudra* and inhale through the right. Hold the breath in then slowly exhale through the left nostril. This *pranayama* is thought to stimulate the *pingala nadi*, purify the cranium and balance the *doshas*.

Chandrabheda (moon activating breath)

Close the right nostril with *Vishnu mudra* and inhale through the left. Retain the inhalation for a moment, and then exhale through the right nostril. This *pranayama* activates the *ida nadi*, calms the nervous system, and releases mental tension.

Nadi Shodhana (energy channel cleansing breath)

Also known as alternate-nostril and balanced breathing, this *pranayama* is performed with *Vishnu mudra* - bend the first two fingers and bring their tips under the muscle of the thumb. Use the thumb to close off right nostril then inhale through the left. At the top of the breath close off the left with the outer two fingers and exhale right. Inhale through the right and close off with the thumb. Exhale through the left and then inhale through the left. Close the left again and keep repeating until the mind is calm and peaceful. The *pranayama* should end with an exhalation on the left. The inhalation and exhalation should be of equal duration with a pause at the midpoints.

Antara Kumbhaka (breath retention after inhalation)

Inhale deeply and fill the lungs completely. Hold the breath in as long as comfortable or for a designated count. For example, "Inhale for a count of six, hold for 11, and then exhale for a count of 8." The *pranayama* of breath retention increases endurance and concentration and regulates the mind.

Bahya Kumbhaka (breath retention after exhalation)

Exhale all of the air from the lungs and hold the breath out for as long as comfortable or for a designated count. This *pranayama* is believed to reduce the metabolic rate, prevent aging and increase concentration.

Bhastrika (bellows breath)

Sit comfortably and inhale, swelling the abdomen with the breath. Pump the abdomen in and out quickly to release and take in breath. Inhalations and exhalations are brief and of equal duration. This *pranayama* creates heat in the body, increases energy and vitality, and strengthens the central nervous system.

Kapalbhati (frontal brain cleansing)

This breathing exercise is also one of the shatkarmas (cleansing techniques) because it clears the mind by bringing in more light and oxygen. This is also referred to as a breath of fire technique because it is done by rapidly pulsing the abdomen with the breath. The belly is relaxed and extends out on inhalation and then it is snapped in on the exhalation. The emphasis is on exhalation and creating a strong contraction in the lower abdominals, while forcing the air out rapidly.

Viloma (ladder breath)

The ladder breath can be performed be interrupting the inhalation or exhalation. The breath should be divided into thirds with a pause in between. For example, "Inhale, pause, inhale, pause, inhale, pause, full exhale." When *viloma* is performed on inhalation, it is more activating, and when performed on exhalation, it is more calming. The exercise is deepened when practiced with *kechari mudra*.

Sheetkari (hissing breath)

Inhale through the teeth, making a hissing sound, and exhale through the nose strongly. The tongue can be placed behind the two front teeth. The benefit of this, *pranayama,* is a cooling of the body. It is believed to make one a *Kamadeva* or god of love.

Sheetali (cooling breath)

Curl the tongue and slowly suck air in through the mouth. Retain the breath, and lower chin to the chest in *jalandhara bandha*. Hold the breath for a count of 20. Then block the right nostril and exhale through the left nostril. The benefits of this *pranayama* include curing an enlarged stomach or spleen and reducing fever, excess bile, hunger and thirst.

Bhramari (humming bee breath)

Place the three central fingers of each hand over the eyelids, the thumbs close off the ears. For as long as possible, exhale through the teeth, making a buzzing sound.

Moorchha (great swooning breath)

Place the hands behind the hips and straighten the arms. Bring the shoulder blades onto the back. Take a deep breath and hold the breath in as you let the head rest back on the shoulders. This *pranayama* is thought to balance the cerebral spinal fluid.

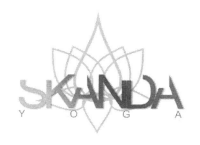

CHAPTER 8

Sun Salutations and Vinyasa

The sun salutation, *surya namaskar*, is a form of dynamic stretching that involves progressive movements with the breath to warm the body, and to create a general opening. It can be performed in many ways, and all are acceptable, but one style or variation may be more advantageous to a practitioner than another. The sun salutation is a physical honoring of the sun, and ideally should be done facing the direction of the sun, to stay in remembrance of its life-supporting energy. It is performed spiritually as a way of building the *Prana* (life force) energy and converting it into *shakti* (spiritual power), while staying in remembrance of the invisible creator. The practice of the mystic is to perform the sun salutation as if they were the sun sending love and support to all of humanity. The spiritual and mystical practice of the sun salutation is far more important than how it is performed physically. The following information details the technique for performing the sun salutation in Skanda Yoga.

Surya Namaskar A [0]
Tadasana with Anjali Mudra (mountain pose with hands in prayer, samasthiti)

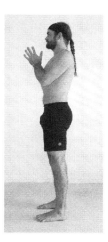

Stand feet hip-distance apart. Hands in *anjali mudra*. Stay in remembrance of the intention for the practice. Inner rotate the top of the thighbones and root them back, as the sitting bones widen apart, scoop the tail bone down and draw the lower belly in. Root down from the hips through the feet, and rise up out of the hips. Lift the ribcage and shoulders up and then curl the shoulders onto the back body. Slide the palate back and open the heart.

Urdhva Hastasana (upward hand pose)

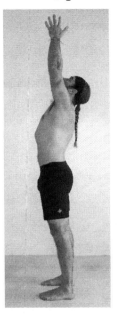

On inhalation, sweep the arms overhead with outer rotation in the top of the arms, so the pinky finger is leading the way. Gaze up at the hands. The thumbs are aligned over the nose. Stretch up as you root down through the legs. On exhalation, dive forward into *uttanasana*, with the arm bones inner rotating, so the shoulder blades stay engaged on the back body.

Uttanasana (intense pose, "standing forward fold")

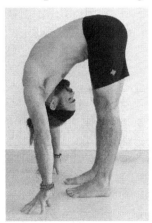

Bow forward and take the head toward the navel, so the lower abdomen lifts and the kidneys widen. There is a 2-inch gap between the top of the thighs and the lower floating ribs. Move the arms and shoulders away from the legs and squeeze the shoulder blades together. Squeeze the leg muscles into the bones and lift them up toward the hips, as you push energy from the hips down through the floor. Do not push energy back or lean back to feel a stretch at the top of the hamstrings. Instead of focusing on the sensation of stretching, aim to recruit more strength in the legs. Use blocks if necessary under the hands to keep the legs straight if tight. If no blocks are available, then keep the knees bent.

Ardha Uttanasana (half intense pose)

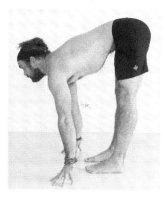

Inhale, lengthen the spine and outer rotate the top of the arm bones, so the creases of the elbows are pointing straight ahead. Push the head up and curl in the upper back. Exhale, step or jump into plank position.

Jump Back

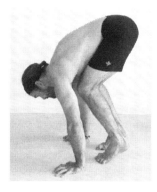 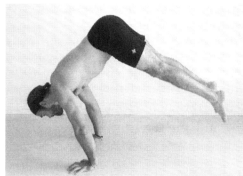

Bend the knees, jump up, and then straighten the legs. Land with the core engaged, arms straight, and the feet in flexion. In Skanda Yoga, we advise students not to jump back into *chaturanga dandasana,* as it is unnecessary to build strength and poses a risk of strain or destabilization for the rotator cuff by the sudden force placed upon the shoulder muscles. *Chaturanga dandasana* may be entered from *uttanasana* if the student can float back without jumping, and the shoulders do not break parallel with the elbows.

Utthita Chaturanga Dandasana (extended four limbed staff pose, "plank pose")

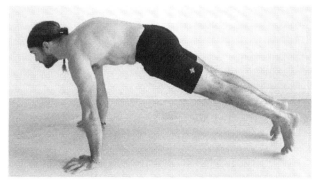

Hold plank on inhalation. Grip or claw with the hands then lean forward onto the tips of the big toes. If that is difficult, then stay on the balls of the feet, but keep extending energy forward. Firm the lower abdomen and round the lower back. Scoop the tailbone and hold the core strong. On exhalation, curl in the upper back, melting the heart down, and slowly descend into *chaturanga dandasana*. The elbows should not touch the ribcage during the descent, and the shoulders should not break parallel with the elbows. The knees can be placed on the floor first to take stress off the shoulders.

Chaturanga Dandasana (four limbed staff pose)

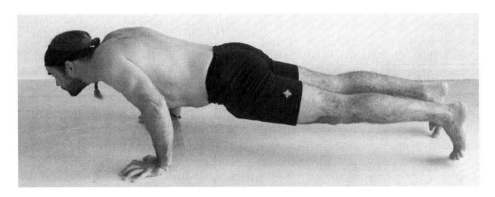

Hold *chaturanga dandasana* briefly at the midpoint of the exhalation before transitioning into *bhujangasana* or *urdhva mukha vrksasana*. The shoulders are lifting away from the floor as the heart descends. The lower abdomen is lifting as the tailbone stays scooping. The head stays pushing up to maintain the curl in the upper back.

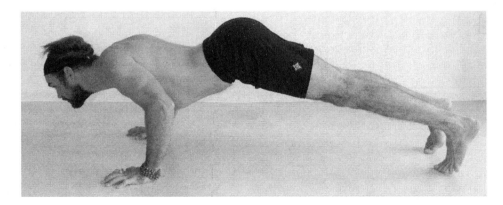

At the end of the exhalation, lift the hips and inner rotate the tops of the thighs. The heels widen apart as energy is pushed out through the balls of the feet. Scoop the tailbone under and push the hips down to lift the upper body into *bhujangasana* or *urdhva mukha vrksasana*. This transition technique may take some practice time before it feels fluid. In the meantime, the transition can be practiced by lowering down flat on the belly, or just flipping the feet over at the end of the descent.

Bhujangasana (cobra pose)

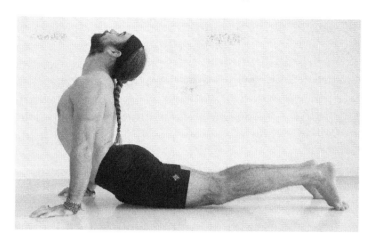

Inhale and lift up into cobra pose. The hips and thighs stay rooted on the floor. Lengthen up and out of the hips, and then curl the shoulders on the back. Pull the hands back to engage the arms and extend the spine forward. Outer rotate the tops of the arms, while the forearms stay inner rotating, and then push the head back. The tops of the toes push down and pull back toward the hips, and the hands pull back toward the hips, then from the hips lengthen out and curl deeeper.

Urdhva Mukha Svanasana (upward facing dog)

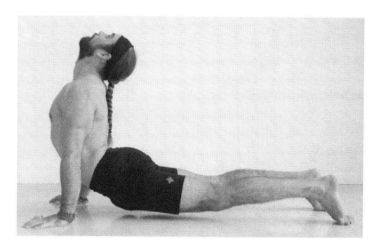

From *bhujangasana*, if the engagement can be held in the upper back without the shoulders rolling forward, then lift the thighs off of the floor into *urdhva mukha svanasna*. The index knuckle roots down as the top of the shoulders angle back. Push the head back, as the hands pull back and feet pull forward.

At the end of the inhalation, transition from *bhujangasana* or *urdhva mukha svanasana* lower back into *chaturanga dandasana* on exhalation.

Chaturanga Dandasana (four limbed staff pose)

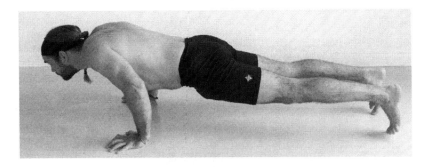

From *chaturanga dandasana,* push back to *adho mukha svanasana* at the end of the exhalation. If this transition is difficult, then modify by placing the knees on the floor.

Adho Mukha Svanasana (downward facing dog)

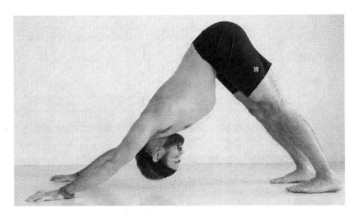

Hold *adho mukha svanasana* for five breaths. Roll the thighs in and outer rotate the arms, and then push out in both directions.

Jump Forward

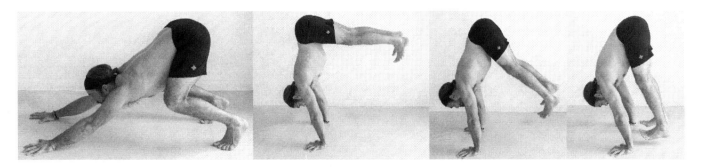

At the end of the 5th exhalation in *adho mukha svanasana,* bend the knees and jump the feet toward the front of the mat. Flex the toes and straighten the legs as soon as the feet spring off of the floor. Lift the hips over the shoulders, and then lightly set the feet back down.

Ardha Uttanasana (extended intense pose)

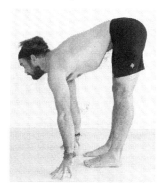

Inhale, lengthen the spine and squeeze the leg muscle into the bones.

Uttanasana (intense pose)

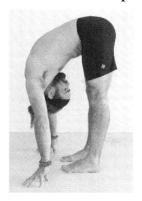

Exhale and bow into a forward bend. Squeeze the shoulder blades on the back and lift them toward the hips. Lift the belly up, and push energy down through the legs.

Urdhva Hastasana (upward hand pose)

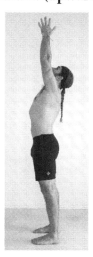

On inhalation, root down through the feet and sweep the arms over head.

Tadasana with Anjali Mudra (samasthiti)

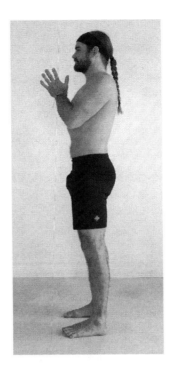

On exhalation, return to *samasthiti*.

Surya Namaskar A

The following description of the sun salutation is with breath and basic instruction only.

1. Come to *samasthiti* at the front of the mat with hands in prayer position. Exhale, root down through the legs and release the hands.
2. Inhale, sweep the arms overhead.
3. Exhale, dive forward.
4. Inhale, lengthen the spine.
5. Exhale, step or jump back into plank.
6. Inhale, hold plank and strengthen the core.
7. Exhale, lower to *chaturanga dandasana*.
8. Inhale, press up into *bhujangasana* or *urdhva mukha svanasana*.
9. Exhale, lower back down into *chaturanga dandasana*.
10. Press back into *adho mukha svanasana* at the end of the exhale, and hold for five deep *ujjayi* breaths. At the end of the 5th exhalation, bend the knees and step or jump to the front of the mat.
11. Inhale, lengthen the spine.
12. Exhale, bow to the heart.
13. Inhale, squeeze the legs together, root down through the feet, and rise up.
14. Exhale, return to *samasthiti* with hands in prayer position.

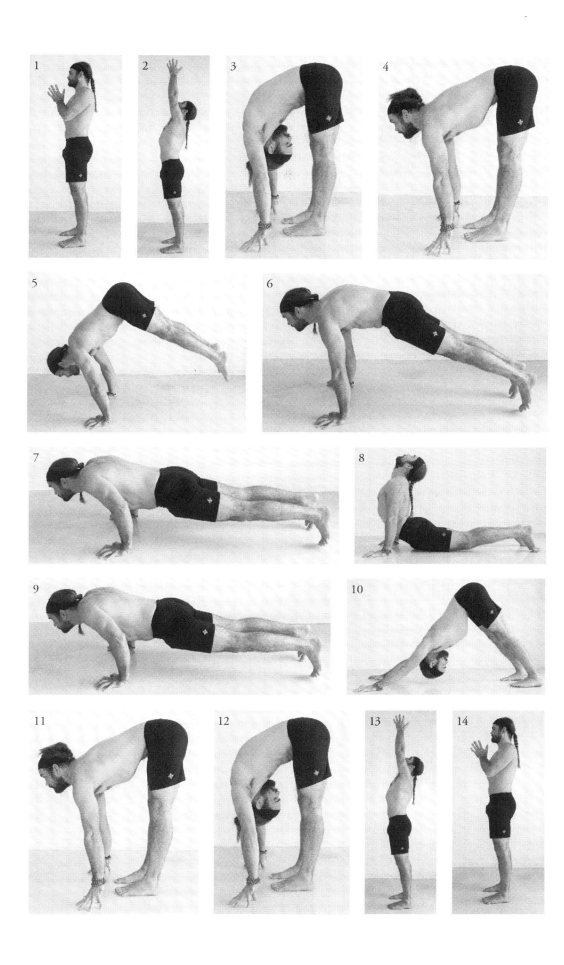

Surya Namaskar B [00]

Surya namaskar B incorporates *utkatasana* instead of *urdhva hastasana* as in *surya namaskar A*. *Virabhadrasana I* is also performed on the right and left sides with a *vinyasa* in between. In Skanda Yoga classes, *surya namaskar B* is practiced with both standard and dynamic forms of alignment. The following images and descriptions of *surya namaskar B* are for dynamic alignment practice. If the sun salute is to be performed traditionally or with standard alignment, then the feet should be together in *uttanasana* and *utkatasana*, and the back foot is flat in *virabhadrasana I*. Plank pose is still held with an inhalation, instead of descending immediately with exhalation.

Utkatasana (fierce pose, "chair pose")

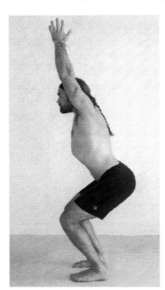

On exhalation, bend the knees and lower the hips. On inhalation, sweep the arms overhead. Firm the lower abdomen and squeeze the ribcage in.

Virabhadrasana I (warrior pose I, standard and dynamic technique)

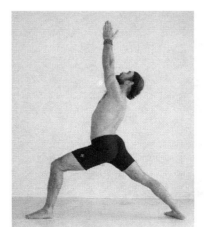 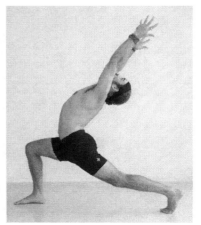

On inhalation, step one foot up from down dog to the front of the mat. Bend the forward knee over the ankle and sweep the arms overhead. If performing a traditional *surya namaskar B* with the back foot flat, then hold for one breath and exit on exhalation. If performing Skanda style *surya namaskar B* with the back heel elevated, then hold the pose for five breaths.

Basic instructions for *surya namaskar B*:

1. Start in *tadasana* with the hands in prayer position.

2. Exhale into squatting and sweep the arms overhead on the inhalation.

3. Exhale, dive forward into *uttanasana*.

4. Inhale, lengthen the spine.

5. Exhale, step or jump back into plank.

6. Inhale, hold plank and strengthen the core.

7. Exhale, lower into *chaturanga dandasana*.

8. Inhale, lift into *bhujangasana* or *urdhva mukha svanasana*.

9. Exhale, flow back into *adho mukha svanasana*.

10. Inhale, step the right foot into *virabhadrasana I* with the back foot flat or with the heel up. Hold for five breaths.

11. Exhale, step back into plank and hold plank. Inhale, strengthen the core.

12. Exhale, lower into *chaturanga dandasana*.

13. Inhale, lift into *bhujangasana* or *urdhva mukha svanasana*.

14. Exhale, flow back into *adho mukha svanasana*.

15. Inhale, step the left foot into *virabhadrasana I* with the back foot flat or with the heel up. Hold for five breaths.

16. Exhale, step back into plank and hold plank. Inhale, lift the lower belly up and in.

17. Exhale, lower into *chaturanga dandasana*.

18. Inhale, lift into *bhujangasana* or *urdhva mukha svanasana*.

19. Exhale, flow back into *adho mukha svanasana* and hold for five breaths. At the end of the 5th exhale, step or jump the feet to the front of the mat.

20. Inhale, lengthen the spine.

21. Exhale, bow into *uttanasana* and squat into *utkatasana* at end of exhale.

22. Inhale, sweep arms overhead.

23. Exhale, stand and return to *samasthiti*.

The following images are of a dynamic *surya namaskar B* performed with feet hip-distance apart and the back heel is lifting in *virabhadrasana I*.

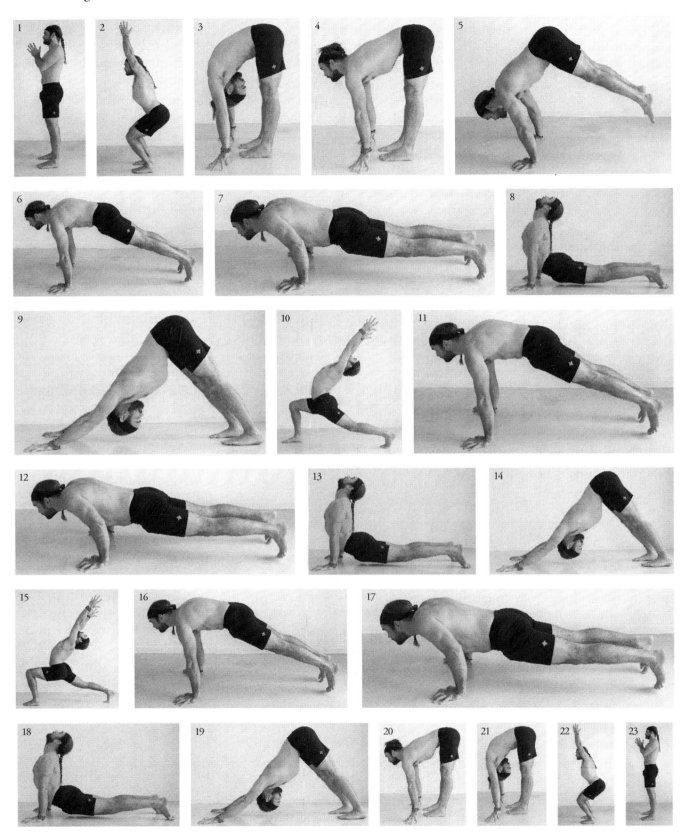

Vinyasa

Flowing between sets of poses or between the right and left sides of poses performs a *vinyasa*. It consists of stepping, jumping, or floating back into plank or *chaturanga dandasana* from a standing or sitting position, inhaling up to cobra/up dog, and exhaling into down dog, and then jumping into the next pose. The difference between a sun salutation and a *vinyasa* is that the former always starts and returns into *tadasana*. A *vinyasa* can start from sitting or standing, but is initiated by flowing with the breath from plank or *chaturanga dandasana*, and entering *bhujangasana/urdhva mukha svanasana* on inhalation, and transitioning to *adho mukha vrksasana* on exhalation, and then entering the next pose on inhalation, which could be stepping the opposite foot up or jumping through to sitting. The following techniques are represented to enhance *vinyasa* transitions.

Feet Transitioning in Vinyasa or Surya Namskar

When starting a *vinyasa* from *utthita chaturanga dandasana* (elevated four angle staff or "plank" pose), the weight of the body is supported equally between the hands and the toes of the feet. As the weight shifts forward to begin the transition, it moves into the hands and this draws the feet more vertical (figure 8.3). By lifting onto the tips of the big toes with remaining toes flexed and flared out to the sides, energy is drawn up through the body and into the shoulder girdle. This action protects the muscles and tendons that stabilize the shoulder joints by enabling them to curl back during the descent into four-angle staff pose or *chaturanga dandasana*.

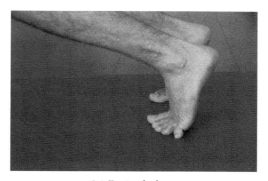

8.1 Feet in plank pose

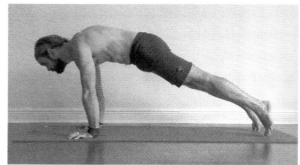

8.2 Shifting weight into hands to begin lowering down from plank pose into chaturanga dandasana

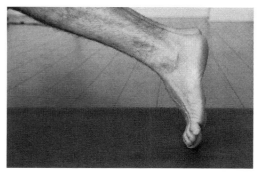

8.3 Foot becomes vertical

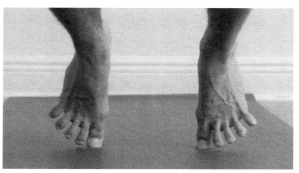

8.4 Weight transfers onto big toes

Utthita Chaturanga Dandasana

Enter plank pose on inhalation. Lean forward and engage the lower body. On exhalation, soften in the upper back and melt the heart down, and then descend into *chaturanga dandasana*.

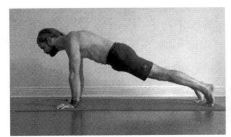

8.5 entering plank.

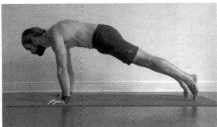

8.6 the lower body engages on inhalation

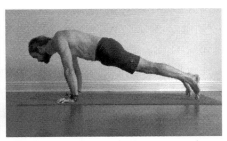

8.7 upper body descends on exhalation to initiate descent

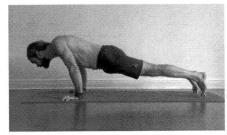

8.8 lowering into chaturanga dandasana

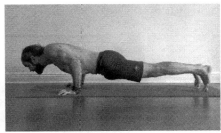

8.9 holding chaturanga dandasana

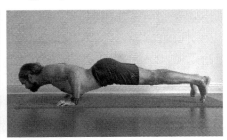

8.10 lifting hips at the end of exhalation to gain momentum to lift into bhujangasana or urdhva mukha svanasana

Chaturanga Dandasana

Four limbed staff pose can be modified if correct positioning cannot be held with integrity. The tops of the shoulders should not break parallel with the elbows. A block can be placed under the shoulders to ensure that they do not break parallel by touching the block. If they do touch the block or the shoulders break parallel with the shoulders, then it is recommended to only lower a few inches down or to rest the knees down.

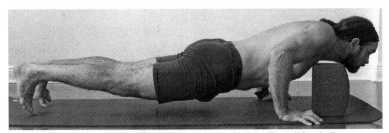

8.11 chaturanga dandasana with block so the arms don't break parallel with elbows

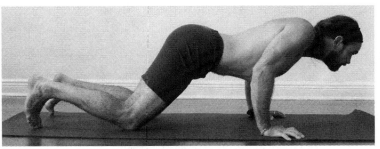

8.12 chaturanga dandasana modification

Lolasana & Tolasana

Chaturanga *dandasana* can be entered from sitting poses or by lifting into *tolasana* or *lolasana*, and then swinging through to initiate a *vinyasa*. Place the hands in front on the hips and curl the shoulders onto the back. Then press down and lift up. Swing the legs through the arms to enter *chaturanga dandasana*.

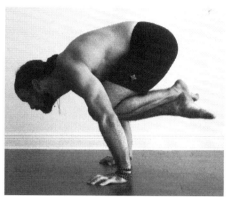

8.13 Ankles cross to lift

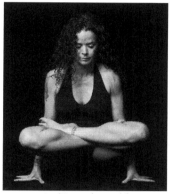

8.14 Legs in lotus to lift

Jump Through

Jumping from down dog into sitting performs a jump through. The ankles are crossed in mid-air or the legs are kept straight. Either technique is acceptable to enter the next pose. Start by bending the knees from down dog as shown in image 8.15, then jump and cross ankles like in *lolasana*, then lower to sitting, and extend the legs straight.

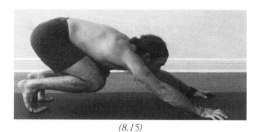

(8.15)

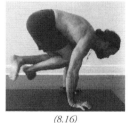

(8.16)

To jump through with legs straight, bend the knees as in image 8.15, and then lean forward coming onto the tips of the big toes, as in image 8.17. Spring off the toes and kick the legs through the arms. The legs straighten fully with the feet in flexion. Lower down into *dandasana*.

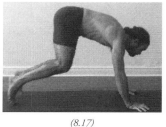

(8.17)

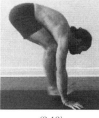

(8.18)

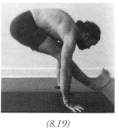

(8.19)

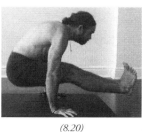

(8.20)

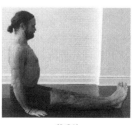

(8.21)

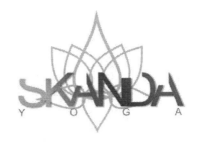

CHAPTER 9

Asanas

There are 840,000 *asanas*. The following section aims only to highlight the major ones used in the Skanda Yoga class sequences.

The *drishti* or gazing point in asana can be different for each practitioner in the same pose. Attention should be focused where there is no strain. It can be a spot on the floor for balance, the big toe, tip of the nose, or the third eye. It doesn't necessarily matter where it is just as long as it is practiced. By stabilizing the gaze, we strengthen our concentration and bring balance to the nervous system. If the eyes wander during the practice, then it can create an unconscious pattern of stress. If the eyes are closed, then it creates more relaxation and drops the heart and respiratory rate. The *drishti* is practiced to maintain focus by linking action and perception in the moment. There are nine gazing points referred to as the *nava drishtis*.

1. *Nasagari* – gaze at the tip of the nose
2. *Ajna Chakra* – gaze at the space between the eyebrows
3. *Nabi Chakra* – gaze at the navel
4. *Hastagrai* – gaze at the hand
5. *Padhayoragai* – gaze at the toes
6. *Parsva Drishti* – gaze to the distance at the right side
7. *Parsva Drishti* – gaze to the distance to the left side
8. *Angusta Ma Dyai* – gaze at the thumbs
9. *Urdhva Drishti* – gaze up to the sky

All of the poses should be held for a minimum of 5-13 breaths to receive the therapeutic benefits. The benefits become more pronounced if the time is extended, but it should be not be held to extreme lengths that tire the body.

It should be noted that the instructions accompanying each *asana* do not cover foundation, *bandhas*, *spanda*, balancing actions, or stretching techniques. It does not cover the difference between performing the pose in standard or dynamic alignment. Those are all covered in detail in the previous chapters. Further, those techniques should first be practiced with the basic poses listed in the beginning of the book prior to incorporating them into additional *asanas*.

The instructions given are for setting up, entering and exiting the pose, as well as refining techniques that are specific to the pose. They do not serve to replace instruction from a live teacher, as the pose is experienced and performed differently depending upon the body type of the practitioner. When practicing, it is important to listen to the body's feedback first; if something doesn't feel right, then exit the pose. The breath will let you know. If you can relax and deepen the exhalation, then you can stay in the pose. If the body cannot breathe fully, then that is a signal that you should not be there. The key is to practice with consistency. What may be impossible one day will become routine in the future, and that is the magic of the practice. Do not be attached to any of the results. It is not about the pose, but the experience that is cultivated. The more time we spend in *asana*, the more healing, relaxation, and strength of spirit is gained.

It is not possible to do the same pose all day every day. Enjoy it when it comes and create a sacred space, and then let it dissolve, so you can re-create it again later. Most importantly, stay in remembrance of your true Self as an aspect of the Divine consciousness, and perceive through the illusion of separation.

Standing Poses

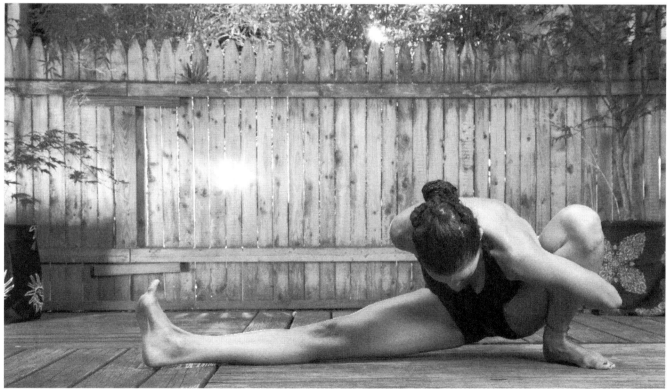

photo by Mauricio Velez

Standing poses build strength in the legs and create a general opening in the hips. They also prepare the body for arm balances and deeper backbends. Standing poses activate the lower *chakras* and create stability physically as well as energetically. They are especially beneficial when used therapeutically to recover from injuries and surgeries, and also for building confidence and strength of spirit to overcome limitations. All standing poses can be modified or supported with props or a wall, so that they are accessible to any practitioner.

The following poses can be entered from many possible positions, but the technique descriptions are written from the perspective of a *vinyasa* class.

1. Tadasana with anjali mudra (mountain pose with prayer seal)

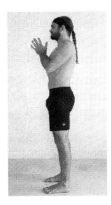

Come to standing with the feet together or hip-distance apart. In either position, the outer edge of the heel should be aligned with the outer edge of the fourth toe. Root energy down through the four corners of the feet to distribute the weight evenly. Squeeze the shins toward the central axis, then inner rotate the top of the thighbones and root them back into the hamstrings. Firm the lower abdomen and scoop the tailbone. Tone and lift the pelvic floor. Lift the shoulders toward the ears then curl them onto the back. Lift and open the heart. Slide the lower jawbone back to align over the central axis. Stand strong and firm like a mountain.

Benefits: This pose tones the leg muscles, improves posture and, relieves sciatica. It initiates a state of concentration and prepares the mind for the practice.
Chakra: root

2. Urdhva Hastasana (upward hand pose)

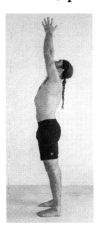

From *tadasana,* release the hands beside the hips on exhalation, and then outer rotate the arms as they reach overhead on inhalation. Gaze up as the head tilts back. Align the tips of the thumbs over the tip of the nose, and root energy from the hips down through the feet.

Benefits: This pose opens the lungs and deepens the breath. It tones spinal nerves and stretches the abdominal organs.
Chakra: root, throat

3. Uttanasana (intense pose)

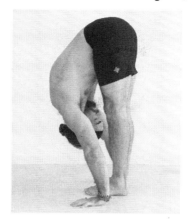

From *urdhva hastasana,* fold forward and place the hands in front or beside the feet. Deepen the forward bend on exhalation, taking the head toward the knees. Squeeze the shins in, and move the thighbones apart and back. Lift the quadriceps and abdominal muscles up, and maintain the shoulder blades lifting up the back away from the ears.

Benefits: This pose lengthens the hamstrings, improves blood circulation, and reduces fatigue and anxiety. It stimulates the liver, spleen, and kidneys. It can be performed to relieve stomach pain during menstrual periods.
Contraindications: People with back pain or herniated disks should bend knees or not fold forward fully.
Modification: Place the hands on blocks or a chair.
Chakra: root, sacral

4. Ardha Uttanasana (half intense pose)

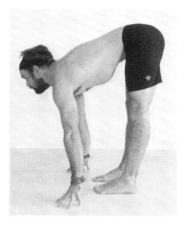

Lengthen the spine and outer rotate the top of the arm bones, so the creases of the elbows are pointing straight ahead. Push the head up and curl in the upper back.

Benefits: This pose extends the spine and tones the spinal nerves. It prepares the body to enter plank or *chaturanga dandasana* with good alignment.
Contraindications: Avoid pushing the head up if have a neck injury.
Modification: Place hands on blocks to keep the legs straight.
Chakra: root, throat

5. Parivrtta Uttanasana (revolved intense pose)

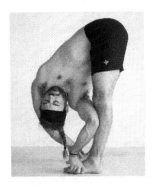

From *uttanasana,* place the fingers of the opposite hand palm face up under the opposite foot. Grab the other foot with the free hand with the palm facing in. Push the head up into the top arm to deepen the twist.

Benefits: This pose lengthens the back muscles and tones the abdominal organs. It improves digestion.
Contraindications: Avoid if cannot keep both legs straight or have a lumbar herniation.
Modification: Place both hands in fingertip position in front of the feet. Reach one hand across and grab the outside of the shin. Pull the chest to the side so it is centered over that leg. Another alternative is to place one hand on the floor underneath the head. Reach the other arm behind the back. If the left arm is behind the back, then bend the right knee and deepen the twist. A block can be placed under the hand if the hamstrings are tight.
***Chakra*:** root, solar plexus

6. Hasta Padangusthasana (hand to big toe pose)

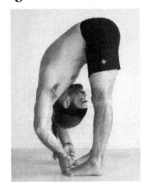

From *uttanasana,* grab the big toes with the first two fingers of the hands. Pull up on the toes and push the toes down into the fingers. Bend the elbows out to the side and move them forward away from the legs. Engage the shoulders and lift them up the back away from the ears.

Benefits: This pose lengthens the hamstrings, improves blood circulation, and reduces fatigue and anxiety. It stimulates the liver, spleen, and kidneys. It can be performed to relieve stomach pain during menstrual periods. This pose also creates strength in the fingers, legs, and upper back.
Contraindications: People with back pain or herniated disks should bend knees or not fold forward fully. Do not bring head between knees with a slipped disc.
Modification: Bend the knees.
***Chakra*:** root, sacral

7. Padahastasana (feet on hands pose)

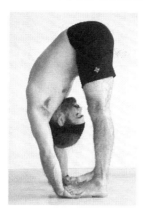

From *uttanasana,* place the palms of the hands under the balls of the feet. Pull up with the hands, as the feet push down. Engage the shoulders and lift them up the back away from the ears.

Benefits: This pose lengthens the hamstrings, improves blood circulation, and reduces fatigue and anxiety. It stimulates the liver, spleen, and kidneys. It can be performed to relieve stomach pain during menstrual periods. It builds strength in the legs and upper back.
Contraindications: People with back pain or herniated disks should bend knees or not fold forward fully. Do not bring head between knees with a slipped disc.
Modification: Bend the knees.
Chakra: root, sacral

8. Karmasana (action pose)

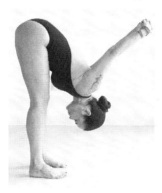

From *uttanasana,* separate the feet to hip-distance apart, and then clasp hands behind the back. Squeeze the arms and shoulder blades together. Extend the wrists overhead and move the shoulders up the back away from the ears.

Benefits: This pose strengthens the infraspinatus rotator cuff muscle and releases tension in the deltoids. It opens the chest and releases neck tension.
Contraindications: Avoid with acute shoulder pain.
Modification: Hold a strap between the hands if cannot keep the arms straight.
Chakra: root, sacral, throat

9. Parivrtta Karmasana (revolved action pose)

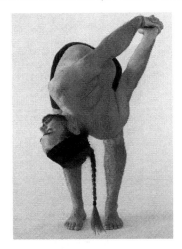

From *karmasana*, bend one knee and rest one shoulder on top of the thigh. Outer rotate the opposite shoulder and twist to gaze up at the ceiling.

Benefits: This pose strengthens the infraspinatus rotator cuff muscle and releases tension in the deltoids. It opens the chest and releases lower back tension.

Contraindications: Avoid if have lumbar herniation.

Modification: Hold a strap between the hands if cannot keep the arms straight.

Chakra: root, solar plexus

10. Utkatasana (fierce pose)

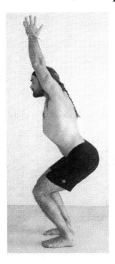

From *tadasana*, bend the knees, squat down, and sweep the arms overhead. Keep the hips heavy and descending. Actively move the arms back in line with the ears.

Benefits: This pose builds strength in the legs, abdominals, and the back. Regular practice can prevent the occurrence of sciatica.

Contraindications: Avoid with low blood pressure, insomnia, and headaches.

Chakra: root, sacral

11. Ardha Utkatasana (half fierce pose)

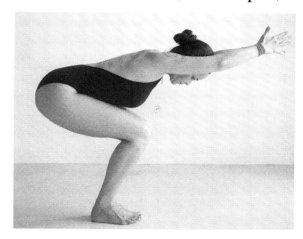

From *utkatasana,* bow half-way forward so the torso, arms, and thighs are parallel with the floor. Keep the arms and shoulders lifting above the ears and release the heart down.

Benefits: This pose builds strength in the legs, shoulders, and the upper back.
Contraindications: Avoid with low blood pressure, insomnia, and headaches.
Chakra: root, sacral

12. Parivrtta Utkatasana I (revolved fierce pose)

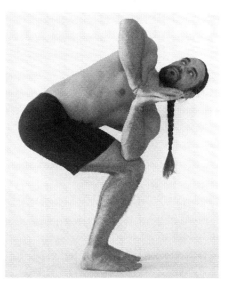

From *utkatasana,* twist and hook one elbow on the outside of the opposite thigh. Press into the hands and deepen the twist.

Benefits: This pose builds strength in the legs and tones the internal organs. It stimulates the pancreas and is useful in treating diabetes. It also maintains regularity.
Contraindications: Avoid with low blood pressure, insomnia, and headaches.
Chakra: root, sacral

13. Parivrtta Utkatasana II (revolved fierce pose II)

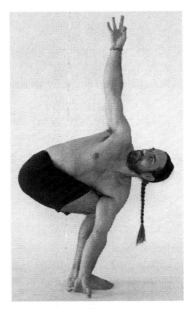

From *parivrtta utkatasana,* extend one hand to the floor. Outer rotate the shoulder and reach the opposite arm up. Press the bottom arm into the leg and deepen the twist.

Benefits: This variation opens the chest.
Chakra: root, sacral

14. Vanarasana I (monkey tail pose I, "lunge position")

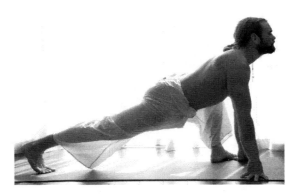

Step one foot up to the outside edge of the mat and bring both arms on the inside of the leg. Place the hands in ridgetop or fingertips position. Keep the arms straight and outer rotate the tops of the arms. Pull the shoulders down the back and extend the heart forward. Inner rotate the top thigh of the back leg and squeeze it into the midline as it lifts away from the floor.

Benefits: This pose opens the hips and prepares the body for the practice.
Modification: Place the back knee on the floor if the hips are tight.
Chakra: root, throat

15. Vanarasana II (monkey tail pose II)

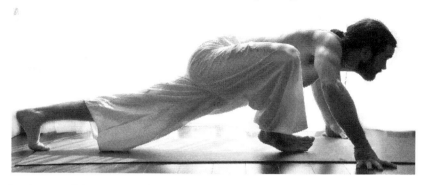

Step one foot up to the front of the mat and take the hands forward in an elevated position. Bend the elbows up to engage the back body. Push the head up and slowly lower the chest down. Deepen the pose by flexing the forward foot and rocking onto the outside edge. Push down through the outside edge of the foot, so the heel slightly lifts to keep ankle, shin, and knee aligned. Widen the forward knee out to the side to create more opening for the hip.

Benefits: This pose opens the hips and the heart.
Modification: Place the back knee on the floor if the hips are tight.
Chakra: root, heart

16. Vanarasana III (monkey tail pose III)

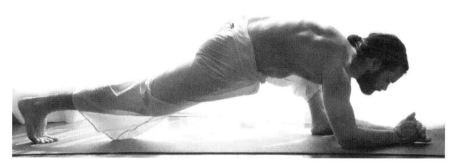

Step one foot up to the front of the mat and point the foot out to the side a few degrees, bow down, and come onto one or both forearms. Lift the back leg up and firm the lower abdominals.

Benefits: This pose opens the outer hip of the forward leg and creates strength in the back leg.
Modification: Place the back knee on the floor if the hips are tight.
Chakra: root, sacral

17. Somachandrasana I (elixir of the moon pose I)

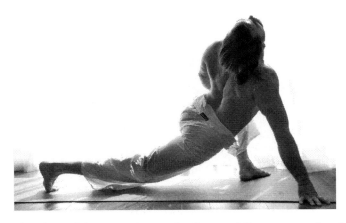

Step one foot up to the outside edge of the mat. Point the forward foot out to the side 45 degrees and place the hand at the top of the thigh. Bend the forward knee deep, as you open the heart, throat, and take the head back.

Benefits: This pose opens the front hip of the back leg and creates strength in the back body. It prepares the body for the practice.
Modification: Place the back knee on the floor if the hips are tight.
Chakra: root, heart

18. Somachandrasana II (elixir of the moon pose II)

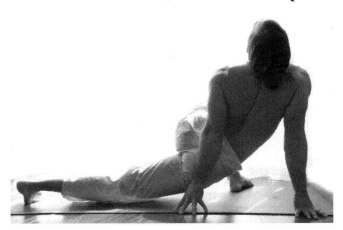

From *somachandrasana I* position, reach the arm of the expanding leg behind the back for the floor on fingertips. Keep the back leg straight and strong. The heel can angle to the side or rock onto the outside edge of the foot for goofy-foot to deepen the opening.

Benefits: This variation creates a greater opening in the outer hip of the back leg and releases tension in the IT band.
Modification: Place the back knee on the floor if the hips are tight.
Chakra: root, heart

19. Somachandrasana III (elixir of the moon pose III)

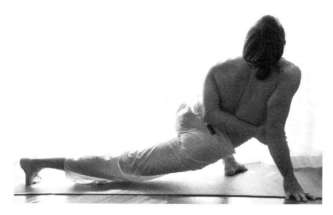

From *somachandrasana II* position, reach the arm of the expanding leg behind the back and grab the elbow. Bend the supporting arm and pull against it as you curl back over the forearm. The pose can be deepened by inner rotating the back thigh and rocking onto the outside edge of the foot for goofy-foot.

Benefits: This variation creates a greater opening in the chest and shoulders.
Modification: Place the back knee on the floor if the hips are tight.
Chakra: root, heart

20. Somachandrasana IV (elixir of the moon pose IV)

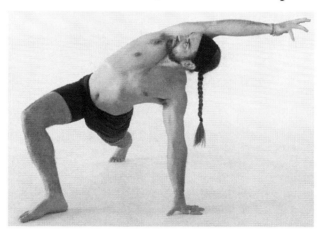

Step one foot up into a lunge and point the foot out to the side 45 degrees. Place one hand out to the side with outer rotation of arm bone. Keep the back leg straight and strong then bend the forward knee deep. Sweep the top arm overhead parallel with the floor with the pinky finger hooking under. Push the head into the arm to deepen the opening.

Benefits: This variation builds strength in the legs and in the arms.
Modification: Place the back knee on the floor if the hips are tight.
Chakra: root, heart

21. Somachandrasana V (elixir of the moon pose V)

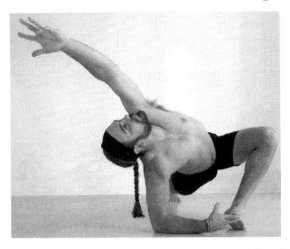

Assume *somachandrasana I* position and come onto one forearm and hook the big toe with the first two fingers, palm face-up. Sweep the top arm back overhead with the palm face-down and the pinky finger hooking under to keep the arm outer rotating. Push down through the outer edge of the foot and lift the inner edge. Widen the knee out to the side and extend the hips forward and down. Keep the forward foot strong, so it does not sickle or buckle at the ankle.

Benefits: This variation builds strength in the legs and opens the hips.
Modification: Place the back knee on the floor if the hips are tight.
Chakra: root, sacral

22. Subramanyasana (Subramanya's pose)

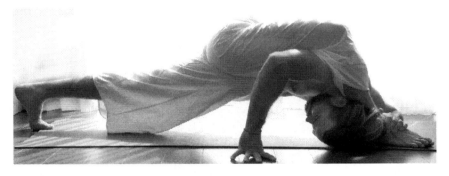

Step one foot up to the front of the mat and grab the ankle with the opposite hand. Rest the elbow down and pull the head towards the foot or under the leg. Reach the leading arm through and push the shoulder up into the leg to take the head deeper. Subramanya is another name for Skanda, and means that he has knowledge of Brahman.

Benefits: This pose opens the hips and creates strength in the neck.
Modification: Place the back knee on the floor if the hips are tight.
Chakra: root, brow

23. Anjaneyasana (Anjaney's pose, "monkey lunge")

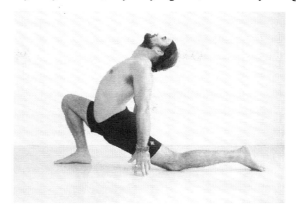

Step one foot up into a lunge position and place the stabilizing knee on the floor. Lift the ribs and shoulders toward the ears, and then curl the shoulders back, so the bottom tips of the shoulder blades lift up into the heart. Reach the fingertips for the floor, and extend the hips forward and down. Anjaney was the first name given to Hanuman from his mother Anjana.

Benefits: This pose opens the hips and releases tension in the hip flexors. It tones the back and stretches the abdominal muscles. It can also help with sciatica and respiratory ailments.
Contraindications: Avoid with cardiac conditions.
Modification: Place the hands on the hips if the fingers don't reach the floor.
Chakra: root, heart

24. Adho Mukha Anjaneyasana (downward facing Anjaney's pose)

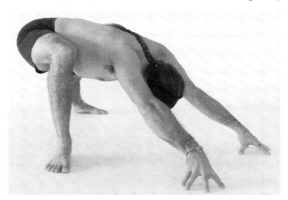

Step one foot up into a lunge position and turn the back heel down and in. Place the hands out to the side in an elevated position. Keep the arm bones lifting and outer rotating. Strengthen the back leg, inner rotate the top of the thigh, and then widen the sitting bones back and apart.

Benefits: This pose builds strength in the legs and opens the hips. It tones the back and increases circulation between the shoulder blades.
Modification: Place the hands on blocks if the spine rounds.
Chakra: root, sacral

25. Vrksasana (tree pose)

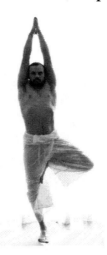

From *tadasana,* lift one leg up and turn the knee out to the side. Place the foot against the inner thigh and squeeze the two together. Draw the belly in, and scoop the tailbone under. Reach the arms overhead and root down through the grounding leg as you extend up out of the hips. Stretch the shoulders and arms up.

Benefits: This pose strengthens the feet, ankles, and legs. It improves balance and concentration. It also relieves sciatica and reduces flat feet.
Contraindications: Avoid with low blood pressure, insomnia, and headaches.
Modification: Place the hands on the hips if become unstable with arms overhead.
Chakra: root, sacral

26. Parsva Vrksasana (side tree pose)

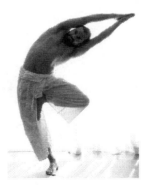

From *vrksasana,* root down through the standing leg, lift up out of the hips, and bow to the side of the bent leg. Keep deepening the twist as you increase the side bend. Press the foot against the inner thigh and press the thigh into the foot to hold the engagement in the legs and to stabilize the balance.

Benefits: This pose stretches the obliques, intercostals, and anterior serratus muscles. It improves balance and concentration.
Contraindications: Avoid with low blood pressure, insomnia and headaches.
Chakra: root, sacral

27. Vakra Vrksasana (bent tree pose)

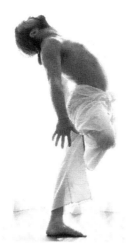

From *vrksasana,* extend the hips forward and the heart up, and then take the head back. Reach the arms down for the floor with hands free or clasped.

Benefits: This pose tones the back muscles and stretches the abdominal muscles. It improves balance and concentration.
Contraindications: Avoid with low blood pressure, insomnia, and headaches.
Chakra: root, heart

28. Adho Mukha Svanasana (downward facing dog pose)

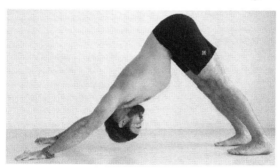

Enter the pose from a *vinyasa* or from an all-fours position. Push down through the hands to actively lift the arms and shoulders away from the floor. Keep the arm bones actively lifting and outer rotating. Widen the shoulders and collarbones apart. Open the heart and extend it toward the thighs. Squeeze the lower ribcage in and firm the lower abdominals. Engage the leg muscles into the bones and push the tops of the thighbones back. Extend energy from the hips down through the heels.

Benefits: This pose strengthens the arms and legs. It relieves fatigue and balances the nervous system.
Contraindications: Avoid if have carpal tunnel syndrome.
Modification: Bend the knees if the spine rounds. The hands can be placed on a chair if have a wrist or shoulder injury.
Chakra: root, heart

29. Parivrtta Eka Hasta Adho Mukha Svanasana (revolved one hand down dog pose)

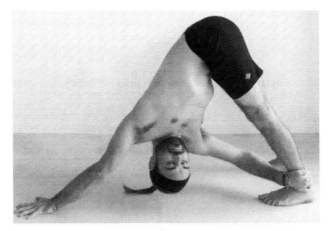

From down dog, reach one hand across and grab the opposite ankle. Let the shoulder blade sink into the back, and then push out through the hand to deepen the twist. Keep the hips level and both thighs pushing back evenly.

Benefits: This pose strengthens the arms and legs. It tones the internal organs.
Contraindications: Avoid if have carpal tunnel syndrome.
Modification: Walk the hands and feet closer together if cannot reach the ankle.
Chakra: root, solar plexus

30. Parivrtta Eka Hasta Eka Pada Adho Mukha Svanasana (revolved one hand one foot down dog)

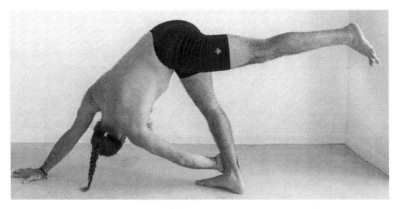

From down dog, reach one hand across and grab the opposite ankle. Lift one leg parallel with the floor and squeeze it into the midline. The heel of the grounding foot can turn in to help stabilize the balance for the lifting leg.

Benefits: This pose strengthens the arms and legs. It tones the internal organs. It improves balance and concentration.
Contraindications: Avoid if have carpal tunnel syndrome.
Modification: Walk the hands and feet closer together if cannot reach the ankle.
Chakra: root, solar plexus

31. Parivrtta Eka Pada Adho Mukha Svanasana (revolved one foot down dog)

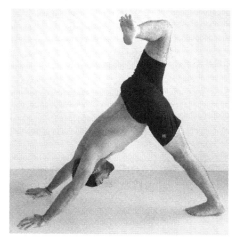

From down dog, lift one leg, bend the knee, and then twist to open the hip. Maintain the upper back level. Lift the arm of the grounding leg away from the thigh, and extend the heart toward the leg. Looking for the lifting foot under the arm will help to maintain the shoulders level.

Benefits: This pose strengthens the arms and legs. It tones the internal organs. It opens the front of the hips and prepares the body for the practice.
Contraindications: Avoid if have carpal tunnel syndrome.
Chakra: root, heart

32. Eka Pada Dhanur Adho Mukha Svanasana (one foot bow down dog pose, "Mad Dog")

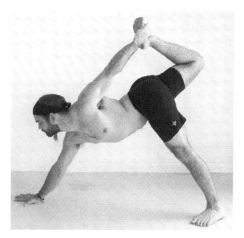

From down dog, lift one leg up and point it toward the head. The opposite hand reaches for the inside of the opposite foot. Kick the leg back and lift the arm up. Push the head up and melt the heart. The ankle of the grounding leg can turn in slightly for more stability.

Benefits: This pose strengthens the arms, legs, and back. It improves balance and concentration.
Contraindications: Avoid if have carpal tunnel syndrome.
Chakra: root, heart

33. Vira Adho Mukha Svanasana (powerful downward facing dog, "Turbo Dog")

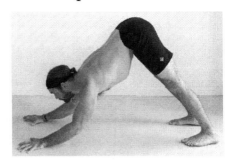

From down dog, bend the elbows down toward the mat, so they are hovering a few inches off the floor. Squeeze the arms, shoulders, and upper back into the center. Push the head up and root the thighs back. From turbo dog, slide through into a *vinyasa* or jump into crow pose. This pose is one of the best preparations for building strength to perform arm balances, as well as strengthening and stabilizing the rotator cuff muscles.

Benefits: This pose strengthens the arms and upper back.
Contraindications: Avoid if have carpal tunnel syndrome.
Chakra: root, heart

34. Virabhadrasana I (warrior I pose)

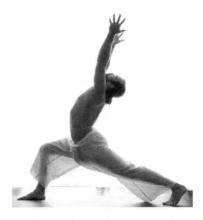

Step one foot forward to the front of the mat from down dog pose. Place the back foot flat for more stability, or lift the heel to square the hips forward to create more opening. Bend the forward leg at a 90-degree angle and align the outer edge of the knee with the outside edge of the foot. Draw the lower abdomen in and hold the core strong as the arms move back overhead. Pull the shoulders down the back and outer rotate the tops of the arms and shoulders. Lift the heart up, curl in the upper back, and then reach through the hands.

Benefits: This pose expands the chest and lungs. It strengthens the legs, shoulders, and back muscles. It also creates vigor, enthusiasm, and confidence.
Contraindications: Avoid with high blood pressure or cardiac conditions.
Modification: Place the back heel against a wall to increase stability and strength recruited. Place a block between the hands to squeeze the arms into the center, which stabilizes the rotator cuff and synergistically engages *muladhara chakra*.
Chakra: root, heart

35. Virabhadrasana I (warrior I pose variation, one hand behind head)

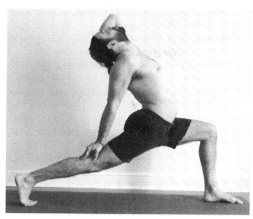

Assume *virabhadrasana I* position and place one hand on the hamstrings of the back leg. On inhalation, lift the leg up into the hand and then push from the hip through the back heel. On exhalation, walk the fingers down the leg toward the calf and take the pose deeper. When you can't go any further, bend the top arm and place the hand behind the head. The arm bone is beside the cheekbone. Press the head back into the hand, lift the heart up, and curl more in the upper back.

Benefits: This pose builds strength in the neck and the stabilizing leg.
Contraindications: Avoid with high blood pressure, cardiac conditions, neck injury, or psoas strain.
Modification: Place the back heel against a wall to increase stability and strength recruited.
Chakra: root, heart

36. Virabhadrasana I (warrior I pose variation, two hands behind head)

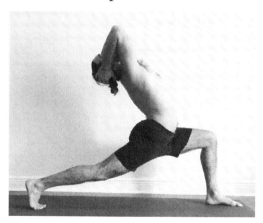

Assume *virabhadrasana I* position and place both hands behind the head. Pinch the head with the forearms and push the head back into the hands. Curl in the upper back and lift the heart up.

Benefits: This pose builds strength in the neck and expands the chest.
Contraindications: Avoid with high blood pressure, cardiac conditions. Avoid with neck injury.
Modification: Place the back heel against a wall to increase stability and strength recruitment.
Chakra: root, heart

37. Virabhadrasana I (warrior I pose variation, wrists crossed)

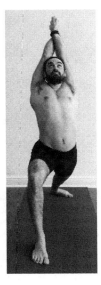

Step one foot forward to the front of the mat from down dog pose. Turn the back heel down and in. Bend the forward knee at a 90-degree angle and reach both arms straight ahead. Cross the same wrist as the leading leg on top of the other wrist (for example, if the right leg is in front, then cross the right wrist on top of the left). The palms and fingers are pressed flat together. Bring the biceps behind the ears. Press the head back into the top of the arm bones to create more opening for the upper back.

Benefits: This pose creates strength in the legs and the arms. It opens the shoulder girdle.
Contraindications: Avoid if have a shoulder injury.
Modification: Place the hands in prayer position in front of the chest.
Chakra: root, throat

38. Uttana Virabhadrasana I (intense warrior I pose)

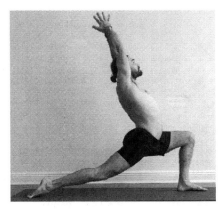

Step one foot forward to the front of the mat from down dog pose and rest the back knee on the floor. Place both hands on the forward thigh and bend the knee deep to extend the hips forward and down. Spread the toes of the back foot and press down strong through the outside edge of the foot. Lift the knee off of the floor, draw the belly in, scoop the tailbone, and then extend the arms overhead. Place the hands flat together and squeeze the arms into the head.

Benefits: This pose creates strength in the legs and the arms.

Contraindications: Avoid if have a shoulder or hip flexor injury.

Modification: Keep the back knee on the floor if the pose is unstable. Place a block between the hands to squeeze into if the elbows want to bend with the hands flat together.

Chakra: root, throat

39. Garuda Virabhadrasana (eagle warrior pose)

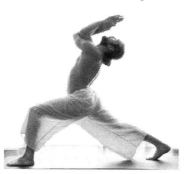

Assume *virabhadrasana I* pose and wrap the arms in eagle position with the arm of the back leg on top. Reach the arms overhead as the forward leg bends deep.

Benefits: This pose creates strength in the legs and stretches the rotator cuff.

Contraindications: Avoid if have a shoulder injury.

Modification: Place the hands in prayer position in front of the chest.

Chakra: root, heart

40. Atmanjali Virabhadrasana (warrior pose with hands in reverse prayer)

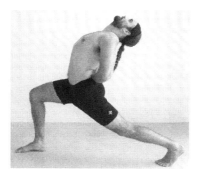

Assume *virabhadrasana I* pose and place the hands in reverse prayer position. Push the outside edge of the hands into the spine and curl over the hands. Pull the elbows and shoulders down, and lift the heart up. If having the hands in reverse prayer position is too difficult, then clasp elbows behind the back instead.

Benefits: This variation creates strength in the legs and opens the wrists.

Contraindications: Avoid if have a wrist injury.

Modification: Clasp elbows behind the back.

Chakra: root, heart

41. Baddha Hasta Virabhadrasana (bound hands warrior pose)

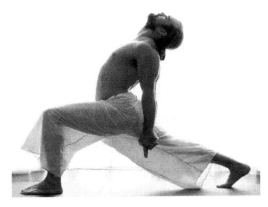

Assume *virabhadrasana I* pose and clasp hands behind the back and lift the ribcage up, then squeeze the shoulder blades together on the back. Slide the palate back, and then push the head back. Reach the hands for the floor to stretch the chest. Push down through the forward foot and pull the leg back concentrically to engage the hamstrings, then bend the forward leg and go deeper. Maintain the back leg lifting away from the floor and inner rotating.

Benefits: This pose expands the lungs and opens the chest. It creates strength in the legs and stretches the shoulders.
Contraindications: Avoid with high blood pressure or cardiac conditions.
Chakra: root, sacral

42. Utthita Baddha Hasta Virabhadrasana (extended bound hands warrior pose)

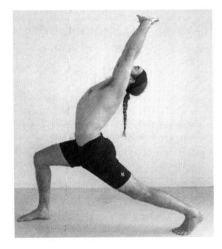

Assume *virabhadrasana I* pose and clasp hands. Extend the arms overhead with the palms face up. Squeeze the arms toward each other and push energy out from the shoulders through the hands.

Benefits: This pose creates strength in the legs and opens the shoulders.
Contraindications: Avoid with high blood pressure, cardiac conditions, or shoulder injuries.
Chakra: root, sacral

43. Virabhadrasana II (warrior II pose)

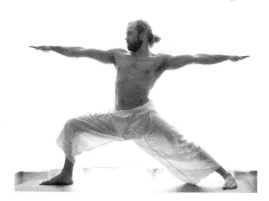

Step one foot up to the front of the mat from down dog, so the ankle is aligned with the wrists. Keep the forward knee bent at a 90-degree angle, and take the back foot flat to the floor. The forward knee stays aligned with the outer edge of the forward foot. Reach the arms out over the legs, so they are parallel with the floor. Draw the lower abdomen in and scoop the tailbone under.

Benefits: This pose focuses the mind, and strengthens the arms and legs. It also creates energy, enthusiasm, and confidence.
Contraindications: Avoid with high blood pressure or cardiac conditions.
Modification: Place the back heel against a wall to increase stability and strength recruited.
Chakra: root, sacral

44. Parsva Virabhadrasana (side warrior pose)

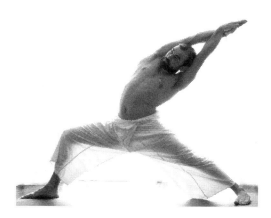

From *virabhadrasana* I variation, lean over the back leg, and extend energy forward. Use the bottom arm to pull the top arm down. Push the head up into the top arm and deepen the twist as you lean back. Lift the ribcage up to stretch the side of the body.

Benefits: This pose creates strength in the legs and stretches the side body. It also opens the shoulders.
Contraindications: Avoid if shoulder injury.
Modification: Don't cross wrists and perform one of the following pose variations.
Chakra: root, sacral

45. Parsva Virabhadrasana (side warrior pose variations)

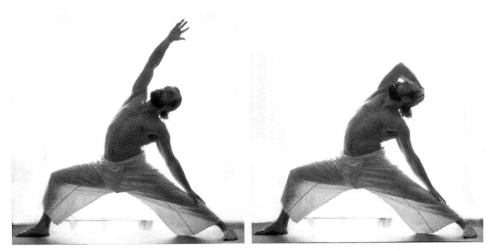

From *virabhadrasana II*, reach one hand down the grounding leg, and reach the opposite arm overhead. Lift up out of the hips and stretch the ribcage up. The expanding arm can then bend to grab the base of the skull. Push the head back to stretch the triceps deeper.

Benefits: This pose creates strength in the legs and stretches the side body.
Contraindications: Avoid with high blood pressure or cardiac conditions.
Chakra: root, sacral

46. Virabhadrasana III (warrior III pose)

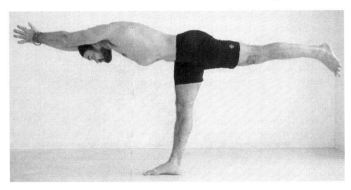

Assume *virabhadrasana I* position and stand up on the forward leg. Extend the arms and the back leg parallel with the floor. Inner rotate the top of the thigh of the lifting leg and squeeze it into the midline to activate the adductor muscle. Actively lift the arms and shoulders above the ears, and descend the heart toward the floor.

Benefits: This pose develops balance and concentration. It tones the abdominal area and generates inner heat. It strengthens the feet, ankles, and legs.
Contraindications: Avoid with high blood pressure or cardiac conditions.
Modification: Place the hands overhead against a wall to increase stability. The hands can be placed behind the head to build neck strength, or bring them into reverse prayer position behind the back to open the wrists.
Chakra: root, sacral

47. Veerastambhasana (warrior Veerastambha's pose, "humble warrior")

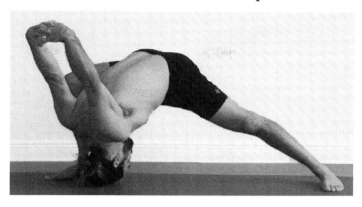

From *baddha hasta virabhadrasana,* bow forward and extend the wrists overhead toward the floor, as you take the head toward the foot. Keep the upper back engaged by lifting the shoulders toward the hips.

Benefits: This pose creates strength in the legs and opens the hips. It stretches the shoulders and releases neck tension.
Contraindications: Avoid with high blood pressure, cardiac conditions, or sciatica.
Modification: Hold a strap between the hands.
Chakra: root, throat

48. Salamba Utthita Parsvakonasana (supported side angle with elbow on thigh & hand on block)

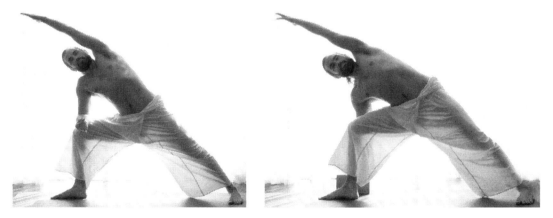

Enter the pose from down dog or from standing in warrior II position. Extend forward and rest the bottom arm on the extending leg or place the hand on a block. Reach the top arm overhead at a 45-degree angle. Extend energy from the back heel through the reaching hand.

Benefits: This pose creates strength in the legs and opens the hips. It opens the chest and expands lung capacity. Relieves sciatic and arthritic pain. Prepares the body for the full pose *utthita parsvakonasana.*
Contraindications: Avoid if suffering from insomnia, high or low blood pressure, or headaches. Avoid twisting the neck if have a neck injury.
Chakra: root, sacral

49. Utthita Parsvakonasana (extended side angle)

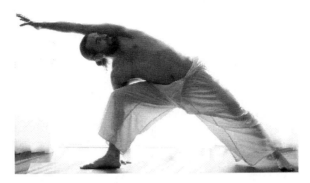

Step one foot up to the front of the mat from down dog, with the ankle aligned with the wrists, and place the back foot flat. Engage *uddiyana* and *mula bandha*, and then deepen the twist reaching the top arm overhead at a 45-degree angle or parallel with the floor. The back thigh stays rooting back and inner rotating, as the forward thigh is descending and outer rotating. Both of the arm bones outer rotate to create more opening of the heart.

Benefits: This pose creates strength in the legs and opens the hips. It opens the chest and expands lung capacity. Relieves sciatic and arthritic pain. Prepares the body for sitting poses.

Contraindications: Avoid if suffering from insomnia, high or low blood pressure, or headaches. Avoid twisting the neck if have an injury.

Modification: Place the grounding hand on the inside of the leg if have a lower back injury or suffering from piriformis syndrome.

Chakra: root, sacral

50. Parsvakonasana (side angle pose variation with one hand behind the head)

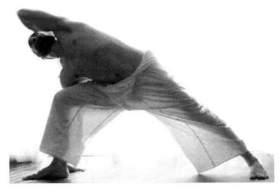

From *utthita parsvakonasana,* bend the top arm and grab the base of the skull. Push the head back into the hand as the heart extends forward. Keep the arm bone beside the cheekbone, and the elbow pointing straight ahead.

Benefits: This variation opens the upper back and strengthens the neck. It stretches the triceps and latissimus dorsi muscles.

Contraindications: Avoid twisting the neck if have an injury.

Chakra: root, throat

51. Ardha Vira Parsvakonasana (half warrior side angle)

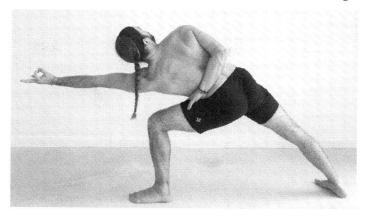

From *utthita parsvakonasana,* wrap the top arm wrap behind the back for the expanding thigh. Reach the lower arm straight ahead in *jnana mudra* with palm face-up. Lift up out of the hips so the torso is in line with the back leg. Resist the arch in the lower back by bringing the top ribcage down and in.

Benefits: This pose creates strength in the legs and generates inner heat.
Contraindications: Avoid twisting the neck if have an injury.
Chakra: root, sacral

52. Vira Parsvakonasana (warrior side angle pose)

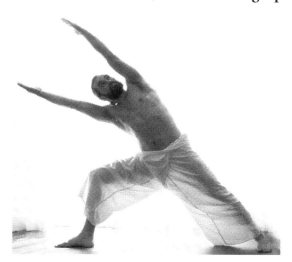

From *utthita parsvakonasana,* reach both arms straight ahead while maintaining the twist in the upper body. The top arm, torso, and back leg are all in line. Hold the core strong, and push through the back leg, as the arms reach.

Benefits: This pose creates strength in the legs and generates inner heat.
Contraindications: Avoid twisting the neck if have an injury.
Chakra: root, sacral

53. Ardha Baddha Parsvakonasana (half bound side angle pose)

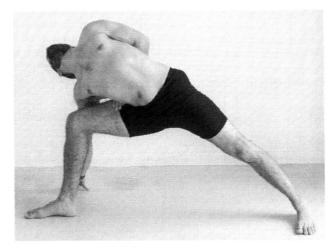

From *utthita parsvakonasana,* bow forward and wrap the top arm behind the back for the thigh of the expanding leg. Push the head into the top of the shoulder blades and extend the heart forward. Curl the shoulder further back then deepen the twist.

Benefits: This pose creates strength in the legs and opens the shoulders.
Contraindications: Avoid if suffering from insomnia, high blood pressure, or headaches. Avoid twisting the neck if have an injury.
Chakra: root, sacral

54. Ardha Baddha Uttana Parsvakonasana (half bound intense side angle pose)

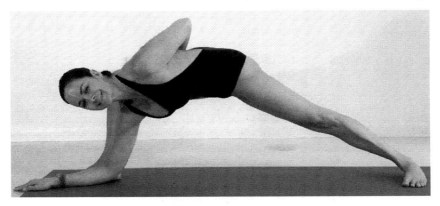

From *ardha baddha parsvakonasana,* bring the grounding arm on the inside of the leg and place the forearm on the floor. Push down through the back foot to keep the leg strong and resisting the floor. Release tension in the forward hip and push the top of the thigh down.

Benefits: This pose creates strength in the legs and opens the hips.
Contraindications: Avoid if suffering from insomnia, high blood pressure, or headaches. Avoid twisting the neck if have an injury.
Chakra: root, sacral

55. Baddha Parsvakonasana (bound side angle pose)

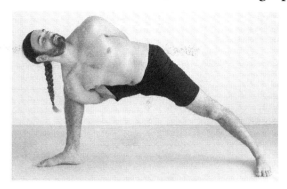

Step one foot to the front of the mat and take the back foot flat to the floor. Wrap the same arm under the expanding leg and grab the top wrist, or clasp fingers of the opposite hand behind the back. Pull the top arm straight, curl the shoulder back, and then push the head back to deepen the rotation.

Benefits: This pose creates strength in the legs and opens the shoulders.
Contraindications: Avoid if suffering from insomnia, high blood pressure, or headaches. Avoid twisting the neck if have an injury.
Modification: Use a strap to bind if unable to clasp hands.
Chakra: root, sacral

56. Raja Baddha Parsvakonasana (kingly bound side angle pose)

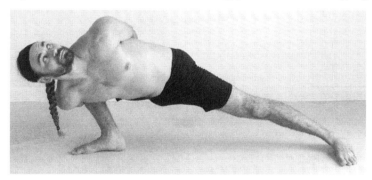

Step one foot to the front of the mat and take the back foot flat to the floor. Wrap the same arm in front of the shin of the expanding leg, and clasp the opposite hand or wrist behind the back. Bend the knee over the toes, as the upper body twists. Press down strong through the outside edge of the back foot to counterbalance the forward extending energy.

Benefits: This pose creates strength in the legs and opens the shoulders. It unravels the *granthis* (psychic knots) that bind the *kundalini shakti* (primal life force energy) from travelling up the spine.
Contraindications: Avoid if suffering from insomnia, high blood pressure, or headaches. Avoid twisting the neck if have an injury. Avoid if have weak or swollen knees.
Modification: Use a strap to bind if unable to clasp hands.
Chakra: root, sacral

57. Parivrtta Parsvakonasana (revolved side angle pose)

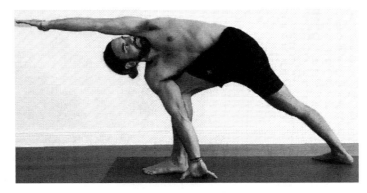

From *virabhadrasana I* or *Anjanyeasana,* twist and take the opposite arm across to the outside of the expanding leg. Outer rotate the arm, so the elbow crease faces out, and place the fingers on the floor beside the foot. Reach the top arm parallel with the floor. Duck the head under the arm and deepen the twist.

Benefits: This pose creates strength in the legs and tones the internal organs. It stretches the back and lengthens the spine. It stimulates the pancreas and prevents constipation.
Contraindications: Avoid if suffering from insomnia, high blood pressure, or headaches. Avoid twisting the neck if have an injury.
Modification: Bring the hands into prayer position if the fingers don't reach the floor.
Chakra: root, solar plexus

58. Parivrtta Baddha Parsvakonasana (revolved bound side angle pose)

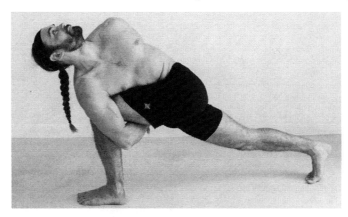

From *utthita parivrtta parsvakonasana,* push the bottom wrist under the expanding leg with the top hand, and then reach behind the back to clasp hands or the top wrist. Curl the shoulder back and deepen the twist. Keep the back leg straight, lifting up, squeezing in, and extending energy from the hip out through the heel.

Benefits: This pose creates strength in the legs and tones the internal organs. It stretches the back, lengthens the spine, and opens the shoulders. It stimulates the pancreas and prevents constipation.
Contraindications: Avoid clasping if have a shoulder injury.
Modification: Use a strap if unable to bind hands.
Chakra: root, solar plexus

59. Utthita Trikonasana (extended triangle pose)

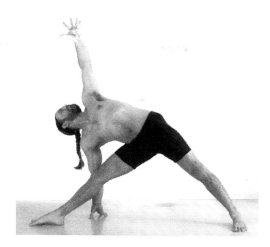

From *utthita parsvakonasana*, or from a lunge position, bow forward to the heart, and then straighten the forward leg as the top of the thigh rotates in. Then outer rotate the top of the thigh and the supporting arm. Firm the lower abdomen firm, scoop the tailbone, and then twist the upper body. Root both thighbones back into the hamstrings, and engage the quadriceps. Lift the thigh muscles up toward the hips, while pushing out through the feet. Bring the top ribcage in and lengthen the lower ribcage as you extend energy from the palate through the crown of the head.

Benefits: This pose creates strength in the legs and pelvis, while lengthening the hamstrings. It stimulates nervous system and the reproductive organs. It improves digestion, and helps alleviate nervousness and anxiety.
Contraindications: Avoid if back muscles strained.
Modification: Place the grounding hand on the inside of the leg to relieve lower back stress and avoid twisting the neck.
Chakra: root, sacral

60. Ardha Vira Trikonasana (half warrior triangle pose)

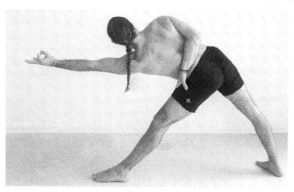

From *utthita trikonasana*, wrap the top arm behind the back, then from the hips push out through the legs, and reach the bottom arm straight ahead in *jnana mudra. Resist the arch in the lower back by bringing the top ribcage down and in.*

Benefits: This pose creates strength in the legs and pelvis. It generates inner heat and strengthens the breath.
Contraindications: Avoid if back muscles strained.
Chakra: root, sacral

61. Vira Trikonasana (warrior triangle pose)

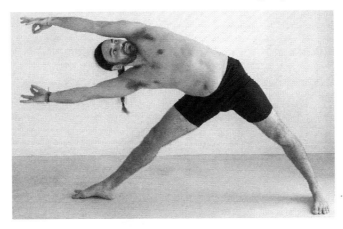

From *utthita trikonasana,* push energy out from the hips down through the feet and reach both arms straight ahead. Release the palate and strengthen the *ujjayi* breath.

Benefits: This pose creates strength in the legs and pelvis. It generates inner heat and strengthens the breath.
Contraindications: Avoid if back muscles are strained.
Chakra: root, sacral

62. Utthita Uttana Trikonasana (extended intense triangle pose)

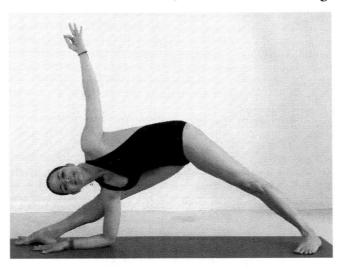

From *utthita trikonasana,* bring the grounding arm on the inside of the expanding leg. Bend the elbow and rest the forearm on the floor. Keep both legs straight and fully engaged.

Benefits: This pose creates strength in the legs and pelvis. It lengthens the hamstrings and opens the hips. It stimulates the nervous system and the reproductive organs. It improves digestion, and helps alleviate nervousness and anxiety.
Contraindications: Avoid if have a pulled or strained hamstring.
Chakra: root, sacral

63. Trikonasana (triangle pose variation)

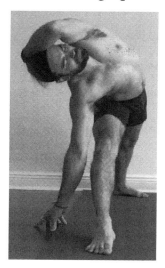

From triangle pose, reach the top arm overhead and parallel with the floor. Keep the arm bone beside the cheekbone then bend the arm and grab the base of the skull. Push the head back into the hand, curl in the upper back, and extend the heart forward.

Benefits: This variation of triangle pose builds strength in the neck and opens the heart. It stretches the side of the body and tones the upper back.

Contraindications: Avoid if the back leg wants to bend or if the top of the thigh moves forward.

Chakra: root, heart

64. Trikonasana (triangle pose variation)

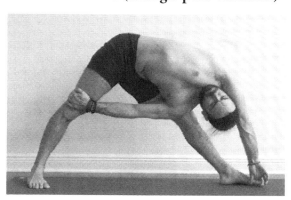

From triangle pose, bring the stabilizing hand on the inside of the shin, then reach the top arm overhead and grab the big toe with the palm face out. Reach the stabilizing hand back and grab the outside edge of the thigh. Pull in on the IT band of the back leg and push the head up into the top arm to deepen the twist. Keep pushing energy from the center out through the periphery.

Benefits: This variation of triangle pose stretches the side body and prepares the body for sage Vishvamitra's pose.

Contraindications: Avoid with hamstring injury.

Modification: Use a strap to hold the foot.

Chakra: root, heart

65. Utthita Parivrtta Trikonasana (extended revolved triangle pose)

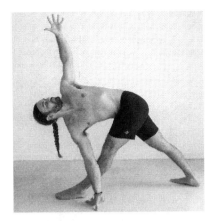

From *utthita trikonasana,* place both hands on the floor and step the back foot in a few inches and turns the toes in, and heel out, so the foot is set at a 60-degree angle. Twist and place the opposite arm across the outer edge of the expanding leg. Outer rotate the arm so the fingers point in. Bend the elbow a little and push the forearm into the shin to increase stability. Pull the forward thigh and hip back, and square the hips forward. Keep both thighbones pushing back and root strongly through the heels. Lengthen out of the hips and deepen the twist.

Benefits: This pose creates strength in the legs and pelvis. It tones the spinal nerves and the internal organs. It improves digestion, and helps with nervousness and anxiety.
Contraindications: Avoid if back muscles strained or if have lumbar herniation.
Modification: Place the grounding hand directly underneath the face to increase stability.
Chakra: root, solar plexus

66. Baddha Trikonasana (bound triangle pose)

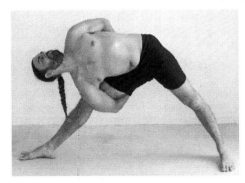

From *utthita trikonasana,* wrap the grounding arm under the expanding leg and clasp hands behind the back. Lean the head back to open the throat, and then outer rotate the top shoulder. Keep both legs straight and active.

Benefits: This pose creates strength in the legs and pelvis. It stimulates the nervous system and the reproductive organs. It improves digestion, and helps with nervousness and anxiety.
Contraindications: Avoid if back muscles strained.
Modification: Use a strap to clasp.
Chakra: root, sacral

67. Parivrtta Baddha Trikonasana (revolved bound triangle pose)

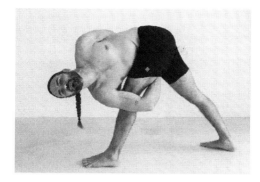

From *utthita parivrtta trikonasana*, bend the forward leg a few inches and pass the wrist between the legs using the top hand. Then re-straighten the leg and clasp hands behind the back. Root both thighbones back and extend energy down through both heels. Square the hips forward and lengthen out of the waistline as you twist. If entering from *parivrtta baddha parsvakonasana*, then step the back foot in a few inches, take the back foot flat, and then straighten the forward leg.

Benefits: This pose creates strength in the legs and pelvis. It tones the spinal nerves and the internal organs. It improves digestion, and helps with nervousness and anxiety.
Contraindications: Avoid if back muscles strained or lumbar spine herniated. Avoid if shoulder injured.
Modification: Use a strap to clasp.
Chakra: root, solar plexus

68. Baddha Eka Pada Uttanasana (bound one foot intense pose)

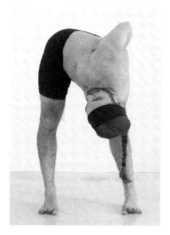

From *uttanasana*, take the feet slightly wider than hip distance apart. Reach one arm between the legs and the other hand behind the back to clasp. Push both thighbones back, straighten the legs, and then deepen the twist.

Benefits: This pose releases lower back tension and opens the shoulders.
Contraindications: Avoid if shoulder injured.
Modification: Use a strap to clasp.
Chakra: root, solar plexus

69. Parivrtta Baddha Eka Pada Uttanasana (revolved bound one foot intense pose)

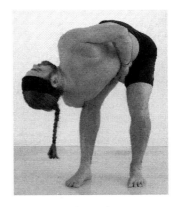

From *uttanasana,* take the feet slightly wider than hip distance apart. Twist and reach one arm around the outside of the opposite leg. Reach the free arm behind the back and clasp hands. Straighten the bound leg and keep the free leg slightly bent. Lift the hip of the bound leg and pull it back to deepen the twist.

Benefits: This pose releases lower back tension and opens the shoulders. It tones the internal organs and improves digestion.
Contraindications: Avoid if shoulder injured.
Modification: Use a strap to clasp.
Chakra: root, solar plexus

70. Utthita Ardha Chandrasana (extended half moon)

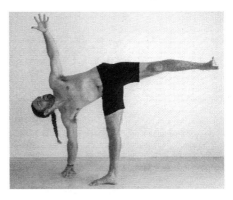

From *utthita trikonasana,* take the top hand to your hip and bend the forward leg. Place the grounding hand in front of you six to eight inches and slightly off to the side. Step up on the forward foot and lift the back leg parallel with the floor. Reach the top hand up and deepen the twist. Extend energy from the hips out through the heels. Gaze at the floor or straight ahead. If the pose is stable then look up toward the ceiling.

Benefits: This pose strengthens the legs and abdomen. It improves concentration, coordination, and balance. It helps alleviate stress, anxiety, fatigue, sciatica, and menstrual pain.
Contraindications: Avoid with low blood pressure, headache, or insomnia.
Modification: Use a block under the hand to help stabilize.
Chakra: root, sacral

71. Utthita Parivrtta Ardha Chandrasana (extended revolved half moon)

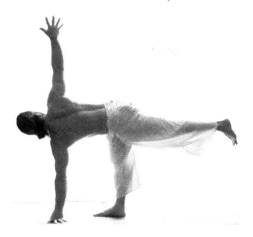

From *utthita ardha chandrasana,* take the top hand down and reach the bottom hand up. Inner rotate the lifting leg and outer rotate the standing leg to square the hips. Squeeze the inner thighs together to stabilize the pose. Extend energy from the hips out through the heels.

Benefits: This pose creates strength in the legs and pelvis. It improves concentration, coordination, and balance. It helps alleviate stress, anxiety, fatigue, sciatica, and menstrual pain. It improves digestion and prevents irregularity.
Contraindications: Avoid if lower back strained or if have lumbar herniation.
Modification: Place a block under the hand to keep the grounding leg straight.
Chakra: root, solar plexus

72. Vira Ardha Chandrasana (warrior half moon)

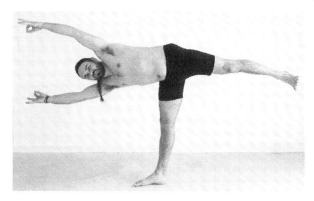

From *utthita ardha chandrasana,* reach the top arm straight ahead parallel with the floor. Grab the ankle of the standing leg with the lower arm, and then slowly slide the hand up the leg until the balance is sustained. Reach the lower arm straight ahead and strengthen the core to hold the balance.

Benefits: This pose creates strength in the legs and pelvis. It improves concentration, coordination, and balance. It generates inner heat for the practice.
Contraindications: Avoid if lower back strained.
Chakra: root, sacral

73. Baddha Ardha Chandrasana (bound half moon)

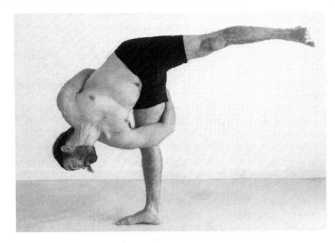

From *baddha trikonasana,* bend the knee, lean forward, and lift the back leg up parallel with the floor. Keep the forward leg slightly bent until the top leg reaches parallel, then straighten the leg fully.

Benefits: This pose creates strength in the legs and opens the shoulders. It improves concentration, coordination, and balance.
Contraindications: Avoid if lower back strained or if have lumbar herniation.
Modification: Place a block under the hand to keep the grounding leg straight.
Chakra: root, sacral

74. Parivrtta Baddha Ardha Chandrasana (revolved bound half moon)

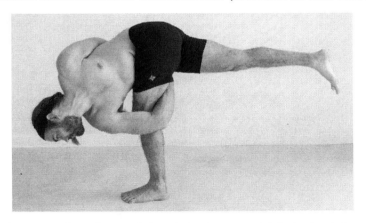

From *parivrtta baddha trikonasana,* lean forward, bend the knee, and lift the back leg up parallel with the floor. Straighten the standing leg and keep the inner thighs squeezing in toward the midline to stabilize the balance.

Benefits: This pose creates strength in the legs and pelvis. It improves concentration, coordination, and balance. It helps alleviate stress, anxiety, fatigue, and menstrual pain. It improves digestion and prevents irregularity.
Contraindications: Avoid if lower back strained or if have lumbar herniation.
Modification: Use a strap to clasp.
Chakra: root, solar plexus

75. Svarga Dvijasana (bird of paradise)

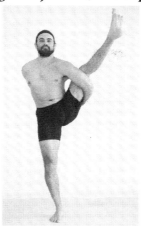

From *baddha eka pada uttanasana,* shift the weight to the opposite foot, and pick up the bound leg. Stand upright then bow forward, inner rotate the bound leg, and then straighten it fully. Draw the belly in, scoop the tailbone, and then push energy out from the hips through the heels.

Benefits: This pose creates strength in the legs and opens the hips. It improves concentration, coordination, and balance.
Contraindications: Avoid if hamstring pulled or strained.
Modification: Keep the leg bent if the hamstring is injured.
***Chakra*:** root, sacral

76. Parivrtta Svarga Dvijasana (revolved bird of paradise)

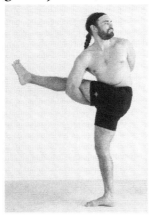

From *parivrtta baddha eka pada uttanasana,* shift the weight to the opposite foot, and pick up the bound leg. Twist and look back over the shoulder, and then extend the leg straight.

Benefits: This pose creates strength in the legs and opens the hips. It improves concentration, coordination, and balance.
Contraindications: Avoid if lumbar spine herniated.
Modification: Use a strap to clasp or grab the outside edge of the foot with the opposite hand, and then twist reaching the opposite hand straight back behind you.
***Chakra*:** root, solar plexus

77. Ardha Chandra Chapasana (sugarcane pose)

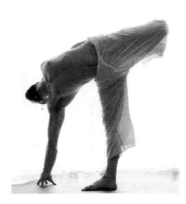

From *utthita ardha chandrasana,* bend the top leg and bring the knee to the chest. Grab the outside edge of the foot, and roll the shoulder back, as you kick the leg back. Then the head pushes back into the top of the shoulder blades, and the heart extends forward.

Benefits: This pose creates strength in the legs and opens the front of the hips. It improves concentration, coordination, and balance.
Contraindications: Avoid with high blood pressure, lower back pain, or pulled hamstring.
Modification: Place a block under the grounding hand to keep the standing leg straight.
Chakra: root, heart

78. Nindra Eka Pada Dhanurasana (standing one foot bow pose)

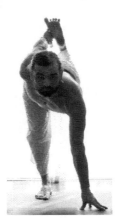

From *utthita parivrtta ardha chandrasana,* bend the top leg and reach back with the opposite hand to grab the inside edge of the foot. Keep the hips and chest squared forward with no twist, then kick the leg straight back, and lift it higher. Push the head straight up and melt the heart down.

Benefits: This pose creates strength in the legs and opens the front of the hips. It tones the spinal nerves and creates back body strength.
Contraindications: Avoid with high blood pressure, lower back pain, or a pulled hamstring.
Modification: Place a block under the grounding hand to keep the standing leg straight.
Chakra: root, heart

79. Ardha Baddha Padma Vrksasana (half bound lotus tree pose)

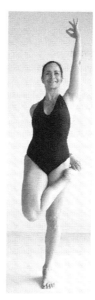

From *tadasana,* bring one foot into half lotus and then reach behind the back with the same arm to grab the foot. Release tension in the hip and bring the knee toward the midline, and then stretch the free hand up and smile.

Benefits: This pose opens the hips and shoulders.
Contraindications: Avoid if have a strained medial collateral ligament.
Modification: Use a strap to hold the foot.
Chakra: root, sacral

80. Ardha Baddha Padmottanasana (half bound lotus stretched out pose)

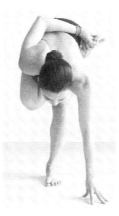

From *ardha baddha padma vrksasana,* fold forward and place the hand on the floor. Release tension from the hip and let the knee drop in toward the midline.

Benefits: This pose opens the hips and shoulders. It calms the nervous system and reduces stress.
Contraindications: Avoid if have a strained medial collateral ligament.
Modification: Use a strap to hold the foot.
Chakra: root, sacral

81. Utthita Hasta Padangusthasana I (extended hand to big toe pose I)

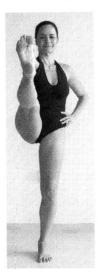

From *tadasana,* lift one knee up and hook the big toe from the outside of the leg with the first two fingers of the hand. Extend the leg straight and then bow forward over the leg. Bend the elbow out to the side, pull the shoulder down the back, and extend the heart forward.

Benefits: This pose creates strength in the legs and lengthens the hamstrings. It improves balance and concentration.
Contraindications: Avoid if have sciatica.
Modification: Use a strap to hold the foot and/or a wall to place the free hand on to stabilize.
Chakra: root, sacral

82. Utthita Hasta Padangusthasana II (extended hand to big toe pose II)

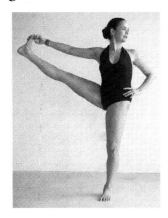

Assume *utthita hasta padangusthasana I,* position and lift back upright, outer rotate the elevated leg, and extend it out to side. Micro-bend the elbow and use the strength of the arm to elevate the leg higher. Twist the neck and gaze in the opposite direction of the elevated leg.

Benefits: This pose creates strength in the legs and lengthens the hamstrings. It improves balance and concentration.
Contraindications: Avoid if have sciatica.
Modification: Use a strap to hold the foot and/or a wall to place the free hand on to stabilize.
Chakra: root, sacral

83. Utthita Hasta Padangusthasana III (extended hand to big toe pose III)

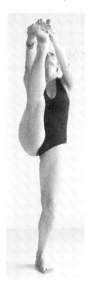

From *utthita hasta padangusthasana II,* grab the foot with both hands and kick the leg down to engage the leg muscles, then lean back to lift the leg higher.

Benefits: This pose creates strength in the legs and lengthens the hamstrings. It improves balance and concentration.
Contraindications: Avoid if have sciatica.
Modification: Use a strap to hold the foot and/or a wall to place the free hand on to stabilize.
***Chakra*:** root, sacral

84. Utthita Hasta Padangusthasana IV (extended hand to big toe pose IV)

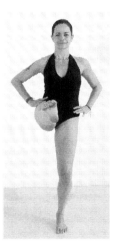

From *utthita hasta padangusthasana III,* place both hands on the hips, point the foot, and hold the leg up as long as possible. When you start to reach your edge, lean the torso back and lift the heart up.

Benefits: This pose creates strength in the legs. It improves balance and concentration.
Contraindications: Avoid if have a knee injury.
***Chakra*:** root, sacral

85. Vira Utthita Hasta Padangusthasana (powerful extended hand to foot, "Skanda squat")

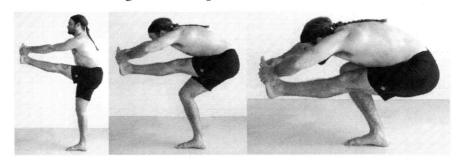

From *utthita hasta padangusthasana,* grab the foot of the expanding leg with both hands. Draw the leg bone and the arm bones back into the center, and then bend the stabiliziling leg. Squat down and bring the arms, chest, and thigh parallel with the floor. Stand back up and repeat until failure. Focus on keeping the stabilizing knee aligned with the outer edge of the foot during the descent and ascent.

Benefits: This pose creates strength in the legs and stabilizes the knees. It improves balance and concentration. It develops vigor and enthusiasm, while generating internal heat.
Contraindications: Avoid if have sciatica or a knee injury.
Modification: Use a strap to hold the foot.
Chakra: root, sacral

86. Urdhva Prasarita Ekapadasana (upward stretched out one foot pose, "standing splits")

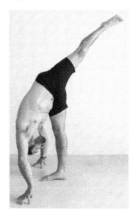

From *utthita ardha chandrasana* or *utthita parivrtta ardha chandrasana,* bring both hands to the floor and outer rotate the hip of the expanding leg. Inner rotate the thigh to take the leg higher, and push energy from the hip out through the mound of the big toe. Bow toward the leg, but keep the arms and shoulders lifting away to open the heart. If the pose can be deepened, then grab the outside of the shin with the opposite hand and pull it toward the center as you bow deeper.

Benefits: This pose creates strength in the legs and lengthens the hamstrings. It stimulates the liver and kidneys.
Contraindications: Avoid if have lower back or ankle injuries.
Modification: Place blocks under the hands to keep the standing leg straight.
Chakra: root, sacral

87. Parsvottanasana (intense side stretch pose)

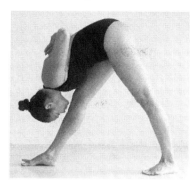

From *tadasana,* bring the hands into *atmanjali mudra* (hands in reverse prayer position) or clasp elbows behind the back. Step one foot 2.5-3 feet back. Place the back foot at a 30-degree angle. Square the hips forward and root both thighs back evenly. If entering the pose from *atmanjali virabhadrasnana,* then step the back foot forward a few inches and turn the heel down and in. Square the hips forward and bow down over the expanding leg.

Benefits: This pose creates strength in the legs. It opens the shoulders and wrists. It reduces flat feet and improves digestion.
Contraindications: Avoid if have a lower back injury or high blood pressure.
Modification: Use a strap to hold the foot.
Chakra: root, sacral

88. Prasarita Padottanasana I (extended wide leg pose I)

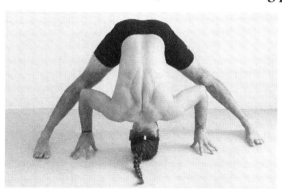

Extend the legs wide with the outer edges of feet parallel with the outer edges of the mat, or turn the toes in and heels out to create more opening if tighter. Place the crown of the head on the floor with the elbows pulling back toward the armpits, and engage the shoulder blades on the back. Squeeze the leg muscles to the bones and lift them up toward the hips. From the hips, push energy out through the feet.

Benefits: This pose strengthens inner thighs and hamstrings. It tones the abdominal organs and improves digestion. Good for headaches, fatigue, and mild depression.
Contraindications: Avoid if have a lower back injury or high blood pressure.
Modification: Place the hands on blocks.
Chakra: root, sacral

89. Prasarita Padottanasana II (extended wide leg pose II)

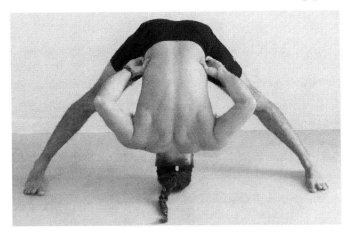

Assume *prasarita padottanasana I* position and place the three central fingers on the inside of the iliac crests. Press into the abdomen with the fingers, and use the strength of the core to take the crown of the head to the floor.

Benefits: This pose strengthens inner thighs, hamstrings, and abdomen. It tones the internal organs and improves digestion. Good for headaches, fatigue, and mild depression.
Contraindications: Avoid if have a lower back injury or high blood pressure.
Modification: Place the hands on blocks.
Chakra: root, sacral

90. Prasarita Padottanasana III (extended wide leg pose III)

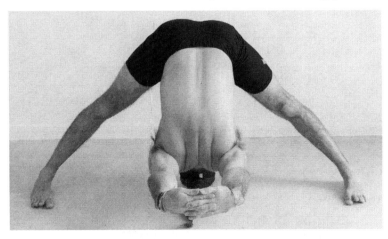

From *prasarita padottanasana II* clasp hands behind the back and fold forward. Engage the upper back and lift the shoulders up toward the hips, and then extend the wrists overhead for the floor.

Benefits: This pose strengthens inner thighs, hamstrings, and abdomen. It opens the chest and stretches the shoulders. Good for headaches, fatigue, and mild depression.
Contraindications: Avoid if have a lower back injury or high blood pressure.
Modification: Use a strap between the hands.
Chakra: root, throat

91. Prasarita Padottanasana IV (extended wide leg pose IV)

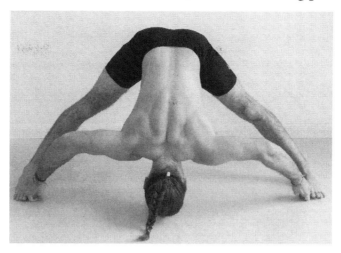

From *prasarita padottanasana III,* fold forward and clasp the big toes with the first two fingers of the hands with palms facing in. Bend the elbows out to the side and pull up, as the legs and big toes push down.

Benefits: This pose strengthens inner thighs, hamstrings, and upper back. It is good for headaches, fatigue, and mild depression.
Contraindications: Avoid if have a lower back injury or high blood pressure.
Modification: Use a strap between the hands.
Chakra: root, sacral

92. Prasarita Padottanasana V (extended wide leg pose V)

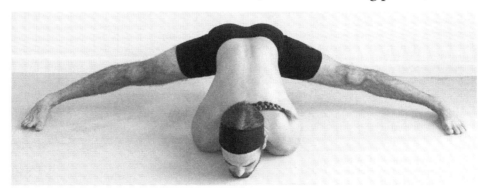

From *prasarita padottanasana IV,* take the feet as wide as you can and go as deep as you can. Reach the arms under the legs and clasp hands. Place the chin on the floor and stretch the neck forward.

Benefits: This pose lengthens the inner thighs and hamstrings. It is good for headaches, fatigue, and mild depression.
Contraindications: Avoid if there is more weight on the chin than the arms.
Modification: Place the forearms under the shoulders and use them for support.
Chakra: root, throat

93. Vira Prasarita Padottanasana (warrior extended leg pose, "warrior splits")

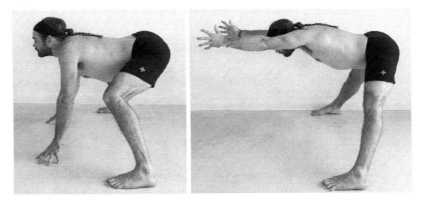

Assume *prasarita padottanasana I* position and bring the hands under the shoulders. Bend the knees and arch the spine. Push the head up and tilt the pelvis down. Squeeze the inner thighs together and inner rotate the thighbones, and then straighten the legs. Lean the hips back and reach both arms straight ahead.

Benefits: This pose strengthens the inner thighs, hamstrings, and abdominals. It is good for generating inner heat.
Contraindications: Avoid if have an adductor muscle injury.
Chakra: root, sacral

94. Parivrtta Prasarita Padottanasana I (revolved extended leg pose I)

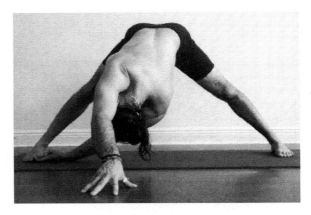

Assume *prasarita padottanasana I* position and reach the arms straight ahead on fingertips. Lift the shoulders away from the floor and reach one hand under to hook the opposite big toe with the first two fingers and the palm facing up. Duck the head under the arm and push it up to deepen the twist.

Benefits: This pose strengthens the inner thighs and hamstrings. It lengthens the back muscles and tones the internal organs. It is good for digestion.
Contraindications: Avoid if have an adductor muscle injury.
Modification: Bring the feet closer together or use a strap to hook the foot. Another alternative is to place one hand under the face without reaching for the foot, and then reach the other hand behind the back. Place a block under the hand to keep the spine parallel with the floor if the hamstrings are tight.
Chakra: root, solar plexus

95. Parivrtta Prasarita Padottanasana II (revolved extended leg pose II)

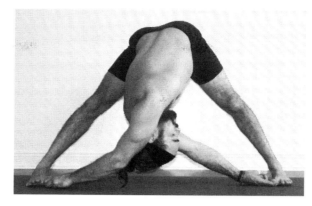

From *parivrtta prasarita padottanasana I,* bend both knees and hook the other big toe with the extending hand palm facing down. Duck the head under the top arm and then re-straighten the legs to deepen the twist.

Benefits: This pose strengthens the inner thighs and hamstrings. It lengthens the back muscles, stretches the side body, and tones the internal organs. It is good for digestion.
Contraindications: Avoid if have an adductor muscle injury.
Chakra: root, solar plexus

96. Tittibhasana II (insect pose II)

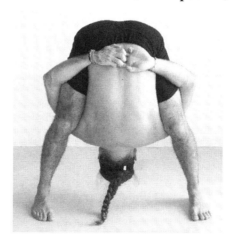

From *uttanasana,* take the feet slightly wider than hip distance and reach both arms between the legs and clasp hands behind the back. If the clasp is not possible, then use a strap or hold the ankles. Use the strength of the arms and legs to pull the chest deeper between the legs.

Benefits: This pose strengthens the legs, opens the hips, and lengthens the hamstrings. It stretches the shoulders. It lengthens the back muscles, stretches the side body, and tones the internal organs. It calms the nervous system.
Contraindications: Avoid if have high blood pressure or a hamstring injury.
Modification: Use a strap to clasp hands or hold on to the ankles.
Chakra: root, sacral

97. Tittibhasana III (insect pose III)

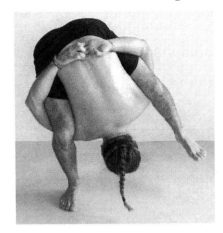

From *tittibhasana II,* shift the weight to one foot and lift the opposite foot up on inhalation. Place the foot down on exhalation. Repeat on the other side, and take five steps forward and five steps backward with the breath.

Benefits: This variation strengthens the feet, ankles, and legs. It improves balance and coordination.
Contraindications: Avoid if have high blood pressure. Avoid if have an ankle or a hamstring injury.
Modification: Use a strap to clasp hands.
Chakra: root, sacral

98. Tittibhasana IV (insect pose IV)

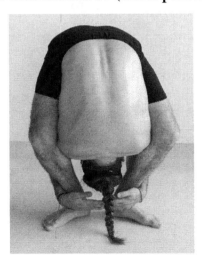

From *tittibhasana II,* turn the feet out to the side and bring the heels together. Reach the arms behind the legs and wrap the hands in front to clasp over the ankles. The head ducks under to deepen the forward bend.

Benefits: This variation strengthens the feet and ankles. It improves balance and coordination. It stretches the back and neck.
Contraindications: Avoid if have high blood pressure or lower spine herniation.
Modification: Use a strap to clasp hands.
Chakra: root, sacral

99. Pashasana (noose pose)

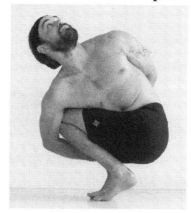

Squat down with the feet and knees together. Place one hand behind you for support and then reach the opposite hand up toward the ceiling and lengthen the side body. Bow forward and wrap the elevated arm around the outside of the opposite thigh. Reach the supporting hand behind the back and clasp hands. Pull the shoulder back and deepen the twist. If twisting around both legs is difficult, then use a strap, or wrap the arm in between the legs and clasp hands. The knees then squeeze together and pinch the shoulder. Once the balance is sustained, begin to let the hips and heels lower down.

Benefits: This pose strengthens the feet, ankles, and inner thighs. It tones the internal organs and improves digestion. It develops balance and concentration.
Contraindications: Avoid if have ankle injury or lower spine herniation.
Modification: Use a strap to clasp hands or clasp from in between the legs.
Chakra: root, sacral

100. Malasana (garland pose)

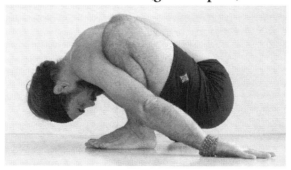

Squat down with the feet together and the knees wide apart, and then bow forward between the legs. Reach the arms back and place the hands on the floor behind you palms face up. Reach the hands behind the back and clasp to deepen the pose.

Benefits: This pose strengthens the feet and ankles. It opens the hips and stretches the shoulders. It tones the internal organs and relieves lower back stress.
Contraindications: Avoid if have knee injury.
Modification: Use a strap to clasp hands behind the back.
Chakra: root, sacral

101. Ardha Malasana I (half garland pose I)

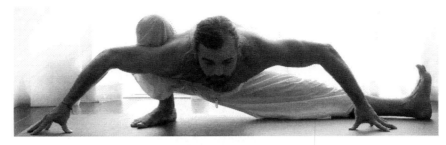

Assume *prasarita padattonasana I* position and bend one knee and shift the body over to that side. Outer rotate the straight leg and point the toes up toward the ceiling. Place the hands wide apart on fingertips or ridgetop position. Bend the elbows up and lift the shoulders up away from the floor. Push the head up and curl in the upper back, and then bow forward and place the head on the floor.

Benefits: This pose strengthens the feet and ankles. It opens the hips, lengthens the hamstrings, and relieves lower back stress.
Contraindications: Avoid if have knee injury.
Modification: Use blocks under the hands to keep the foot flat, or place one hand behind the straight leg and elevate the torso.
Chakra: root, sacral

102. Baddha Ardha Malasana (bound half garland pose)

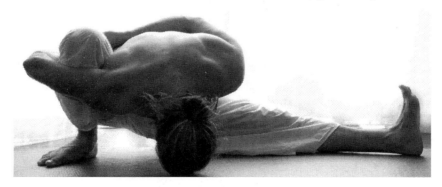

From *ardha malasana,* bow forward and wrap the arm in front of the shin and clasp hands behind the back. Squeeze the arms into the bent leg and pull the head towards the floor.

Benefits: This pose strengthens the feet and ankles. It opens the hips, lengthens the hamstrings, and relieves lower back stress.
Contraindications: Avoid if have knee injury.
Modification: Use a strap to clasp hands behind the back.
Chakra: root, sacral

103. Ardha Malasana II (half garland pose II)

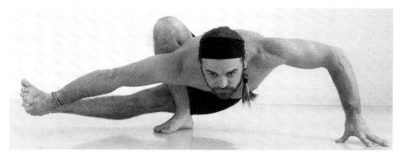

From *urdhva prasarita ekapadasana,* swing the top leg out to the side behind you. Grab the outside of the foot with the opposite hand. Squat down and lift the leg with the arm. Outer rotate the hip and release it toward the floor.

Benefits: This pose strengthens the feet and ankles. It opens the hips, stretches the IT band and outer hip rotators. It relieves lower back stress.
Contraindications: Avoid if have knee injury.
Modification: Use a strap to hold the foot.
Chakra: root, solar plexus

104. Garudasana I (eagle pose)

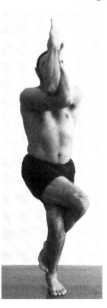

From *tadasana,* wrap one leg over the other and cross the ankle behind the leg, or point the foot toward the floor. Wrap the same arm as the top leg under the opposite arm, then bring the palms together and stretch the arms up.

Benefits: This pose strengthens the feet and ankles. It opens the hips, stretches the IT band and outer hip rotators. It detoxes the body by placing pressure on the lymphatic glands. It improves balance and concentration.
Contraindications: Avoid if have knee injury.
Modification: Point the foot toward the floor instead of crossing behind the leg.
Chakra: root, sacral

105. Garudasana II (eagle pose II)

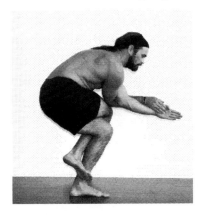

From *garudasana I* position, bow forward and rest the bottom elbow on the top thigh or lower knee. Extend the arms toward the floor to stretch the tops of the shoulders.

Benefits: This pose strengthens the feet and ankles. It opens the hips, stretches the IT band, outer hip rotators, and shoulders. It detoxes the body by placing pressure on the lymphatic glands. It improves balance and concentration.
Contraindications: Avoid if have knee injury.
Modification: Point the foot toward the floor instead of crossing behind the leg.
Chakra: root, sacral

106. Urdhva Kaliasana (upward facing goddess pose)

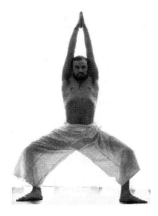

Take a wide leg stance with the knees bent and the ankles directly under the knees. Turn the feet out to the side so that the inner edges of the feet are parallel with the side of the mat. Draw the lower abdomen in and scoop the tailbone. Sweep the arms overhead with palms flat and squeeze the arms into the midline. Hold the core strong and let the hips sink down, and then pull the knees apart toward the outside edges of the feet.

Benefits: This pose strengthens the legs, abdominal muscles, and shoulders. It opens the hips and inner thigh muscles. It develops awareness of the center.
Contraindications: Avoid if have adductor muscle injury.
Modification: Clasp elbows behind the back.
Chakra: root, sacral

107. Shankarasana (sage Shankara's pose, "conqueror of the four corners")

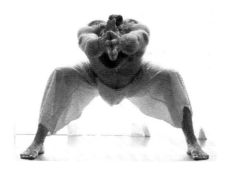

From *urdhva Kaliasana,* point the feet forward, bow forward, and reach the arms straight ahead parallel with the floor. Lift the arms and shoulders above the ears. Squeeze into the head, curl in the upper back, and lower the heart toward the floor.

Benefits: This pose strengthens the legs, abdominal muscles, and shoulders. It opens the hips and inner thigh muscles. It develops awareness of the center.
Contraindications: Avoid if have adductor muscle injury.
Modification: Place the hands on a chair to maintain stability and upper back integration.
Chakra: root, sacral

108. Nindra Hindolasana (standing baby cradle)

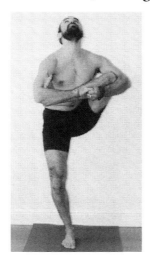

From *tadasana,* place one foot on top of the opposite knee. Flex the foot to keep the ankle, shin, and knee aligned. Squat halfway down and clasp hands in *Ganesha mudra* over the front of the shin. Curl in the upper back to bring the leg close to the chest, and then pick up the leg. Pull the leg in tight and lean back to deepen the opening.

Benefits: This pose strengthens the legs and opens the hips. It releases piriformis tension. It improves balance and concentration.
Contraindications: Avoid if have a knee injury.
Modification: Use a strap to clasp hands, or just hold the knee and ankle with the hands.
Chakra: root, sacral

109. Nindra Vayu Muktyasana (standing wind releasing pose)

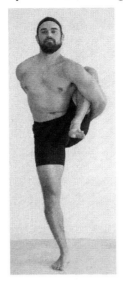

From *tadasana,* bend one leg up and hold the top of the ankle with the opposite hand. Bow forward and wrap the free arm in front of the shin, then clasp hands behind the back. Squeeze the arm into the bound leg and root down through the standing foot.

Benefits: This pose strengthens the legs, opens the hips, and stretches the shoulders. It improves balance and concentration.
Contraindications: Avoid if have a shoulder injury.
Modification: Use a strap to clasp hands.
Chakra: root, sacral

110. Nindra Vayu Mukttonasana (standing wind releasing face to knee pose)

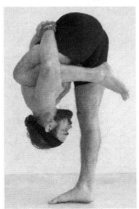

From *nindra vayu muktyasana,* bow forward and bring the face to the knee. Hold the pose and then stand back up.

Benefits: This pose strengthens the legs, opens the hips, and stretches the shoulders. It improves balance and concentration.
Contraindications: Avoid if have high blood pressure, headache, or shoulder injury.
Modification: Use a strap to clasp hands.
Chakra: root, sacral

111. Nindra Ardha Bhekasana (standing half frog pose)

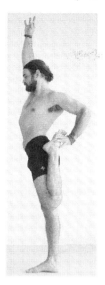

From *tadasana,* bend one leg behind and pinch the big toe between the thumb and index finger. Pivot the hand on top, widen the elbow, and then bring the foot to the outer edge of the hip. Draw the belly in, scoop the tailbone under, and extend energy out through the knee. Press the foot forward to the side of the hip and reach the free hand up toward the ceiling, or reach behind the back for the top of the foot.

Benefits: This pose strengthens the legs and opens the shoulders. It releases tension in the quadriceps and hip flexors. It improves balance and concentration.
Contraindications: Avoid if have high blood pressure, headache, or shoulder injury.
Modification: Use a strap to clasp the foot.
Chakra: root, sacral

112. Ruchikasana (sage Ruchika's pose)

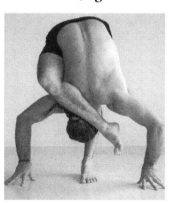

From *eka pada sirsasana,* rock forward and place the hands and the free foot on the floor. Straighten the leg and bow forward. Push the head up and bend the arms out to the side, or clasp hands overhead like in *gomukhasana.*

Benefits: This pose strengthens the legs and opens the hips. It improves balance and concentration.
Contraindications: Avoid if have high blood pressure or headache.
Modification: Use a strap to clasp hands.
Chakra: root, sacral

113. Durvasana (sage Durvasa's pose)

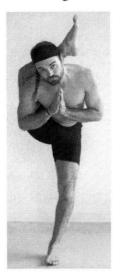

From *Ruchikasana,* stand up and bring the hands into *anjali mudra.* Maintain pressure of the head pressing into the leg.

Benefits: This pose strengthens the legs and opens the hips. It relieves varicose veins and tones the reproductive organs. It improves balance and concentration.

Contraindications: Avoid if have high blood pressure or headache.

Modification: Hold on to the foot from standing and bring it up towards the head. Lean back into a wall and use a partner for additional support.

Chakra: root, throat

114. Nindra Baddha Yoga Dandasana (standing bound yogi's staff pose)

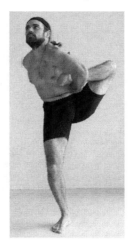

From *yoga dandasana,* rock forward over the opposite foot and come to standing, and then bind hands behind the back.

Benefits: This pose strengthens the legs and opens the hips. It relieves varicose veins and tones the reproductive organs. It improves balance and concentration.

Contraindications: Avoid if have a knee injury.

Modification: Use a strap to clasp hands behind the back.

Chakra: root, sacral

115. Natarajasana (lord of the dance pose)

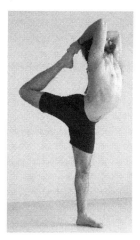

From *tadasana,* bend one leg behind you and grab the big toe, or the inside edge of the foot with the palm face up and elbow pointing down. Squeeze your knees together, draw the belly in, and scoop the tailbone under. Kick down into your hand to engage the top of the thigh. Then pivot the elbow up to the ceiling and turn the palm down to grab the top of the foot. Reach the opposite arm overhead and clasp the foot with both hands.

Benefits: This pose strengthens the legs and opens the hips. It stretches the quadriceps and hip flexors. It tones the back and stimulates the spinal nerves, kidneys, and adrenals. It improves balance and concentration.
Contraindications: Avoid if have a knee or ankle injury.
Modification: Use a strap to clasp the foot overhead.
Chakra: root, heart

116. Baddha Natarajasana (bound lord of the dance pose)

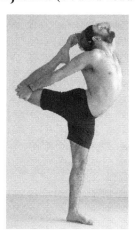

From *natarajasana,* reach the same arm as the elevated leg back and grab the knee. Lift the knee up and extend the heart forward.

Benefits: This pose strengthens the legs and opens the hips. It stretches the quadriceps and hip flexors. It tones the back and stimulates the spinal nerves, kidneys, and adrenals. It improves balance and concentration.
Contraindications: Avoid if have a knee or ankle injury.
Modification: Use a strap to clasp the foot overhead.
Chakra: root, heart

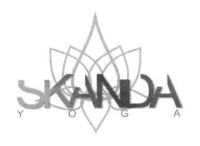

CHAPTER 10

Inversions

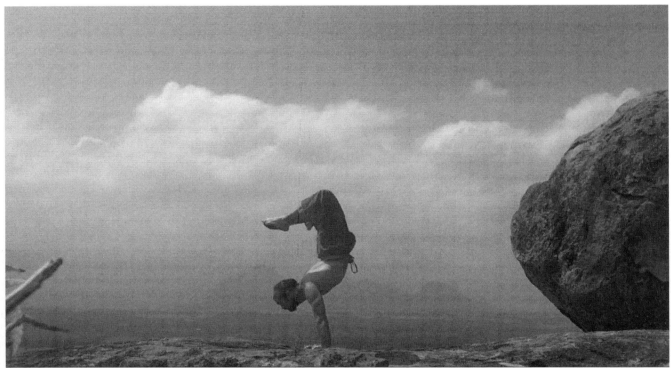

Palani, India

Inversions are the hardest to perform, but offer the greatest benefits. Personally, it took me a year before I figured out how to do a headstand and five years before I could do a handstand. The key is persistence. Keep practicing with patience and you will see improvement in the forms. Yoga makes the impossible possible.

Inverting the body has numerous health benefits. It increases circulation throughout the body, removes stagnant fluids, and reduces swelling. The brain becomes more oxygenated, improving focus and concentration. Shoulder stand places pressure on the major lymphatic glands, which forces the toxins out into the bloodstream. When it is held for an extended period, it is beneficial for detoxification.

Although there are numerous benefits, there are also contraindications. All inversions should be avoided if one has high blood pressure or glaucoma. Handstands should be avoided if there is a wrist injury, or modified with an alternate hand position. All inversions should be avoided after the second trimester. All inversions should be avoided during menstruation. Handstands and forearm stand should be avoided if there is a rotator cuff injury. Headstand and inverted ear pressure should be avoided if there is a neck injury. Shoulder stand should be avoided if the cervical spine is herniated or kyphotic.

117. Sirsasana I (headstand I)

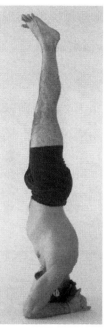

Set the hands in a *tamasic*, *rajasic*, or *sattvic* position. Place the crown of the head down or come more toward the hairline to increase curvature and support in the neck. Lift the knees and walk the feet in to bring the hips over the shoulders. Kick or press the legs up. Push the arms and the creases of the wrists down into the floor. Lift the shoulders away from the ears. Squeeze the lower abdomen and ribcage in and scoop the tailbone to extend energy up through the heels. Activate the feet in *pada bandha*, but let the feet fluctuate between a flex and a point to stabilize the balance. Focus on pushing from the palate through the crown of the head.

Benefits: This pose increases blood flow to the brain and stimulates the pineal and pituitary endocrine glands. It strengthens the lungs by helping to relieve colds, coughs, tonsillitis, halitosis and palpitations. It relieves anxiety and mild depression. Headstand helps with insomnia and headaches. It is recommended for prevention of asthma, hay fever, diabetes and menopausal imbalance. All of the following headstand positions have these benefits.

Contraindications: Avoid with cervical conditions, high blood pressure, heart disease, cerebral thrombosis, arteriosclerosiscoma, chronic catarrh, chronic constipation, kidney problems, sever near-sightedness, chronic glaucoma, and inflammation of the ears or any form of hemorrhage in the head. Should not be practiced during pregnancy after second trimester or menstruation. All of the following headstand positions have these contraindications.

Modification: A blanket can be placed under the head and over the arms for more support. A wall can be used to find balance.

Chakra: brow, crown

118. Sirsasana II or Utripada Sirsasana (headstand II or tri-pod headstand)

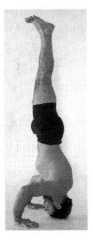

Place the hands and head in an equidistant triangle. Pull the elbows in toward the armpits and bring the shoulder blades flat on the back. Lift the knees and walk the feet in to bring the hips over the shoulders. Kick or press the legs up. Place as much weight into the hands as possible, while keeping the shoulder blades engaged on the back and lifting away from the floor. Push from the palate through the crown of the head.

Benefits: This headstand builds strength in the arms, shoulders, and neck.
Contraindications: Avoid until *sirsasana I* position can be held without the wall for one minute.
Modification: A headstand table can be used to strengthen the arms without weighting the head.
Chakra: brow, crown

119. Sirsasana III (headstand III)

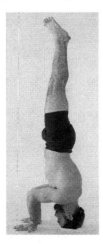

From *sirsasana II,* place one hand and then the other in a reverse position, and then bring the hands closer together. Press down into the hands to maintain the engagement in the upper back. Extend energy from the palate through the crown of the head.

Benefits: This headstand builds strength in the arms, shoulders, and neck. It improves balance and stability.
Contraindications: Avoid until *sirsasana II* position can be held without the wall for one minute.
Chakra: brow, crown

120. Salamba Sirsasana I (supported headstand I)

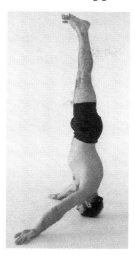

Assume *sirsasana I* position and extend the arms in front of you at a 45-degree angle. Place the hands palms face up. Press down into the floor with the back of the palms to lift the arms and shoulders up. Squeeze into the midline to hold the balance.

Benefits: This headstand builds strength in the arms, shoulders, and neck. It improves balance and stability.
Contraindications: Avoid until *sirsasana II* position can be held without the wall for one minute.
***Chakra*:** brow, crown

121. Salamba Sirsasana II (supported headstand II)

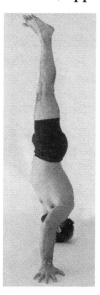

Assume *sirsasana I* position and extend the arms directly out to the side. Place the hands palms face down. Press the hands down into the floor, and squeeze the legs together to stabilize.

Benefits: This headstand builds strength in the arms, shoulders, and neck. It improves balance and stability.
Contraindications: Avoid until *salamba sirsasana I* position can be held without the wall for one minute.
***Chakra*:** brow, crown

122. Baddha Sirsasana (bound headstand)

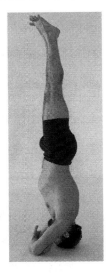

Assume *sirsasana I* position and stack the forearms in front of the forehead. Push the arms into the floor and lift the shoulders up the back.

Benefits: This headstand builds strength in the shoulders and neck. It improves balance and stability.
Contraindications: Avoid until *salamba sirsasana I* position can be held without the wall for one minute.
Chakra: brow, crown

123. Bhujamadya Sirsasana (elbow supported headstand)

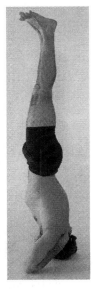

Assume *sirsasana I* position and reach the hands up and pinch the trapezius muscles. Push the elbows down and lift the shoulders up the back.

Benefits: This headstand builds strength in the shoulders and neck. It improves balance and stability.
Contraindications: Avoid until *sirsasana II* position can be held without the wall for one minute.
Chakra: brow, crown

124. Garuda Sirsasana (eagle headstand)

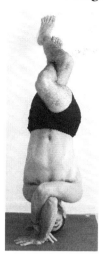

Start by wrapping the arms in eagle position and place the top hand flat to the floor. The other hand is in ridgetop or fingertip position. Take the legs wide apart and walk them in. Lift the hips over the head and then lean forward until the feet lift. Find balance first with the feet hovering off the floor, and then lift the legs and wrap them into eagle position.

Benefits: This headstand builds strength in the shoulders, neck, and abdominal muscles. It improves balance and stability.
Contraindications: Avoid until *sirsasana I* position can be held without the wall for five minutes.
Chakra: brow, crown

125. Niralamba Sirsasana (unsupported headstand)

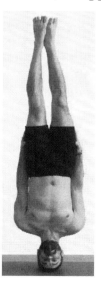

Assume *sirsasana I* position and push down from the roof of the mouth through the crown of the head, and then reach the hands up beside the hips. Squeeze into the midline to stabilize.

Benefits: This headstand builds strength in the neck. It improves balance and stability.
Contraindications: Avoid until *sirsasana I* position can be held without the wall for five minutes.
Chakra: brow, crown

126. Parivrtta Pada Sirsasana (revolved feet headstand)

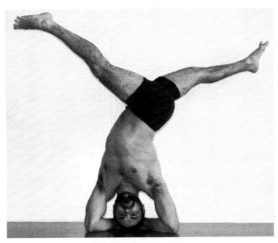

Assume *sirsasana I* position and take the legs wide apart and twist the legs. When you can't twist any further, bend the knees, and then deepen the twist. Straighten the legs and push from the hips out through the heels.

Benefits: This headstand builds strength in the neck. It tones the abdominal muscles and stimulates the internal organs. It improves balance and stability.

Contraindications: Avoid until *sirsasana I* position can be held without the wall for one minute.

Chakra: solar plexus, crown

127. Padma Sirsasana (lotus headstand)

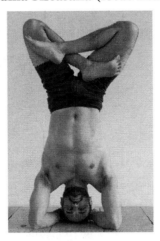

From headstand, point one foot and slide it down the opposite thigh. Twist toward the side of the bent leg and point the knee away from you to create space for the top foot. Point the top foot, snap it down over the top shin into lotus position, and then flex the feet.

Benefits: This headstand builds strength in the arms, shoulders, and neck. It tones the abdominal muscles. It opens the hips, and promotes healing for reproductive organ disorders.

Contraindications: Avoid until lotus position can be held for one minute sitting. Avoid if the medial collateral ligament of the knee is injured.

Chakra: brow, crown

128. Parivrtta Padma Sirsasana (twisting lotus headstand)

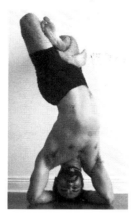

From *padma sirsasana,* twist the legs in one direction and arch the spine to open the hips. Then twist in the other direction.

Benefits: This headstand builds strength in the arms, shoulders, and neck. It tones the abdominal muscles and stimulates the internal organs. It opens the hips, and promotes healing for reproductive organ disorders.
Contraindications: Avoid until lotus position can be held for one minute sitting. Avoid if the medial collateral ligament of the knee is injured.
Chakra: solar plexus, crown

129. Sirsasana Vinyasa (headstand leg raises)

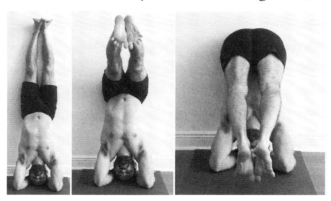

Place hands in a *tamasic, rajasic,* or *sattvic* clasp. Place the head four to six inches from the wall. Lift the knees and walk the feet in until the hips touch the wall or the feet lift. Inner rotate the thighs to elevate the legs to the wall. Flex the feet and push the hips into the wall. Lower the legs back down toward the floor. If the hips start to pull away from the wall, then point the feet and lift the legs back up. Repeat as many times as able. With practice, it can be performed without the wall.

Benefits: This exercise builds strength in the neck, shoulders, lower back, hip flexors, and abdominal muscles.
Contraindications: Avoid with neck injury. Avoid during menstruation or pregnancy second trimester.
Modification: Perform on a headstand table to avoid stressing the neck. If you don't have access to a headstand table, then you can make one out of stacked blocks and a couple of blankets to pad the shoulders.
Chakra: sacral, crown

130. Sirsa Pindasana (headstand womb pose)

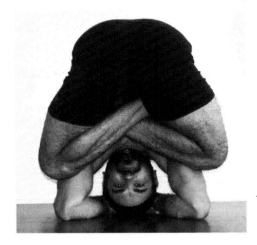

From *padma sirsasana,* lower the legs down onto the arms. Rest there and then lift the legs back up.

Benefits: This headstand builds strength in the arms, shoulders, and neck. It tones the abdominal muscles and stimulates the internal organs. It opens the hips, and promotes healing for reproductive organ disorders.
Contraindications: Avoid until lotus position can be held for one minute sitting. Avoid if the medial collateral ligament of the knee is injured.
Chakra: brow, crown

131. Zizumarasana (dolphin pose)

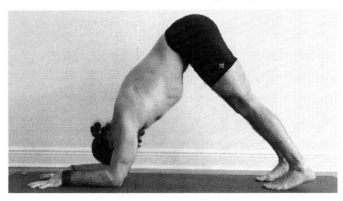

Start from an all-fours position with the elbows under the shoulders and the knees just beyond the hips. Lift the knees and straighten the legs. Push the thigh bones back and extend energy down through the heels.

Benefits: This pose prepares the body for *pincha mayurasana,* and it is a good alternative for inversions if have a wrist injury. It strengthens the shoulders and upper back.
Contraindications: Avoid with legs straight if the lower back rounds.
Modification: Bend the knees to take tension from the back and relieve the arms from over exertion.
Chakra: root, sacral

132. Pincha Mayaurasana (peacock tail feather pose, "forearm stand prep")

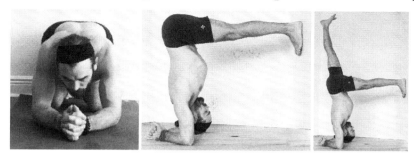

Start with the feet against the wall and the elbows under the shoulders. Clasp hands in a *rajasic* position as if for headstand with the pinky fingers extended forward. Extend the shoulders toward the ears and then curl in the upper back. Lift the knees and step the feet up the wall. Take the chin toward the chest to release the neck and open the chest. From here extend one leg up toward the ceiling. Hold for a couple of breaths and then switch.

Benefits: This preparation for forearm stand strengthens the arms and shoulders. It develops confidence and enthusiasm.
Contraindications: Avoid during menstruation or pregnancy second trimester.
Modification: Place the forearms on blocks to create more space to lift if the head touches the floor when the neck relaxes.
Chakra: heart, throat

133. Pincha Mayurasana (peacock tail feather pose, "forearm stand")

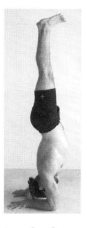

Place the hands in a *rajasic, tamasic,* or *sattvic* position for forearm stand from all fours on the mat. Relax the neck before kicking up, lengthen the shoulders toward the ears, and then curl them onto the back. Lift the knees and walk the feet in. Lift one leg up, inner rotate the thigh, and squeeze it into the midline, then kick up. If the head pushes up too soon, it will lead to over arching in the lower back. Work on taking the engagement out of the neck and into the core. Firm the lower abdomen and squeeze the ribcage in. Scoop the tailbone strong, and engage the gluteal muscles.

Benefits: This pose develops shoulder and back strength. It tones the spine and the abdominal muscles. It helps relieve stress and mild depression. Increases vitality and builds confidence.
Contraindications: Avoid with high blood pressure, heart conditions, vertigo, cerebral thrombosis, chronic catarrh, or menstruation. Avoid if have neck or shoulder injury.
Modification: Place a block between the hands to recruit more strength in the hands and arms to hold the alignment of the elbows under the shoulders.
Chakra: sacral, brow

134. Pincha Mayurasana (peacock tail feather pose with *tamasic* hands, "Forearm stand palms face up")

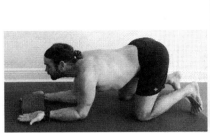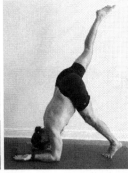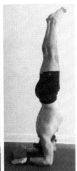

Start with the knees under the hips and the elbows under the shoulders. Place the hands palms face up (a block is optional). Press the backs of the hands down and outer rotate the arm bones, attempting to bring the thumbs to the floor. Lift the hips and step one foot halfway up. Look towards the foot on the floor and relax the neck. Kick up to bring both legs perpendicular to the floor. Separate the heels, draw the belly in, and extend the tailbone up through the heels.

Benefits: This technique increases balance and stability in *pincha mayurasana*.
Contraindications: Avoid with neck injury. Avoid during menstruation or pregnancy second trimester.
Modification: Lift into dolphin pose with the feet against the wall.
Chakra: sacral, crown

135. Padma Pincha Mayurasana (lotus peacock tail feather pose)

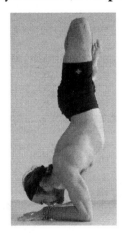

From *pincha mayurasana,* bend one leg and point the foot. Slide it down in front of the opposite thigh. Push the outer edge of the foot into the thigh and extend the knee away to create clearance for the other foot. Then kick the top foot into lotus position.

Benefits: This pose develops shoulder and back strength. It tones the spine and the abdominal muscles. It helps relieve stress and mild depression. Increases vitality and builds confidence.
Contraindications: Avoid until lotus position can be held for one minute sitting. Avoid if the medial collateral ligament of the knee is injured.
Modification: Place a block between the hands to recruit more strength in the hands and arms to hold the alignment of the elbows under the shoulders.
Chakra: sacral, brow

136. Karandavasana (duck pose)

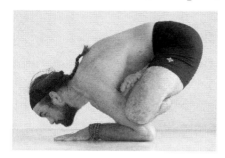

From padma *pincha mayurasana,* hinge at the hips and slowly lower the legs down onto the triceps. Hold for five breaths, and then lift back up by squeezing the legs together. After the legs have moved past parallel, then push the outer edges of the feet into the legs and extend energy out through the knees. Repeat as many times as possible.

Benefits: This pose develops shoulder, back, and neck strength. It tones the spine and the abdominal muscles. It helps relieve stress and mild depression. Increases vitality and builds confidence.

Contraindications: Avoid until lotus position can be held for one minute sitting. Avoid if the medial collateral ligament of the knee is injured.

Modification: Skip lotus position with the legs and place the legs over the upper arms like in *bakasana.*

Chakra: sacral, brow

137. Eka Hasta Shayanasana (one hand resting pose)

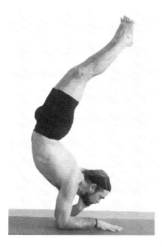

From *pincha mayurasana,* extend the legs over the head and then lift one hand to the chin. Curl in the upper back and descend the heart toward the floor. When the balance is held work on bringing both hands to the chin for full *shayanasana.*

Benefits: This pose develops shoulder, back, and neck strength. It tones the spine and the abdominal muscles. It helps relieve stress and mild depression. Increases vitality and builds confidence.

Contraindications: Avoid until *pincha mayurasana* can be held for one minute without a wall. Avoid if have high blood pressure or a neck injury.

Chakra: throat, brow

138. Shayanasana (pose of repose)

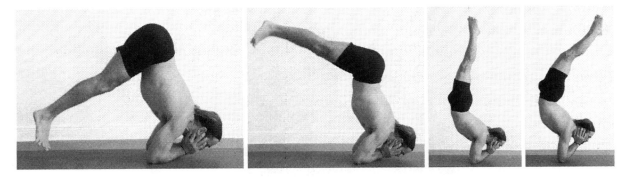

This pose can be entered from *pincha mayurasana* by bringing one hand to the chin and then the next. Pre-set the hands on the chin from kneeling to press up. Straighten the legs, lean forward, and inner rotate the thighs to lift the legs up. Push down through the elbows to lift the shoulders away from the floor.

Benefits: This pose develops shoulder, back, and neck strength. It tones the spine and the abdominal muscles. It helps relieve stress and mild depression. Increases vitality and builds confidence.
Contraindications: Avoid until *pincha mayurasana* can be held for one minute without a wall. Avoid if have high blood pressure or a neck injury.
Chakra: throat, brow

139. Vrischikasana I (scorpion pose I)

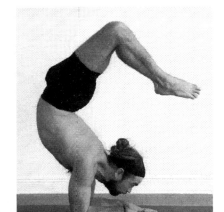

From *pincha mayurasana,* bend the knees and scoop the tailbone up. Push the head up and curl in the upper back. Squeeze the big toes together and engage the inner thighs. Melt the heart down and reach the feet for the back of the head.

Benefits: This pose develops shoulder, back, and neck strength. It tones the spine and the abdominal muscles. It improves circulation in the lower limbs and is good for treating varicose veins. It improves balance and concentration.
Contraindications: Avoid until *pincha mayurasana* can be held for one minute without a wall. Avoid if have high blood pressure, vertigo, cerebral thrombosis, chronic catarrh, menstruation, or heart disease.
Modification: Place a block between the hands to hold the arms in alignment.
Chakra: heart, brow

140. Susiravat Vrischikasana (open space scorpion pose, "hollow back")

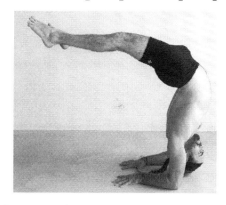

From *pincha mayurasana,* keep the legs straight and take the curve out of the neck. Scoop the tailbone up and slowly lower the legs into a backbend. The head and chest move away at the same rate in the opposite direction. Push the chin into the chest and keep the extension forward to hold the balance.

Benefits: This pose develops shoulder and back strength. It tones the spine and the abdominal muscles. It creates an opening in the chest and the upper back. It improves balance and concentration.

Contraindications: Avoid until *vrischikasana I* position can be held for one minute without a wall. Avoid if have high blood pressure, vertigo, cerebral thrombosis, chronic catarrh, menstruation, or heart disease.

Modification: Place a block between the hands to hold the arms in alignment.

Chakra: heart, throat

141. Garuda Pincha Mayurasana (eagle peacock tail feather pose)

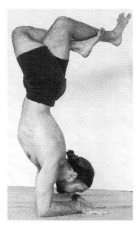

Kick up into forearm stand, with or without the support of a wall. Wrap one leg in front of the other and hook the ankle behind the calf muscle for eagle legs. Push the head up and look for the hands. Tap the wall with the big toe to find balance.

Benefits: This pose develops shoulder and back strength. It improves balance and concentration.

Contraindications: Avoid until *vrischikasana I* position can be held for one minute without a wall. Avoid if have high blood pressure, vertigo, cerebral thrombosis, chronic catarrh, menstruation, or heart disease.

Modification: Place a block between the hands to hold the arms in alignment.

Chakra: heart, throat

142. Visama Pincha Mayurasana (uneven peacock tail feather pose)

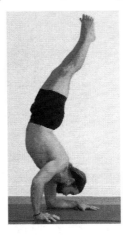

Place one forearm parallel with outer edge of mat and the opposite hand in line with the elbow. The elbow that is lifted is the same leg that lifts to kick up into the pose. If the right elbow is up, then the right leg lifts, and then kick off floor with the left foot. This centers the weight over the grounded arm. Squeeze the elevated elbow in toward the ribcage to stabilize.

Benefits: This pose develops strength in the arms and back. It tones the spine and the abdominal muscles. It improves balance and concentration.

Contraindications: Avoid until *vrischikasana I* position can be held for one minute without a wall. Avoid if have high blood pressure, vertigo, cerebral thrombosis, chronic catarrh, menstruation, or heart disease.

Chakra: heart, throat

143. Parivrtta Visama Pincha Mayurasana (revolved uneven forearm stand)

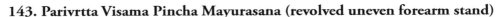

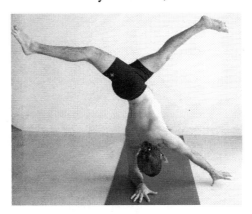

From *visama pincha mayurasana,* spread the legs and twist the leg of the grounding arm across the front of the body. The hand of the elevated arm reaches out to the side on fingertips, and then the thumb holds the balance.

Benefits: This pose develops strength in the arms and back. It tones the spine and the abdominal muscles. It improves balance and concentration.

Contraindications: Avoid until *vrischikasana I* position can be held for one minute without a wall. Avoid if have high blood pressure, vertigo, cerebral thrombosis, chronic catarrh, menstruation, or heart disease.

Chakra: solar plexus, brow

144. Visama Vrischikasana (uneven scorpion pose)

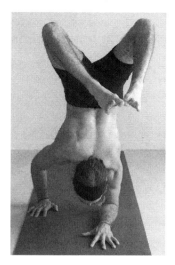

From *visama pincha mayurasana,* bend both legs toward the head. Push the head up and curl the heart forward.

Benefits: This pose develops strength in the arms and back. It tones the spine and the abdominal muscles. It improves balance and concentration.

Contraindications: Avoid until *vrischikasana I* position can be held for one minute without a wall. Avoid if have high blood pressure, vertigo, cerebral thrombosis, chronic catarrh, menstruation, or heart disease.

Chakra: heart, brow

145. Visama Vrischikasana (uneven scorpion pose variation)

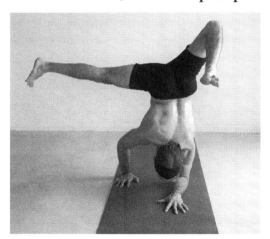

From *visama vrischikasana,* extend one leg out to the side of the elevated elbow. From here, the legs can be lowered into an *eka pada Koundinyasana* variation, or a *parsva bakasana* variation.

Benefits: This pose develops strength in the arms and back. It tones the spine and the abdominal muscles. It improves balance and concentration.

Contraindications: Avoid until *vrischikasana I* position can be held for one minute without a wall. Avoid if have high blood pressure, vertigo, cerebral thrombosis, chronic catarrh, menstruation, or heart disease.

Chakra: heart, brow

146. Adho Mukha Vrksasana (downward facing tree, "handstand")

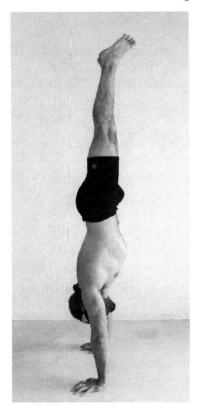

Set the hands in a standard or dynamic alignment position. Press, kick, or jump up. If kicking up, lift one leg, inner rotate the thigh, squeeze it into the midline, and then kick up using the strength of the bottom leg. If jumping up, work on doing it with legs bent, straight, and wide. Spring off of the toes when jumping, and flex or floint in mid-air. Focus on bringing the hips over the shoulders to stabilize. If pressing up, lean forward and slide the toes toward the wrists, until the feet lift. Then, inner rotate the thighbones to take the legs all of the way up.

Emphasize a strong grip or craw with the hands. Use the feet to counterbalance by engaging *pada bandha* while moving towards a flex or point, depending upon the sway of the body. For example, if the feet come over the head toward a back bend, then the feet flex more to straighten back out. If the legs move forward toward the chest, then the feet point to go back up. When the balance is sustained, squeeze the lower abdomen and ribcage in, and then extend energy from the tailbone through the heels.

Benefits: This pose develops strength in the wrists, arms, back, abdominals, and inner thighs. It relieves stress and mild depression. It improves balance and concentration. It develops confidence, courage, and vitality.

Contraindications: Avoid if have high blood pressure, vertigo, cerebral thrombosis, chronic catarrh, menstruation, pregnancy (third trimester), or heart disease.

Modification: Use a wall to help stabilize.

Chakra: sacral, heart

147. Eka Pada Adho Mukha Vrksasana (one foot handstand prep technique)

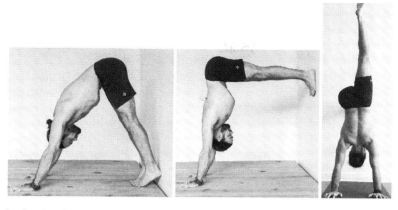

Start in down dog with the heels elevated on the wall. Step one foot up the wall and then the other. Bring the legs parallel with the floor and the hips stacked over the shoulders. Stay here if you are new to handstand until it can be held comfortably. From here, take the chin to the chest to open the upper back, or lift one leg toward the ceiling to begin to work towards the full form of the pose.

Benefits: Builds strength in the arms and upper back. Develops concentration and focus. Increases confidence and vigor. It is beneficial for working towards the full handstand.

Contraindications: Avoid with wrist injury. Avoid during menstruation or pregnancy second trimester.

Modification: Place the hands in fists or ridgetop to avoid aggravating the wrist if injured or to build more strength in the pose.

***Chakra*:** heart

148. Eka Pada Adho Mukha Vrksasana Vinyasa (one foot handstand transition technique)

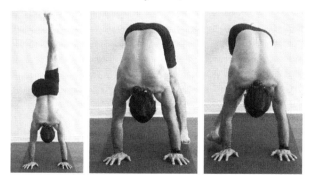

From one foot handstand prep technique, lower the extending leg down to the wrist and extend the leg back up or cross over and touch the other wrist, and then go back up. Repeat up to 13 times. Lower the leg on inhalation and extend back up on exhalation.

Benefits: Builds strength in the hands, arms, abdominals, and upper back. Develops concentration and focus. It is beneficial for working towards kicking up into handstand and holding the balance.

Contraindications: Avoid with wrist injury. Avoid during menstruation or pregnancy second trimester.

Modification: Place the hands in fists or ridgetop to avoid aggravating the wrist if injured or to build more strength in the pose.

***Chakra*:** heart

149. Adho Mukha Vrksasana (handstand balancing technique)

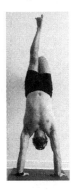

Place hands on the floor, fingertip to elbow distance away from the wall. Kick up and place one foot on the wall with the knee bent. The other leg extends straight up. Squeeze the inner thighs and knees together, and then tap the wall with the foot of bent leg to find stability. This same technique can be used to find the balance in forearm stand and headstand.

Benefits: This preparation for finding balance in *pincha mayurasana* or *adho mukha vrksasana* develops strength and awareness of the center to stabilize the form. It strengthens the arms, shoulders, and inner thighs.
Contraindications: Avoid during menstruation or pregnancy second trimester.
Modification: Use a belt or Infinity Strap for the arms to keep them straight if they want to bend. The prop should be placed just above the elbows.
***Chakra*:** heart, throat

150. Adho Mukha Vrksasana Vinyasa (downward facing tree transition, "handstand leg raises")

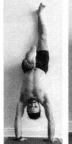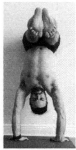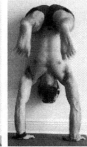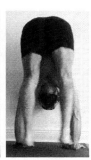

Measure the distance between your thumb and pinky finger when spreading the hand wide. Place the fingers this distance away from the wall. Kick into handstand and rest the hips and legs against the wall. Take the chin to the chest and extend the heart forward. Press one heel into the wall and lower the other leg parallel to the floor. The feet maintain a strong flex or floint to stabilize the form. After performing several raises with each leg, practice on lowering both simultaneously. With the hips leaning into the wall, lower both legs down. After the legs reach parallel, then point the feet and go back up, or press the head into the wall and lower the feet to the wrists. With practice, it can be performed without the wall.

Benefits: Builds strength in the hands, arms, and abdominals.
Contraindications: Avoid with wrist injury. Avoid during menstruation or pregnancy second trimester.
Modification: Place the hands in fists or ridgetop to avoid aggravating the wrist if injured or to build more strength in the pose.
***Chakra*:** heart, throat

151. Adho Mukha Hanuman Vrksasana
(downward facing Hanuman tree pose, "handstand splits at wall")

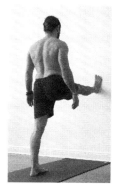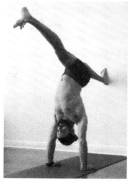

Start by standing with one leg extended parallel with the floor and the foot flat against the wall. Remove the foot from the wall, bow forward, and place the hands on the floor with the fingers aligned with the toes of the standing leg. Prepare for the handstand by first inner rotating the lifting leg and engaging the adductor muscle. Kick up and place a foot flush to the wall. Extend the other leg away from the wall striving for parallel with the floor.

Benefits: Builds strength in the hands, arms, and abdominals. It lengthens the hamstrings and opens the hips.
Contraindications: Avoid with wrist injury. Avoid during menstruation or pregnancy second trimester.
Modification: Place the hands in fists or ridgetop to avoid aggravating the wrist if injured or to build more strength in the pose.
Chakra: heart, throat

152. Adho Mukha Vrksasana (downward tree pose, "press up technique at wall")

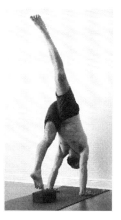

Start by placing a block 2.5-3' from the wall. Place the hands 5-6" away from the wall. Step one foot onto the top of the block. Inner rotate the leg and extend it up toward the ceiling. Lean forward and come onto the tip of the big toe. Hold it here for several breaths and then press or lightly kick up to handstand. Press the trailing leg's heel into the wall and slowly lower the opposite foot toward the block.

Benefits: Builds strength in the hands, arms, and abdominals. Prepares the body to press up with both feet.
Contraindications: Avoid with wrist injury. Avoid during menstruation or pregnancy second trimester.
Modification: Place the hands in fists or ridgetop to avoid aggravating the wrist if injured or to build more strength in the pose.
Chakra: heart, throat

153. Adho Mukha Vrksasana (downward facing tree, "handstand with reverse ridgetops")

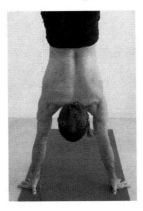

Handstand can also be performed dynamically with reverse ridgetop position. Outer rotate the arms with the thumbs pointing straight ahead in flexion. This takes a lot of strength and effort out of holding the handstand, but may take a long time conditioning the hands to get there. When trying a new hand technique, the legs should walk up the wall first to make sure the form can be maintained. It can be performed also on fists or fingertips.

Benefits: This pose develops strength in the thumbs, hands, wrists, and arms. It improves balance and concentration. It develops confidence, courage, and vitality.

Contraindications: Avoid until *vrischikasana I* position can be held for one minute without a wall. Avoid if have high blood pressure, vertigo, cerebral thrombosis, chronic catarrh, menstruation, or heart disease.

Modification: Use a wall to help stabilize.

Chakra: sacral, heart

154. Vajra and Baddha Hasta Adho Mukha Vrksasana (diamond and bound hands downward facing tree)

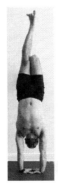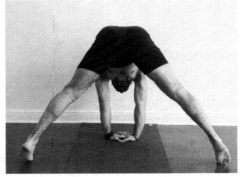

Use a wall for support or practice pressing up without the wall. Set the hands in either diamond or in a bound position. If kicking up, place one foot on the wall and extend the other leg straight up toward the ceiling. If pressing up, start with the legs wider than the hands. Lean the hips over the shoulders and come onto the tips of the big toes. Inner rotate the thighbones and extend all of the way up into handstand.

Benefits: These variations of handstand build strength in the hands and wrists. They increase balance and concentration.

Contraindications: Avoid with wrist injury.

Chakra: heart, solar plexus

155. Prasarita Pada Adho Mukha Vrksasana (extended foot downward facing tree)

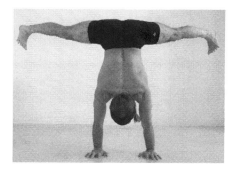

From *adho mukha svanasana,* outer rotate the tops of the shoulders and widen the collarbones apart. Jump the hips over the shoulders and extend the feet wide out to the side. Keep the feet flexed to maintain energy drawing from the feet into the hips. From here, you can twist in either direction for the revolved variation by inner rotating one leg and outer rotating the other.

Benefits: This pose develops strength in the hands, arms, back, and legs. It improves balance and concentration. It develops confidence, courage, and vitality.
Contraindications: Avoid until *adho mukha vrksasana* position can be held for 30 seconds without a wall. Avoid if have high blood pressure, vertigo, cerebral thrombosis, chronic catarrh, menstruation, or heart disease.
Modification: Use a wall to help stabilize.
Chakra: sacral, heart

156. Garuda Adho Mukha Vrksasana (eagle downward facing tree pose)

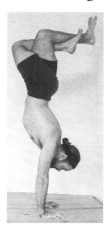

Kick up into handstand with or without the support of a wall. Wrap one leg in front of the other and hook the ankle behind the calf muscle for eagle legs. Push the head up and look for the hands. Tap the wall with the big toe to find balance.

Benefits: This pose develops strength in the hands, arms, and back. It improves balance and concentration.
Contraindications: Avoid if have high blood pressure, vertigo, cerebral thrombosis, chronic catarrh, menstruation, or heart disease.
Modification: Use a wall to help stabilize.
Chakra: sacral, heart

157. Padma Adho Mukha Vrksasana (lotus downward facing tree pose)

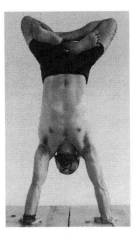

Press up from *urdhva kukkutasana* or kick into handstand and bring the legs into lotus position. Push the head up and squeeze the arms into the center. Outer rotate the top of the shoulders and widen the collarbones apart.

Benefits: This pose develops strength in the hands, arms, and back. It develops balance and concentration.
Contraindications: Avoid if have high blood pressure, vertigo, cerebral thrombosis, chronic catarrh, menstruation, or heart disease.
Chakra: sacral, heart

158. Susiravat Prasarita Adho Mukha Vrksasana (hollowed and spread out downward facing tree, "handstand hollow back prep technique")

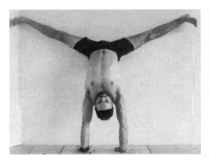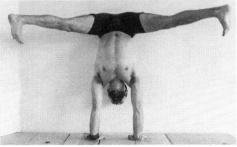

To find the approximate distance to place the hands from the wall, first spread your fingers wide and place the pinky finger at the wall. Then stretch the thumb away from the wall. Mark this space visually and place the tips of the fingers this distance away from the wall. Jump or kick up and rest the hips and thighs into the wall. Flex the feet and take the chin to the chest. Extend the chest forward and then bring the feet off the wall by inner rotating the thighs. After holding the pose with the chin to the chest, push the hips into the wall and take the legs away. Then press the head up towards the wall and take the hips away. From here, release tension in the neck to find balance without the wall.

Benefits: Builds strength in the arms and upper back. It tones the abdominals and inner thighs. It opens the chest and expands the lungs.
Contraindications: Avoid with wrist injury. Avoid during menstruation or pregnancy second trimester.
Modification: Place the hands in fists or ridgetop to avoid aggravating the wrist if injured to build more strength in the pose.
Chakra: heart, throat

159. Eka Hasta Adho Mukha Vrksasana (one arm handstand)

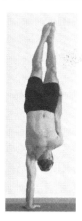

From handstand, shift the weight into one hand and bring the other hand into fingertips or ridgetop position, and then reach the elevated hand up beside the hip. Squeeze the legs into the midline to stabilize the balance. Alternatively, before kicking up, set one hand flat, and the other hand in fingertips position. Then kick up with the leg of the elevated hand leading the way. This will shift the weight into the flat hand. When the balance is held with one hand in fingertips, then lift it off of the floor.

Benefits: This pose develops strength in the hands and arms. It improves balance and concentration. It develops confidence, courage, and vitality.

Contraindications: Avoid until *adho mukha vrksasana* position can be held for 30 seconds without a wall. Avoid if have high blood pressure, vertigo, cerebral thrombosis, chronic catarrh, menstruation, or heart disease.

Modification: Use a wall to help stabilize.

Chakra: sacral, heart

160. Eka Pada Vrischikasana II (one foot scorpion II prep)

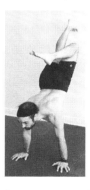

Start from handstand prep at the wall. Lift one leg up toward the ceiling, and then bend the knee and point the foot to the back of the head. Curl the chest forward and push the head up. Hold for a couple breaths and then switch legs.

Benefits: Builds strength in the arms, neck, and upper back. Prepares the spine for backbends.

Contraindications: Avoid with wrist injury. Avoid during menstruation or pregnancy second trimester.

Modification: Place the hands in fists or ridgetop to avoid aggravating the wrist if injured or to build more strength in the pose.

Chakra: heart, throat

161. Tarakasana or Eka Pada Vrischikasana II (demon Taraka's pose or one foot scorpion II)

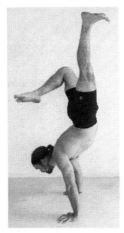

From handstand, bend one leg toward the head, and push the head up. Move the heart forward and down. Keep the other leg extending straight up. From here, work on lowering into *eka pada Koundinyasana II* or *Ashtavakrasana* with the straight leg coming over the arm as you lower down.

Benefits: This pose develops strength in the hands, arms, and back. It improves balance and concentration. It develops confidence, courage, and vitality.
Contraindications: Avoid until *adho mukha vrksasana* position can be held for 30 seconds without a wall. Avoid if have high blood pressure, vertigo, cerebral thrombosis, chronic catarrh, menstruation, or heart disease.
Modification: Use a wall to help stabilize.
Chakra: heart, brow

162. Vrischikasana II (scorpion pose II)

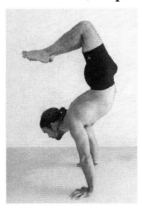

From handstand, bend both legs toward the head and scoop the tailbone up. Push the head up and curl in the upper back.

Benefits: This pose develops strength in the hands, arms, and back. It improves balance and concentration. It develops confidence, courage, and vitality.
Contraindications: Avoid until *adho mukha vrksasana* position can be held for 30 seconds without a wall. Avoid if have high blood pressure, vertigo, cerebral thrombosis, chronic catarrh, menstruation, or heart disease.
Modification: Use a wall to help stabilize.
Chakra: heart, brow

163. Murugan Vinyasa (hero transition, "Superman walkouts")

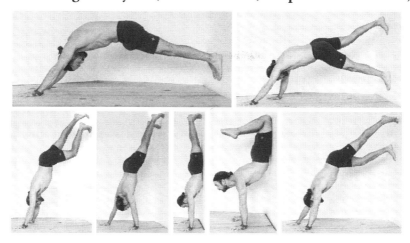

Start from handstand prep position and then walk the hands forward to the front of the mat. The hands are extended in front of the shoulders in an extended plank position. Bring the feet a few inches off the floor and push them into the wall to hold the form. Lift the abdomen and squeeze the lower ribcage in. Stay here for five breaths and then walk the hands in and the feet up the wall. Keep going until the hips and chest reach the wall or rest the thighs into the wall and curl the chest forward into a scorpion position. From here, walk the hands forward into an extended plank and repeat as many times as possible.

Benefits: Builds strength in the hands, arms, abdomen, and upper back. Develops concentration and focus. Increases confidence and vigor. It is beneficial training for all inversions.
Contraindications: Avoid with wrist injury. Avoid during menstruation or pregnancy second trimester.
Modification: Place the hands in fists or ridgetop to avoid aggravating the wrist if injured or to build more strength in the pose.
Chakra: solar plexus, heart

164. Salamba Sarvangasana I (supported shoulder stand pose I)

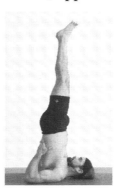

Start from lying flat on the back. Kick the legs overhead and support the hips with the hands holding the lower back. Bring the shoulder blades closer together and push the arms and head down into the floor, so the cervical vertebrae lift up. There should not be any vertebrae touching the floor. If a teacher cannot pass fingers under the neck and between the shoulder blades simultaneously, then a blanket should be used to protect C6 and C7. The shoulders and arms are placed on the blanket with the head on the floor.

Benefits: Creates strength in the upper back, shoulders, and neck. It tones the legs, abdomen, and reproductive organs. Stimulates the thymus, thyroid, and parathyroid endocrine glands. It boosts the immune system and detoxes the body if held for 20 minutes. It relieves mental and emotional stress. It is beneficial for releasing fears, headaches, insomnia, and hypertension. It helps treat asthma, diabetes, colitis, thyroid disorders, impotence, prolapse, menopause, and menstrual disorders. All of the following shoulder stand positions have these benefits.

Contraindications: Avoid if have a neck injury. Avoid if have high blood pressure, vertigo, cerebral thrombosis, chronic catarrh, menstruation, or heart disease. All of the following shoulder stand positions have these contraindications.

Modification: Place blankets under the arms and shoulders with the head hanging off, so the curvature of the neck is enhanced and the vertebrae are off the floor.

Chakra: heart, throat

165. Salamba Sarvangasana II (supported shoulder stand pose II)

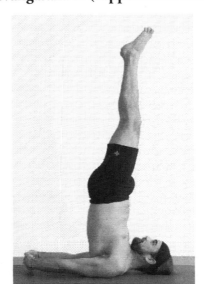

From *salamba sarvangasana,* extend the arms straight and clasp hands. Squeeze the arms together and push them down into the floor.

Benefits: This shoulder stand variation builds more strength in the arms and abdominal muscles. It opens the chest and stretches the shoulders.

Contraindications: Avoid if the neck becomes flat and the cervical vertebrae touch the floor.

Modification: Use a strap between the hands.

Chakra: heart, throat

166. Nirlamba Sarvangasana (unsupported shoulder stand pose)

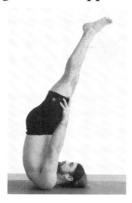

From *salamba sarvangasana,* let the feet come over the head then reach the hands up for the thighs. Keep the head actively pushing back so the neck does not flatten. The shoulder blades push down strong to keep the neck vertebrae off of the floor.

Benefits: This shoulder stand variation builds more strength in the neck and abdominal muscles. It improves balance and concentration.
Contraindications: Avoid if the neck becomes flat and the cervical vertebrae touch the floor.
Modification: Place blankets under the arms and shoulders with the head hanging off, so the curvature of the neck is enhanced and the vertebrae are off the floor.
***Chakra*:** heart, throat

167. Urdhva Padma Sarvangasana (upward lotus shoulder stand pose)

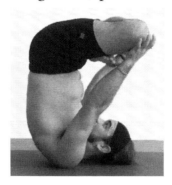

From *salamba sarvangasana,* kick the legs into lotus position or reach up and use one hand to bring the legs into position. Lower the knees onto the hands and push the hands up into the knees. Push the head and shoulders push down into the floor to lift the cervical vertebrae up.

Benefits: This shoulder stand variation builds more strength in the neck and opens the hips. It improves balance and concentration.
Contraindications: Avoid if the neck becomes flat and the cervical vertebrae touch the floor. Avoid until lotus position can be held for one minute sitting. Avoid if the medial collateral ligament of the knee is injured.
Modification: Skip lotus position and bring the legs into *baddha konasana* position, and then place the hands on the knees.
***Chakra*:** heart, throat

168. Pindasana (womb pose)

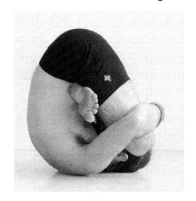

From *urdhva padma sarvangasana,* bring the legs down overhead and clasp hands around the legs. Squeeze the arms into the legs to deepen the opening.

Benefits: This pose tones the spinal nerves. It stretches the upper back and opens the hips. It balances the nervous system.

Contraindications: Avoid if the neck becomes flat and the cervical vertebrae touch the floor. Avoid until lotus position can be held for one minute sitting. Avoid if the medial collateral ligament of the knee is injured.

Modification: Place blankets under the arms and shoulders with the head hanging off, so the curvature of the neck is enhanced and the vertebrae are off the floor.

Chakra: sacral, throat

169. Eka Hasta Parsva Sarvangasana (one hand side shoulder stand pose)

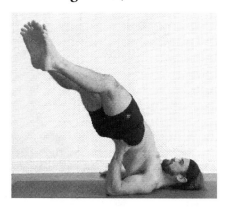

From *salamba sarvangasana,* extend one arm out to the side and twist the hips in the opposite direction. Place the hand of the bent arm on the sacrum, and then the legs slowly move out to the side. Hold the weight of the hips in the hand and descend the legs parallel to the floor.

Benefits: This shoulder stand variation builds strength in the lower abdominals. It relieves lower back stress.

Contraindications: Avoid if the neck becomes flat and the cervical vertebrae touch the floor.

Modification: Place blankets under the arms and shoulders with the head hanging off, so the curvature of the neck is enhanced and the vertebrae are off the floor.

Chakra: sacral, throat

170. Eka Hasta Parsva Padma Sarvangasana (one hand side lotus shoulder stand pose)

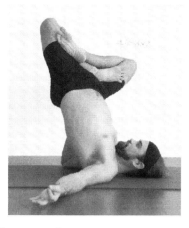

From *salamba sarvangasana,* bring the legs into lotus position. Extend one arm out to the side and twist the hips in the opposite direction. The hand of the bent arm is placed on the sacrum, and then the legs slowly move toward parallel with the floor.

Benefits: This shoulder stand variation builds strength in the lower abdominals and opens the hips. It relieves lower back stress and calms the nervous system.
Contraindications: Avoid if the neck becomes flat and the cervical vertebrae touch the floor.
Modification: Place blankets under the arms and shoulders with the head hanging off, so the curvature of the neck is enhanced and the vertebrae are off the floor.
***Chakra*:** sacral, throat

171. Halasana (plow pose)

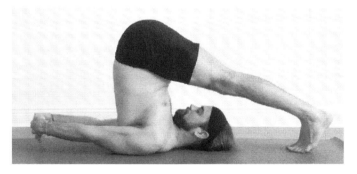

From *sarvangasana,* lower both legs overhead to the floor. Clasp hands behind the back, and then straighten the arms toward the floor.

Benefits: This pose stretches the shoulders and relieves lower back stress. It calms the nervous system, and reduces tension. It stimulates the pancreas, liver, kidneys, thyroid and parathyroid endocrine glands.
Contraindications: Avoid if the neck becomes flat and the cervical vertebrae touch the floor.
Modification: Place blankets under the arms and shoulders with the head hanging off, so the curvature of the neck is enhanced and the vertebrae are off the floor.
***Chakra*:** sacral, throat

172. Supta Urdhva Pada Vajrasana (supine upward foot diamond pose)

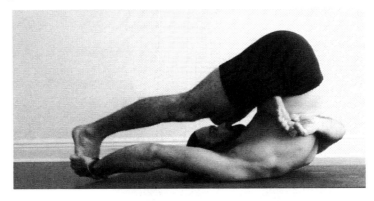

From *ardha badha padma paschimottanasana,* hold onto the bound foot, and roll over backwards on top of the forearm. The straight leg kicks overhead to create momentum. Lift the hips over the shoulders and take the foot to the floor, and then reach for the foot with the free hand. Alternatively, kick the legs overhead first and then reach for the foot behind the back.

Benefits: This pose stretches the shoulders and relieves lower back stress. It calms the nervous system, and reduces tension. It stimulates the pancreas, liver, kidneys, thyroid and parathyroid endocrine glands.
Contraindications: Avoid if the cervical vertebrae touch the floor or if have a neck injury.
Modification: Place blankets under the arms and shoulders with the head hanging off, so the vertebrae are off the floor. Use a strap to hold the foot.
Chakra: sacral, throat

173. Karnapidasana (ear pressure pose)

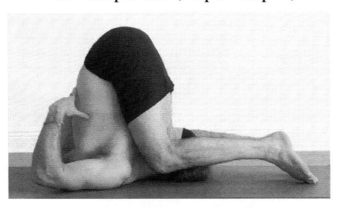

From *halasana,* bend both knees on either side of the head, and lightly pinch the ears. Use the hands to support the lower back.

Benefits: This pose stretches the neck and relieves lower back stress. It calms the nervous system and reduces tension. It stimulates the pancreas, liver, kidneys, thyroid and parathyroid endocrine glands.
Contraindications: Avoid if the cervical vertebrae touch the floor or if have a neck injury. Avoid with spinal conditions.
Modification: Place blankets under the arms and shoulders with the head hanging off, so the cervical vertebrae are off the floor.
Chakra: sacral, throat

174. Parsva Karnapidasana (side ear pressure pose)

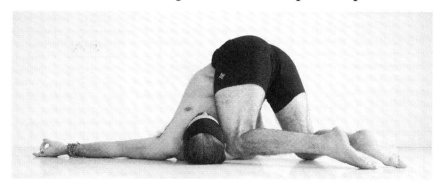

From *karnapidasana,* take the opposite knee to the opposite ear. Support the hip with one hand, and extend the other arm straight to the side. Keep both shoulders flat, and work on taking both knees down to the floor.

Benefits: This pose stretches the shoulders and relieves lower back stress. It calms the nervous system, and reduces tension. It stimulates the pancreas, liver, kidneys, thyroid and parathyroid endocrine glands.
Contraindications: Avoid if the cervical vertebrae touch the floor or if have a neck injury.
Modification: Place blankets under the shoulders and arms with the head hanging off, so the cervical vertebrae are off the floor.
Chakra: solar plexus, throat

175. Shramanasana (ascetic's pose, "wizard's pose")

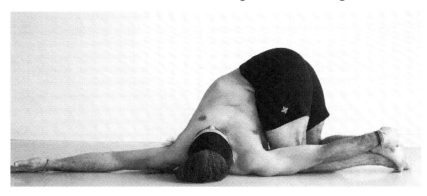

Start from an all-fours position with the hands under the shoulders and knees under the hips. Reach one arm up toward the ceiling and then reach the arm under the other with the shoulder resting on the floor. Bring the opposite knee into the opposite armpit, and then cross the back foot on top of the other. The hand then grabs the ankle of the back leg to stabilize, and the other arm extends straight, so both shoulders and knees are on the ground.

Benefits: This pose stretches the shoulders and relieves lower back stress. It calms the nervous system, and reduces tension. It stimulates the pancreas, liver, kidneys, thyroid and parathyroid endocrine glands.
Contraindications: Avoid if the cervical vertebrae touch the floor or if have a neck injury.
Modification: Keep the knees level with each other and rest the shoulder down.
Chakra: solar plexus, throat

176. Baddha Shramanasana (bound ascetic's pose)

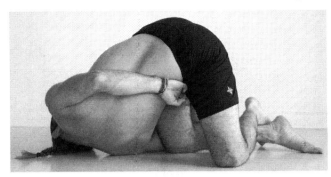

From *shramanasana,* reach the hand that is holding the ankle through the legs, and then reach the other hand behind the back and clasp. Pull against the hands to outer rotate the shoulder and take it to the floor.

Benefits: This pose stretches the shoulders and relieves lower back stress. It calms the nervous system, and reduces tension. It stimulates the pancreas, liver, kidneys, thyroid and parathyroid endocrine glands.
Contraindications: Avoid if the cervical vertebrae touch the floor or if have a neck injury.
Modification: Use a strap to clasp or hold the ankle of the foot on top.
Chakra: solar plexus, throat

177. Viparita Karnapidasana (inverted ear pressure pose)

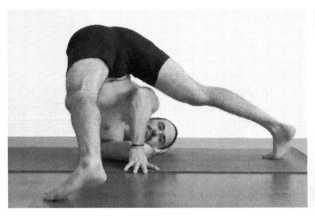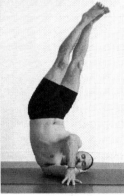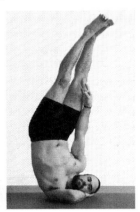

Place one hand on the ear and rest the shoulder down on the floor. The other hand is placed in front of the bent elbow. Lift the hips and turn them down toward the floor. Walk the legs over until the elbow pointing up is in between the legs, then lift the legs up and squeeze them together. When balance is sustained, the free arm reaches up for the legs.

Benefits: This pose strengthens the side body of the latissimus dorsi, intercostals, anterior seratus, and obliques. It develops balance, concentration, and equanimity.
Contraindications: Avoid if have neck injury, high blood pressure, menstruation, or pregnancy.
Modification: Use a partner to assist with the balance.
Chakra: sacral, throat

178. Eka Pada Viparita Karnapidasana (one foot inverted ear pressure pose)

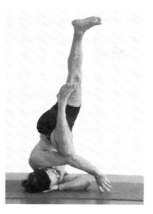

Place one hand on the ear and rest the shoulder down on the floor. The other hand is placed in front of the bent elbow. Lift the hips and turn them down toward the floor. Walk the legs over until the elbow pointing up is in between the legs, and then push the leading knee down into the elevated arm. The trailing leg then lifts straight up toward the ceiling.

Benefits: This pose strengthens the side body of the latissimus dorsi, intercostals, anterior seratus, and obliques. It develops balance, concentration, and equanimity.
Contraindications: Avoid if have neck injury, high blood pressure, menstruation, or pregnancy.
Modification: Use a partner to assist with the balance.
Chakra: sacral, throat

179. Viparita Karnapida Utthita Hasta Padangusthasana (inverted ear pressure extended hand to foot pose)

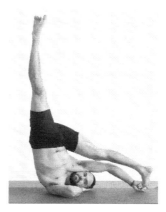

From *eka pada viparita karnapida,* extend the free hand up for the toe of the bent leg, and then extend the leg straight out to the side.

Benefits: This pose strengthens the side body of the latissimus dorsi, intercostals, anterior seratus, and obliques. It opens the hips and lengthens the hamstrings. It develops balance, concentration, and equanimity.
Contraindications: Avoid if have neck injury, high blood pressure, menstruation, or pregnancy.
Modification: Use a partner to assist with the balance.
Chakra: sacral, throat

180. Viparita Karnapida Natarajasana (inverted ear pressure lord of the dance pose)

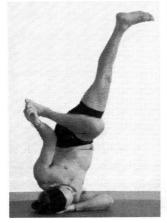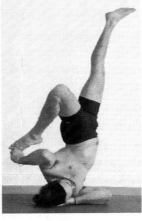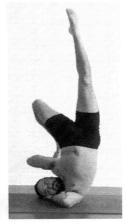

From *viparita karnapida,* bend the same leg as the free arm and grab the inside edge of the foot. Outer rotate the arm, while extending the leg back, and pivot the elbow forward.

Benefits: This pose strengthens the side body of the latissimus dorsi, intercostals, anterior seratus, and obliques. It opens the shoulder and tones the spinal nerves. It develops balance, concentration, and equanimity.
Contraindications: Avoid if have neck injury, high blood pressure, menstruation, or pregnancy.
Modification: Use a strap to hold the foot.
Chakra: heart, throat

181. Viparita Karnapida Urdhva Padmasana (inverted ear pressure lotus pose)

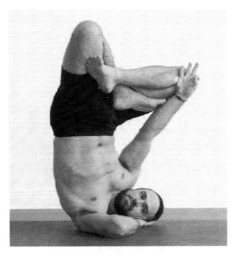

From *viparita karnapida,* kick the legs into lotus, or use the free hand to bring the legs into position. The free hand then extends up in *jnana mudra.*

Benefits: This pose strengthens the side body of the latissimus dorsi, intercostals, anterior seratus, and obliques. It opens the hips and tones the reproductive organs. It develops balance, concentration, and equanimity.
Contraindications: Avoid if have neck injury, high blood pressure, menstruation, or pregnancy.
Chakra: sacral, throat

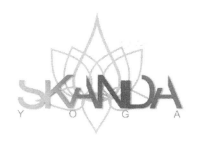

CHAPTER 11

Arm Balances

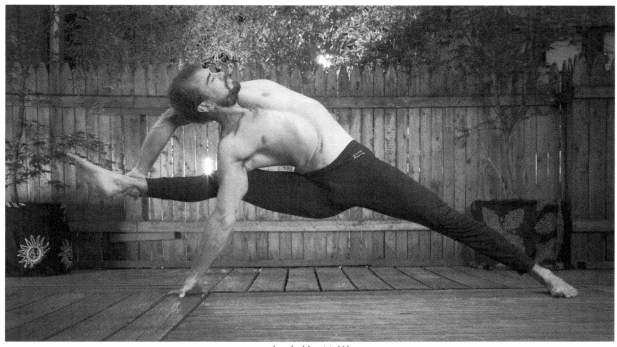

photo by Mauricio Velez

Arm balances are good for building strength and confidence. They require complete focus or you will fall out of the pose. When you achieve an arm balance that you've been working on for a long time, there is an uprising of energy and enthusiasm. In yoga, you want to take the heightened energy off the mat and into the world, so you apply the same determination to other challenges in life. You are capable of more than you can conceive and practicing arm balances is a great way to raise the bar of existence. What is impossible today becomes routine in the future. Remember not to get caught up in striving to attain a pose. Enjoy the process and utilize the energy generated for increasing positivity.

182. Eka Hasta Bhujasana (one hand and arm pose)

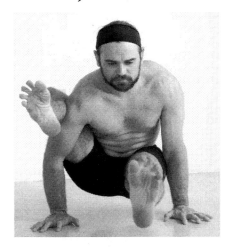

From sitting, bring one leg over one arm. Curl the shoulders back and place the hands in front of the hips. Kick down with the leg that is on top of the arm and then lift the hips. Flex the foot of the straight leg and pull the leg back toward the hip.

Benefits: This pose strengthens the arms and abdominals. It opens the hips and is a good preparation for the following arm balances.
Contraindications: Avoid if have wrist, shoulder, or hip injury.
Modification: Place a block under the hand that doesn't have the leg over the arm, or elevate that hand into ridgetop position.
Chakra: sacral, solar plexus

183. Ashtavakrasana (sage Ashtavakra's pose)

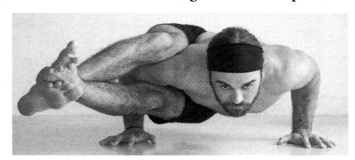

From *eka hasta bhujasana,* bring the ankle of the straight leg on top of the leg that wraps over the arm. Squeeze the legs together, bend both elbows, and bow forward. Push the head up and lift the shoulders away from the floor. Curl in the upper back and melt the heart down.

Benefits: This pose strengthens the arms, wrists, and abdominals.
Contraindications: Avoid if have wrist, elbow, or shoulder injury.
Modification: Place a block under the hand that doesn't have the leg over the arm, or elevate that hand into ridgetop position.
Chakra: sacral, heart

184. Ashtavakrasana (sage Ashtavakra's pose with elevated hands)

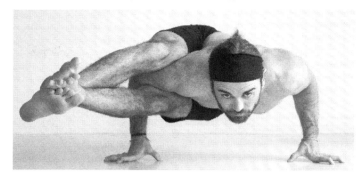

Elevate the hands into ridgetop, or fingertips position, and perform *Ashtavakrasana*.

Benefits: This pose variation creates strength in the hands, arms, and abdominals. It develops balance and concentration.
Contraindications: Avoid if have elbow or shoulder injury.
Modification: Place the hands in fist or fingertip position.
Chakra: sacral, heart

185. Bakasana (crane pose)

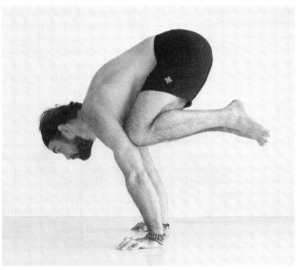

Squat down and place the hands in narrow or wide position under the shoulders and the knees on the outside of the upper arms. Squeeze the legs into the arms, lean forward, and lift the feet with *pada bandha*. Push down through the hands and round the lower back. Slide the legs up the arms until they reach the armpits and the arms are straight.

Benefits: This pose variation creates strength in the hands, arms, and abdominals. It develops balance and concentration.
Contraindications: Avoid if have elbow or shoulder injury.
Modification: This pose can be practiced with the feet on a block. Lean forward and place weight into the hands, and then lift one foot at a time off the block.
Chakra: sacral, heart

186. Bakasana (crane pose with elevated hands)

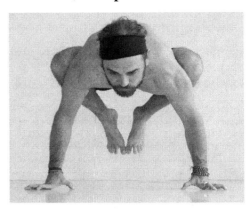

Place the hands in ridgetop position and set the knees over the upper arms. Lean forward, squeeze into the midline, and lift up. Work the thumbs in flexion to stabilize the balance.

Benefits: This pose variation creates strength in the hands, arms, and abdominals. It develops balance and concentration.
Contraindications: Avoid if have elbow or shoulder injury.
Modification: Place the hands in fist or fingertip position.
Chakra: sacral, heart

187. Musti Bakasana (crane pose with fists)

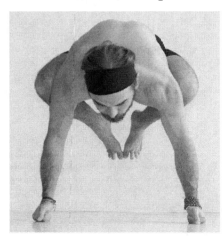

Place the hands into fist position, and the knees over the upper arms. Lean forward, squeeze into the midline, and lift up. The weight should be on the outer three knuckles. If the weight shifts forward, then push the tip of the thumb into the floor to shift the weight to the back of the hand.

Benefits: This pose variation creates strength in the hands, arms, and abdominals. It develops balance and concentration.
Contraindications: Avoid if have elbow or shoulder injury.
Modification: Place a block under the feet as preparation to strengthen the hands.
Chakra: sacral, heart

188. Ardha Bakasana (half crane pose)

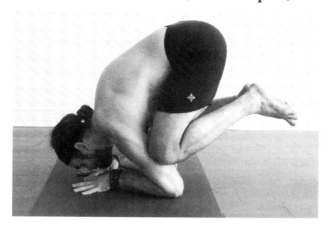

Squat down and place the elbows on the mat under the shoulders. Turn the palms face up and place the back of the forearms on the mat parallel with each other and then turn the palms down. Place the knees on the outside of the arms. Lean forward and squeeze the legs strongly into the arms to lift the feet.

Benefits: This pose variation creates strength in the shoulders, upper back, and inner thighs.
Contraindications: Avoid if have elbow or shoulder injury.
Chakra: root, heart

189. Eka Pada Bakasana I (one foot crane pose I)

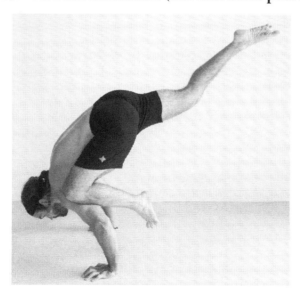

From *bakasana,* push one leg into the arm and kick the foot toward the midline. Extend one leg behind you, squeeze it into the midline, and then lift it higher.

Benefits: This pose variation creates strength in the hands, arms, inner thighs, and abdominals.
Contraindications: Avoid if have elbow or shoulder injury.
Chakra: sacral, heart

223

190. Eka Pada Bakasana II (elevated one foot crane pose II)

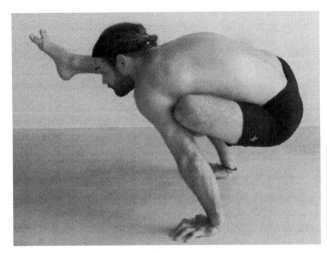

From *bakasana,* push one leg into the arm and kick the foot in toward the midline. Extend the other leg in front and squeeze it into the arm.

Benefits: This pose variation creates strength in the hands, arms, inner thighs, and abdominals.
Contraindications: Avoid if have elbow or shoulder injury.
Chakra: sacral, heart

191. Parsva Bakasana (side crane pose)

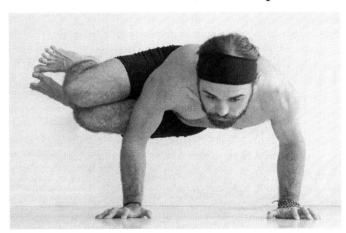

Squat down and twist to the opposite side of one thigh. Hook the elbow on the outside the knee and place the hands in front of you under the shoulders. Lean forward and lift the bottom foot first and then the top foot. It is acceptable for beginners to practice the pose with both elbows on the thigh for more support.

Benefits: This pose variation creates strength in the hands, arms, inner thighs, and abdominals. It tones the internal organs and improves digestion.
Contraindications: Avoid if have elbow or shoulder injury.
Modification: Use a block under the feet and the support of both elbows.
Chakra: solar plexus, heart

192. Musti Parsva Bakasana (side crane pose with fists)

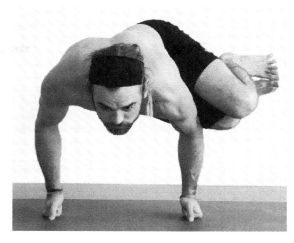

Set the hands into fist position with the thumb in flexion, and perform side crow pose.

Benefits: This pose variation creates strength in the hands, arms, inner thighs, and abdominals. It tones the internal organs and improves digestion.

Contraindications: Avoid if have elbow or shoulder injury. Avoid until can hold *musti bakasana* for 30 seconds.

Chakra: solar plexus, heart

193. Visama Parsva Bakasana I (uneven side crane pose I)

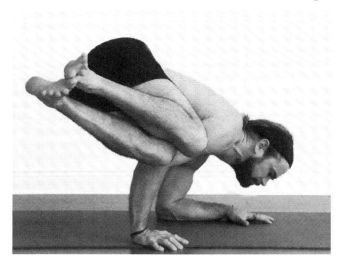

From *parsva bakasana,* lean forward and lower one forearm to the ground. Push down through the forearm and lift the shoulder away from the wrist. This pose can also be entered from *visama pincha mayurasana.*

Benefits: This pose variation creates strength in the hands, arms, inner thighs, and abdominals. It tones the internal organs and improves digestion.

Contraindications: Avoid if have elbow or shoulder injury.

Chakra: solar plexus, heart

194. Visama Parsva Bakasana II (uneven side crane pose II)

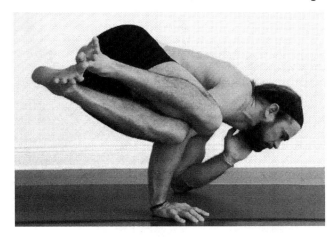

From *visama parsva bakasana,* lift the hand to the chin and rest.

Benefits: This pose variation creates strength in the hands, arms, inner thighs, and abdominals. It tones the internal organs and improves digestion. It develops balance and concentration.

Contraindications: Avoid if have elbow or shoulder injury.

Chakra: solar plexus, heart

195. Trianga Dandasana (three limbed staff pose)

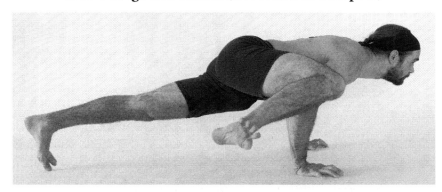

Bring the knee to the outside of the arm and lean forward to come onto the tip of the big toe. Bend the elbows and lower half way down. Keep both shoulders level and parallel with the creases of the elbows.

Benefits: This pose variation creates strength in the hands, arms, and shoulders. It prepares the body for the sage Koundinya series and is a *vinyasa* transition.

Contraindications: Avoid if have elbow or shoulder injury.

Chakra: solar plexus, heart

196. Parashuramasana (eternal warrior pose)

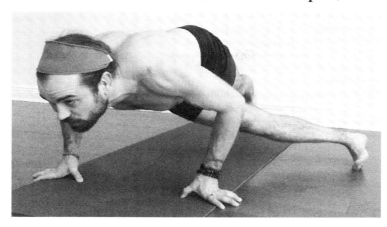

From a plank position, cross one leg in front of the other. Press down through the pinky toe so the heel lifts off of the floor. Lean forward and twist the inner body away from the extending leg. Bend the arms and lower halfway down to bring the shoulders level with the elbows.

Benefits: This pose variation creates strength in the hands, arms, and shoulders. It prepares the body for the sage Koundinya series and is a *vinyasa* transition.

Contraindications: Avoid if have elbow or shoulder injury.

Chakra: solar plexus, heart

197. Dwi Pada Koundinyasana (two foot sage Koundinya pose)

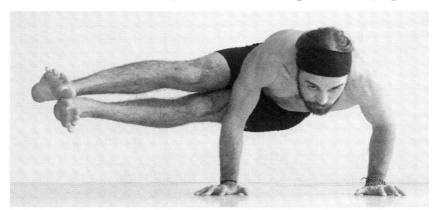

From *parsva bakasana,* extend both legs straight and then flex the toes back toward the face.

Benefits: This pose variation creates strength in the hands, arms, inner thighs, and abdominals. It tones the internal organs and improves digestion. It develops balance and concentration.

Contraindications: Avoid if have elbow or shoulder injury.

Chakra: solar plexus, heart

198. Eka Pada Koundinyasana I (one foot sage Koundinya pose I)

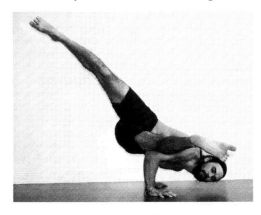

From *dwi pada Koundinyasana,* lift the top leg and take it back. Maintain an inner rotation of the top leg as it lifts.

Benefits: This pose variation creates strength in the hands, arms, inner thighs, and abdominals. It tones the internal organs and improves digestion. It develops balance and concentration.
Contraindications: Avoid if have elbow or shoulder injury.
Modification: Place a block on the floor for the head to rest on, and use the support of both elbows.
Chakra: solar plexus, heart

199. Eka Pada Koundinyasana II (one foot sage Koundinya pose II)

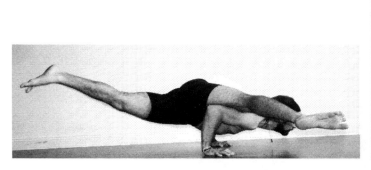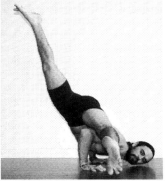

Assume *eka pada Koundinyasana I* position and look toward the foot to shift the weight forward. Bend the top leg and place it over the bottom leg. Slide the bottom leg out and extend it straight behind you. To deepen the pose, inner rotate the forward leg, point the big toe down, and lift the back leg higher.

It is acceptable for beginners to initially use both elbows for support in the *Koundinya* series, but once the strength and stability is achieved, then only one elbow should be used.

Benefits: This pose variation creates strength in the hands, arms, inner thighs, and abdominals. It tones the internal organs and improves digestion. It develops balance and concentration.
Contraindications: Avoid if have elbow or shoulder injury.
Modification: Use the support of both elbows.
Chakra: sacral, heart

200. Eka Pada Koundinyasana (one foot sage Koundinya pose variation, "hummingbird")

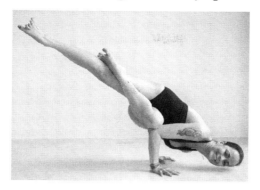

The pose is performed like *eka pada Koundinyasana I* position, except that the bottom leg is bent with the foot on the outside of the lifting leg. Start by stepping one foot into a lunge position and rest the back knee on the floor. Twist and take both arms across to the outside of the thigh. Lean forward onto the hands and lift up. Figure-four the legs, bringing the bottom ankle on top of the lifting leg.

Benefits: This pose variation creates strength in the hands, arms, and abdominals. It tones the internal organs and improves digestion. It develops balance and concentration.
Contraindications: Avoid if have elbow or shoulder injury.
Modification: Place a block under the side of the head.
Chakra: solar plexus, heart

201. Urdhva Navasana (upward boat pose)

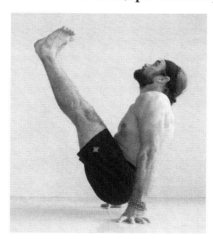

Place the hands beside the hips and curl the shoulders onto the back body. Lift the hips off the floor, lean back, and lift the legs toward the ceiling. Flex the feet and engage the thighs to lengthen out of the hips.

Benefits: This pose creates strength in the arms, abdominals, and hip flexors. It tones the internal organs and improves digestion.
Contraindications: Avoid if have shoulder injury.
Modification: Place blocks under the hands to help initiate lift.
Chakra: sacral, solar plexus

202. Urdhva Ardha Padma Navasana (upward half lotus boat pose)

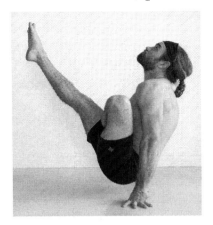

Bring one foot on top of the opposite thigh in half lotus position. Place the hands beside the hips and curl the shoulders onto the back body. Lift up, lean back, and extend the leg as high as possible. Hold the pose for five breaths or use it as a transition into a *vinyasa*.

Benefits: This pose creates strength in the arms, abdominals, and hip flexors. It tones the internal organs and improves digestion.
Contraindications: Avoid if have shoulder injury.
Modification: Place blocks under the hands to help initiate lift.
Chakra: sacral, solar plexus

203. Brahmacharyasana (celibacy pose)

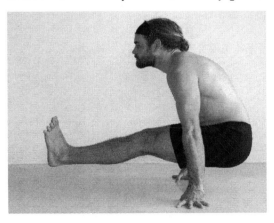

Place the hands beside the hips and curl the shoulders back. Lift the hips and the legs parallel with the floor. Flex the feet and lean the hips back.

Benefits: This pose creates strength in the arms, abdominals, and hip flexors. It tones the internal organs and improves digestion. It develops self-control.
Contraindications: Avoid if have shoulder injury.
Modification: Place blocks under the hands to help initiate lift.
Chakra: sacral, solar plexus

204. Uttana Konasana (intense angle pose)

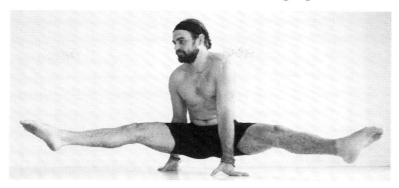

Extend the legs wide from sitting and place one hand to the outside of a hip and the other hand between the legs. Outer rotate the arms and curl the shoulders back. Lift the hips and legs parallel with the floor. Point the feet and extend energy from the hips out through the legs.

Benefits: This pose creates strength in the arms, abdominals, and hip flexors. It tones the internal organs and improves digestion. It develops self-control.
Contraindications: Avoid if have shoulder injury.
Modification: Place blocks under the hands to help initiate lift.
Chakra: sacral, solar plexus

205. Lolasana (pendant pose)

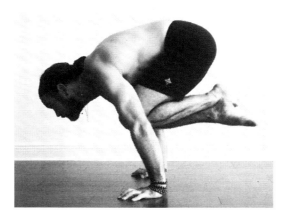

This pose can be held statically or used as a transition in *vinyasa* from seated poses into *chaturanga dandasana*. Start from sitting with the ankles crossed under the hips. Place the hands beside the knees and curl the shoulders back. Press down through the hands and lift the legs to the chest. Stay here for five breaths or kick the legs back into *chaturanga dandasana*.

Benefits: This pose creates strength in the arms, abdominals, and hip flexors. It tones the internal organs and improves digestion. It develops self-control.
Contraindications: Avoid if have shoulder injury.
Modification: Place blocks under the hands to help initiate lift.
Chakra: sacral, solar plexus

206. Galavasana (sage Galava's pose)

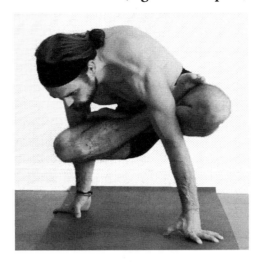

Bring the legs into lotus position. Place one hand between the legs and the other hand outside the hip. Lift up and slide the legs up the arm that is in the center.

Benefits: This pose creates strength in the arms, abdominals, and hip flexors. It tones the internal organs and reproductive organs.

Contraindications: Avoid if have shoulder injury.

Chakra: sacral, heart

207. Musti Galavasana (sage Galava's pose with fists)

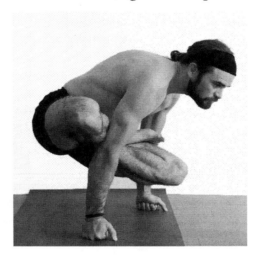

Bring the legs into lotus position. Place the hands in fist position with one between the legs and the other beside the outer hip. Lift the legs and hook them over the elbow.

Benefits: This pose creates strength in the hands, arms, abdominals, and hip flexors. It tones the internal organs and reproductive organs.

Contraindications: Avoid if have shoulder injury.

Chakra: sacral, heart

208. Eka Pada Galavasana (one foot sage Galava's pose)

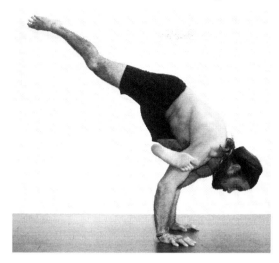

This pose can be entered from squatting or tripod headstand. Place the top of the shin in one armpit and the foot in the opposite armpit. Flex the foot to lock the leg in place. Kick the leg into the arms and lift the back leg up by squeezing it into the center.

Benefits: This pose creates strength in the arms and abdominals. It tones the internal organs and opens the hips.
Contraindications: Avoid if have shoulder injury.
Modification: Place the back foot on a block and tap with the big toe to develop strength to lift up.
Chakra: sacral, heart

209. Eka Pada Galavasana II (one foot sage Galava's pose II)

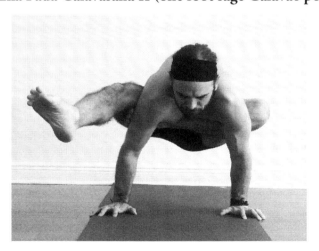

From *eka pada Galavasana I* position, bring the top leg forward and hook it over the foot that is in the armpit. Extend the leg straight ahead and squeeze it in toward the center.

Benefits: This pose creates strength in the arms and opens the hips. It improves balance and concentration.
Contraindications: Avoid if have shoulder injury.
Chakra: sacral, heart

210. Ardha Bhujapidasana (half arm pressure pose)

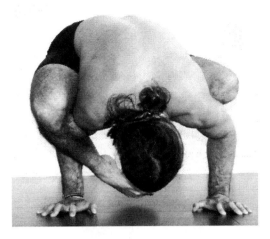

From *eka pada Galavasana II,* bend the leg and point the foot down toward the floor between the hands. Bow forward toward the foot and hold for five breaths.

Benefits: This pose creates strength in the arms and abdominals. It improves balance and concentration.
Contraindications: Avoid if have shoulder injury.
Chakra: sacral, brow

211. Bhujapidasana (arm pressure pose)

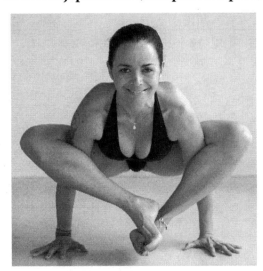

Reach both arms under the legs from squatting or jump the legs over the arms. Sit back on the elbows and hook one foot over the other. Squeeze the legs into the arms, and then bow forward toward the feet.

Benefits: This pose creates strength in the arms and inner thighs.
Contraindications: Avoid if have shoulder or wrist injury.
Modification: Elevate the hands in ridgetop or fist position.
Chakra: sacral, heart

212. Tittibhasana I (insect pose I)

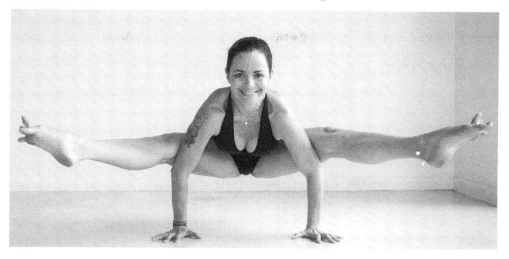

From *bhujapidasana,* extend both legs straight ahead, and then squeeze the legs into the midline.

Benefits: This pose creates strength in the arms and inner thighs.
Contraindications: Avoid if have shoulder or wrist injury.
Modification: Elevate the hands in ridgetop or fist position.
Chakra: sacral, heart

213. Ardha Padma Tittibhasana (half lotus insect pose)

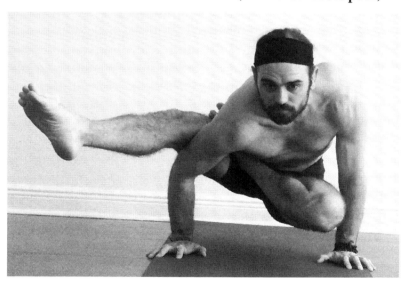

From sitting with one leg in half lotus, lean back and bring the opposite leg over the back of the arm. Then lean forward, place the hands under the shoulders, and lift up. Extend the leg straight and squeeze it in toward the center. Hold for five breaths then kick back into *chaturanga dandasana* and flow through the *vinyasa.*

Benefits: This pose creates strength in the arms, lower abdominals, and hip flexors.
Contraindications: Avoid if have knee injury.
Chakra: sacral, solar plexus

214. Vasisthasana (sage Vasistha's prep pose)

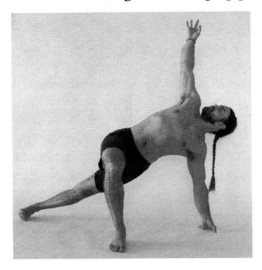

From *adho mukha svanasana,* outer rotate one hand and step one foot halfway up. Point the foot directly out to the side and rock onto the edge of the back foot. Lift the hips, open the heart, and twist.

Benefits: This pose creates strength in the arms.
Contraindications: Avoid if have shoulder or wrist injury.
Modification: Elevate the hand in ridgetop position or perform the pose on the forearm.
Chakra: sacral, heart

215. Vasisthasana (sage Vasistha's pose)

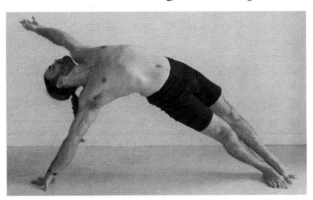

From *adho mukha svanasana,* position the hand for dynamic alignment. Stack one foot on top of the other, lift the hips, and arch the underside of the body. Lean into the back body, open the heart, and take the head back. Place one foot in front of the other to increase stability if needed.

Benefits: This pose creates strength in the arms and tones the lower back and coccyx muscles. Improves balance and concentration.
Contraindications: Avoid if have shoulder or wrist injury.
Modification: Elevate the hand in ridgetop or perform the pose on the forearm.
Chakra: sacral, heart

216. Eka Pada Vasisthasana I (one foot sage Vasistha's pose I)

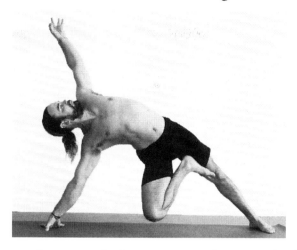

From *Vasisthasana,* lift the bottom foot up and place it against the inner thigh of the top leg. Push the foot into the leg to lift the hip higher and anchor down through the outer edge of the grounding foot.

Benefits: This pose creates strength in the arms and inner thighs.
Contraindications: Avoid if have shoulder or wrist injury.
Modification: Elevate the hand in ridgetop or perform the pose on the forearm.
Chakra: sacral, heart

217. Eka Pada Vasisthasana II (one foot sage Vasistha's pose II)

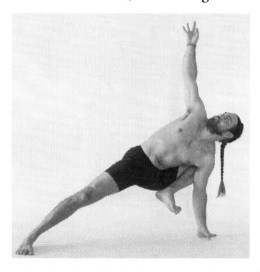

From *trianga dandasana,* pivot onto the hand with the knee trapped over the arm. Turn the back heel down and in and reach the free hand up.

Benefits: This pose creates strength in the arms and inner thighs. It opens the hips and improves balance.
Contraindications: Avoid if have shoulder or wrist injury.
Modification: Hold the foot with the free hand instead of reaching up.
Chakra: sacral, heart

218. Purna Vasisthasana (full sage Vasistha's pose)

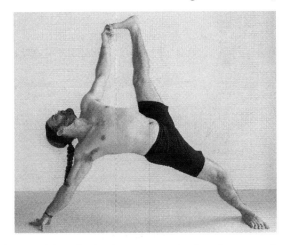

From *Vasisthasana,* lift the top leg and hook the big toe with the first two fingers. Pull the leg and arm bone down, lift the heart up, and then take the head back.

Benefits: This pose creates strength in the arms and legs. It tones the lower back and coccyx muscles. It opens the hips and improves balance.
Contraindications: Avoid if have shoulder or wrist injury.
Modification: Hold the foot with a strap.
Chakra: sacral, heart

219. Camatkarasana (pose of spiritual delight, "wild thing")

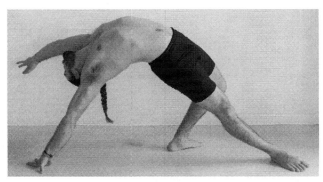

From *Vasisthasana,* step the top foot on the floor behind you with the knee bent and the bottom leg straight. Lift the hips and the heart high, and then curl into a deeper backbend reaching the arm overhead with outer rotation. The pinky finger points toward the floor, not the ceiling, to deepen outer rotation.

Benefits: This pose creates strength in the arms and back. It stretches the abdomen and chest. It opens the hips and improves balance.
Contraindications: Avoid if have shoulder or wrist injury.
Modification: Bend the arm and grab the back of the head to take the pose deeper. Push the head back and curl more in the upper back.
Chakra: sacral, heart

220. Kasyapasana (sage Kasyapa's pose)

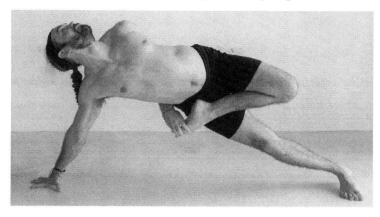

From *Vasisthasana,* bring the top leg into half lotus position. Reach behind the back and grab the foot. The sage Kasyapa was seduced by Maya and fathered the three demons slayed by Skanda.

Benefits: This pose creates strength in the arms. It opens the hips and improves balance. It relieves pain and stiffness in the sacral area.
Contraindications: Avoid if have shoulder or wrist injury.
Modification: Hold the foot with a strap.
Chakra: sacral, heart

221. Kapinjalasana (Chathaka bird prep pose)

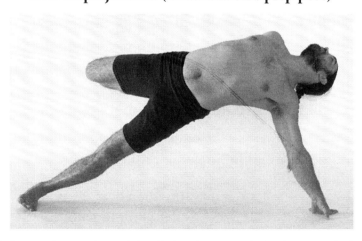

From *Vasisthasana,* bend the top leg and reach back for the top of the foot. Kick the leg back and extend the heart forward. Open the throat and move the head back.

Benefits: This pose creates strength in the arms and back. It opens the front of the hips and improves balance. It relieves pain and stiffness in the sacral area.
Contraindications: Avoid if have shoulder or wrist injury.
Chakra: sacral, heart

222. Kapinjalasana (Chathaka bird pose)

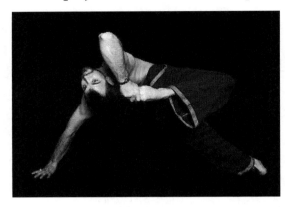

From *Vasisthasana,* bend the top knee and bring it toward the chest. Reach the hand back with the palm face up and grab the outside edge of the foot. Pivot the elbow forward then shift the hand on top of the foot. Kick the leg back and extend the heart forward.

Benefits: This pose creates strength in the arms and back. It opens the front of the hips and improves balance.
Contraindications: Avoid if have shoulder or wrist injury.
Modification: Hold the foot with a strap.
Chakra: sacral, heart

223. Vishvamitrasana (sage Vishvamitra's pose)

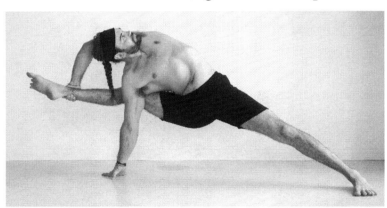

From lunge position, take the back foot flat and reach the arm under the expanding leg. Walk the foot across to the center of the mat until it lifts off of the floor. Grab the big toe, outer edge of the foot, or the outer shin. Bow forward and inner rotate the top of the thigh. Straighten the leg then scoop the tailbone forward. Duck the head under the arm and push it back to deepen the twist. Sage Vishvamitra was the disciple of sage Vasistha.

Benefits: This pose creates strength in the arms and inner thighs. It lengthens the hamstrings and stretches the side body. It improves balance and concentration.
Contraindications: Avoid if have shoulder or wrist injury.
Modification: Hold the foot with a strap.
Chakra: solar plexus, heart

224. Tolasana (scale pose)

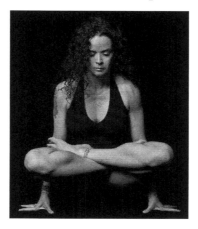

Bring the legs into lotus position and place the hands beside the hips. Outer rotate the arms, curl the shoulders back, and then lift up. Hold the pose with the legs parallel with the floor.

Benefits: This pose creates strength in the arms, abdominals, and hip flexors. It improves balance and concentration. It prepares the body for energy work and meditation.
Contraindications: Avoid if have shoulder or wrist injury.
Chakra: sacral, heart

225. Kukkutasana (rooster pose)

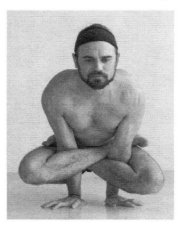

Bring the legs into lotus position and slide the arms through the legs. Bring the hands toward the chin to bring the arms further through and then place them on the floor in front of you. Lean forward and lift up. The rooster is Skanda's other vehicle (*vahana*) next to the peacock. The rooster signals the rising of the new sun, and represents the birth of knowledge and wisdom. Skanda is commonly depicted carrying a flag with the image of a rooster.

Benefits: This pose creates strength in the wrists and arms. It opens the hips, and improves balance and concentration. It tones the reproductive organs.
Contraindications: Avoid if have shoulder or wrist injury.
Chakra: sacral, heart

226. Urdhva Kukkutasana (upward rooster pose)

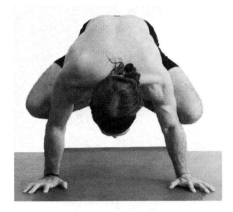

Bring the legs into lotus position and place the hands in front of you. Lean forward, lift the hips, and slide the legs up the arms. Alternatively, from *Galavasana,* swing the bottom knee through the center and hook it on top of the arm. The pose can also be entered from tripod headstand or handstand by hinging at the hips and inner rotating the thighs as you lower down.

Benefits: This pose creates strength in the wrists, arms, abdominals, and hip flexors. It improves balance and concentration. It tones the reproductive organs.

Contraindications: Avoid if have shoulder or wrist injury.

Chakra: sacral, heart

227. Parsva Kukkutasana (side rooster pose)

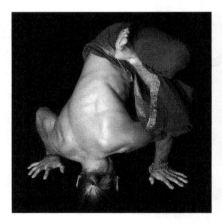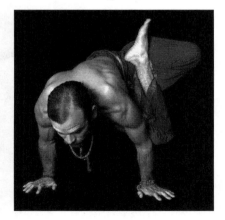

From tripod headstand, bring the legs into lotus position. Lower the legs half of the way down and then twist to hook one knee over the arm. If the left leg is on top in lotus, then twist over the right arm. Roll toward the nose and lift the head.

Benefits: This pose creates strength in the wrists, arms, abdominals, and hip flexors. It improves balance and concentration. It tones the reproductive organs.

Contraindications: Avoid if have shoulder or wrist injury.

Chakra: sacral, solar plexus

228. Hamsasana (swan pose)

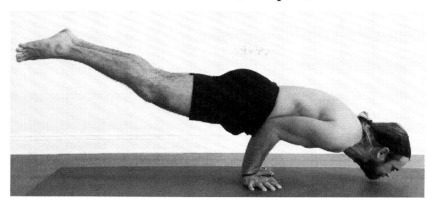

Bring the hands close together with the thumbs a few inches apart, and the fingers angled forward. Hook both elbows on the inside of the iliac crests. Lean forward, lift the head, and then the legs.

Benefits: This pose creates strength in the wrists, arms, and lower back. It improves balance and concentration. It stimulates the pancreas and improves digestion.
Contraindications: Avoid if have shoulder or wrist injury.
Modification: Place the hands on a block.
Chakra: sacral, solar plexus

229. Mayurasana (peacock pose)

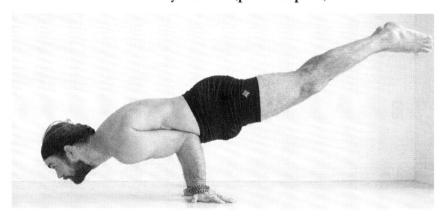

Set the hands close together with the pinky fingers touching and the fingers angled back toward the feet. Bring the elbows toward the navel and rest the head on the floor. Lift the knees and extend the legs straight behind you. Lean forward, lift the head, and then push forward with the toes to lift the legs.

Benefits: This pose creates strength in the wrists, arms, and lower back. It improves balance and concentration. It stimulates the pancreas and improves digestion.
Contraindications: Avoid if have shoulder or wrist injury. Avoid if have high blood pressure, heart condition, hernia, or ulcers.
Modification: Place the hands on a block.
Chakra: sacral, solar plexus

230. Viparita Mayurasana (inverted peacock pose)

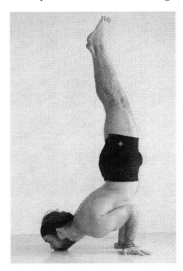

From *mayurasana,* lift the legs straight toward the ceiling and place the chin on the floor.

Benefits: This pose creates strength in the wrists, arms, and lower back. It improves balance and concentration. It stimulates the pancreas and improves digestion.
Contraindications: Avoid if have shoulder or wrist injury. Avoid if have high blood pressure, heart condition, hernia, or ulcers.
Chakra: solar plexus, throat

231. Purna Viparita Mayurasana (full inverted peacock pose)

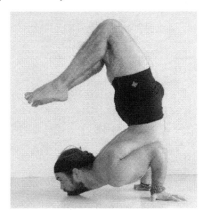

From *viparita mayurasana,* bend both legs and bring the feet toward the head. Release the chest down and stretch the throat forward.

Benefits: This pose creates strength in the wrists, arms, and lower back. It improves balance and concentration. It stimulates the pancreas and improves digestion.
Contraindications: Avoid if have shoulder or wrist injury.
Chakra: solar plexus, throat

232. Musti Padma Mayurasana (fist lotus peacock pose)

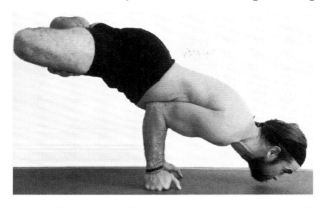

Set the hands into fist position and place them a few inches apart. Bring the elbows toward the navel and rest the head on the floor. Lift the head, and then the knees.

Benefits: This pose creates strength in the wrists, arms, and lower back. It improves balance and concentration. It stimulates the pancreas and improves digestion.
Contraindications: Avoid if have shoulder or wrist injury.
Chakra: solar plexus, throat

233. Viparita Musti Padma Mayurasana (inverted fist lotus peacock pose)

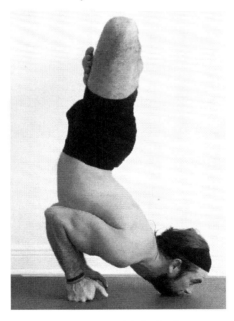

From *musti padma mayurasana,* rest the chin down and lift the knees straight up toward the ceiling.

Benefits: This pose creates strength in the wrists, arms, and lower back. It improves balance and concentration. It stimulates the pancreas and improves digestion.
Contraindications: Avoid if have shoulder or wrist injury.
Chakra: solar plexus, throat

234. Eka Hasta Mayurasana (one hand peacock) or Pungu Mayurasana (wounded peacock)

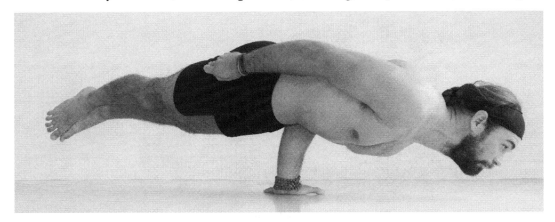

Start with the legs wide and turn one hand out to the side. Lean forward onto the elbow and trap it under the inside of the hip. Place the free hand on fingertips out to the side for support. Lift the legs and squeeze them together. Lift the free hand and bring it beside the hip or reach it straight ahead.

Benefits: This pose creates strength in the wrists, arms, and lower back. It improves balance and concentration. It stimulates the pancreas and improves digestion.

Contraindications: Avoid if have shoulder or wrist injury.

Chakra: sacral, solar plexus

235. Eka Hasta Padma Mayurasana (one hand lotus peacock)

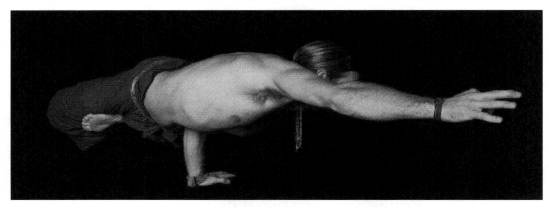

Bring the legs into lotus position and turn one hand out to the side. Lean forward and hook the elbow on the inside of the iliac crest. Lift the legs and then the supporting hand.

Benefits: This pose creates strength in the wrists, arms, and lower back. It improves balance and concentration. It stimulates the pancreas and improves digestion.

Contraindications: Avoid if have shoulder or wrist injury.

Chakra: sacral, solar plexus

236. Chakorasana (moon bird pose)

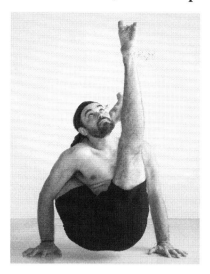

Bring one leg behind the head and place the hands in front of the hips. Push the head up, lift the hips, and extend the straight leg toward the ceiling.

Benefits: This pose creates strength in the arms, abdominals, neck, and lower back. It opens the hips and tones the internal organs.

Contraindications: Avoid if have shoulder or wrist injury. Avoid if have cervical or lumbar herniation.

Chakra: sacral, brow

237. Kala Bhairavasana (destroyer of time pose)

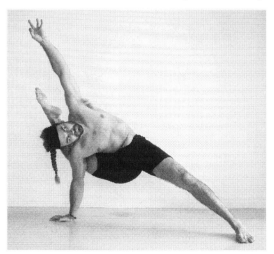

From *chakorasana,* swing the straight leg back through the arms and place the foot on the floor with the heel turned down and in. Pivot onto the arm of the leg behind the head, and lift the other arm toward the ceiling.

Benefits: This pose creates strength in the arms, abdominals, and neck. It opens the hips and tones the internal organs.

Contraindications: Avoid if have shoulder, neck, or wrist injury. Avoid if have cervical or lumbar herniation.

Chakra: sacral, brow

238. Somanathasana (keeper of soma pose)

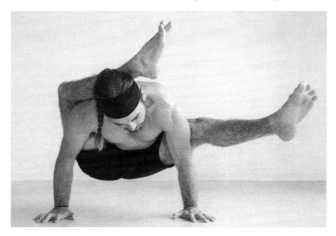

From *kala bhairavasana,* take the top hand to the floor, jump the back leg over the forward arm, and then extend it straight out to the side. From here, return to *chakorasana* or extend the straight leg back and twist into *yoga dandasana II.*

Benefits: This pose creates strength in the arms, abdominals, and neck. It opens the hips, releases lower back tension, and tones the internal organs.
Contraindications: Avoid if have shoulder, neck, or wrist injury. Avoid if have cervical or lumbar herniation.
Chakra: sacral, brow

239. Yoga Dandasana II (yogi's staff pose II)

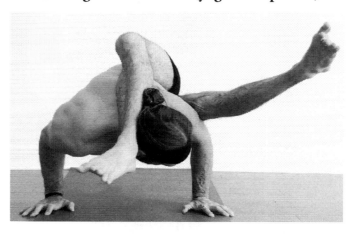

From *chakorasana,* swing the lifting leg back through the arms, and then cross it on top of the opposite arm. Bow forward and extend the leg straight out to the side. The pose can also be entered from *Marichiasana VIII* or *somanathasana.*

Benefits: This pose creates strength in the arms, abdominals, and neck. It opens the hips, releases lower back tension, and tones the internal organs.
Contraindications: Avoid if have shoulder, neck, or wrist injury. Avoid if have cervical or lumbar herniation.
Chakra: solar plexus, brow

240. Dwi Pada Sirsasana II (two feet behind head pose II)

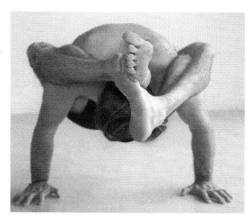

From sitting, bring both legs behind the head and place the hands in front. Push the head up and lift the hips. This pose can also be entered from *somanathasana* by bending the straight leg, crossing ankles, and then ducking the head under.

Benefits: This pose creates strength in the arms, abdominals, and neck. It opens the hips, releases lower back tension, and tones the internal organs.
Contraindications: Avoid if have shoulder, neck, or wrist injury. Avoid if have cervical or lumbar herniation.
Chakra: solar plexus, brow

241. Viranchyasana II (Viranchi's pose II)

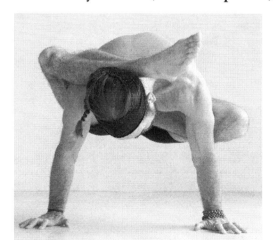

Start from *Viranchyasana I* with one foot in half lotus and the other leg behind the head. Place the hands down and lift the hips up, and then slide the leg in half lotus up the arm. Viranchi or Virancha is another name for Brahma, the creator.

Benefits: This pose creates strength in the arms, abdominals, and neck. It opens the hips, releases lower back tension, and tones the internal organs.
Contraindications: Avoid if have shoulder, neck, or wrist injury. Avoid if have cervical or lumbar herniation.
Chakra: sacral, brow

242. Maksikanagasana I (dragonfly I)

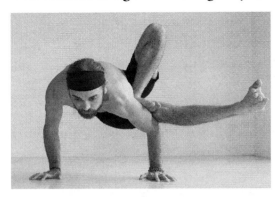

Start with one foot in the armpit from sitting or squatting. Twist and hook the elbow on the outside of the opposite knee. Lean forward, lift the hips, and extend the leg out to the side.

Benefits: This pose creates strength in the arms and abdominals. It opens the hips, releases lower back tension, and tones the internal organs. It improves digestion and stimulates the pancreas.
Contraindications: Avoid if have shoulder, wrist, or knee injury.
Modification: From sitting, rest the forearm on the floor then tilt forward standing up on the opposite arm. Uneven dragonfly (*visama Maksikanagasana*) can be a preparation for the full pose.
Chakra: solar plexus, heart

243. Maksikanagasana II (dragonfly II)

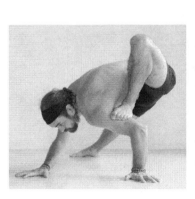 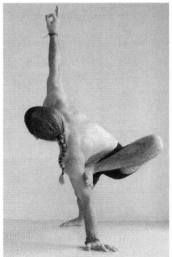

Assume *Maksikanagasana I* position and swing the straight leg back and turn the heel down and in. Twist and extend the free arm up toward the ceiling.

Benefits: This pose creates strength in the arms and abdominals. It opens the hips, releases lower back tension, and tones the internal organs.
Contraindications: Avoid if have shoulder, wrist, or knee injury.
Chakra: sacral, heart

244. Maksikanagasana III (dragonfly III)

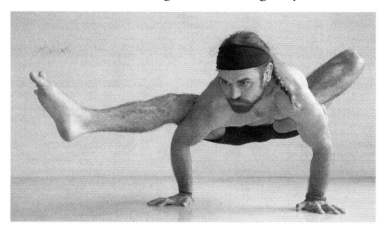

From *Maksikanagasana II,* place the elevated hand down, and then jump or step the back leg over the arm. Lean back and extend the leg out to the side.

Benefits: This pose creates strength in the arms and abdominals. It opens the hips, releases lower back tension, and tones the internal organs.
Contraindications: Avoid if have shoulder, wrist, or knee injury.
Chakra: sacral, heart

245. Maksikanagasana IV (dragonfly IV)

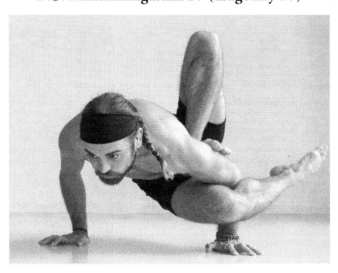

From *Maksikanagasana III,* swing the forward leg back and through the center of the arms. Bend the leg around the arm and point the foot back.

Benefits: This pose creates strength in the arms and abdominals. It opens the hips, releases lower back tension, and tones the internal organs.
Contraindications: Avoid if have shoulder, wrist, or knee injury.
Chakra: sacral, heart

246. Sri Subramanyasana (Subramanya's auspicious pose)

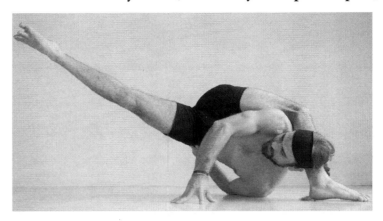

Start from a lunge and hook the head under the expanding leg. Reach the arm through and place the fingertips on the floor, then twist and support the hip with the other hand. Shift your weight forward into the foot that is behind the head and lift the back leg up. Subramanya is another name for Skanda and means that he has knowledge of Brahman, the ultimate reality underlying all phenomena.

Benefits: This pose creates strength in the arms, abdominals, and neck. It opens the hips, releases lower back tension, and tones the internal organs. It improves balance and concentration.

Contraindications: Avoid if have a hamstring injury. Avoid if have cervical or lumbar herniation.

Chakra: brow, crown

247. Valgulasana (bat pose)

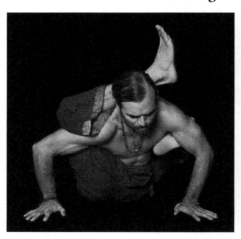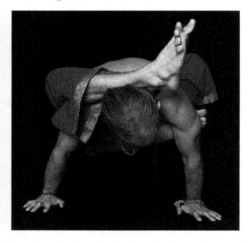

Start with one foot in the armpit and then bring the other foot behind the head. Lean forward and press up. Push the head up strong into the top leg and activate *pada bandha*.

Benefits: This pose creates strength in the arms, abdominals, and neck. It opens the hips, releases lower back tension, and tones the internal organs. It improves balance and concentration.

Contraindications: Avoid if have shoulder, wrist, hip, or knee injury. Avoid if have cervical or lumbar herniation.

Chakra: sacral, brow

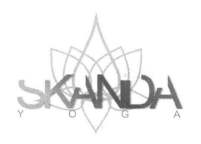

CHAPTER 12

Backbends

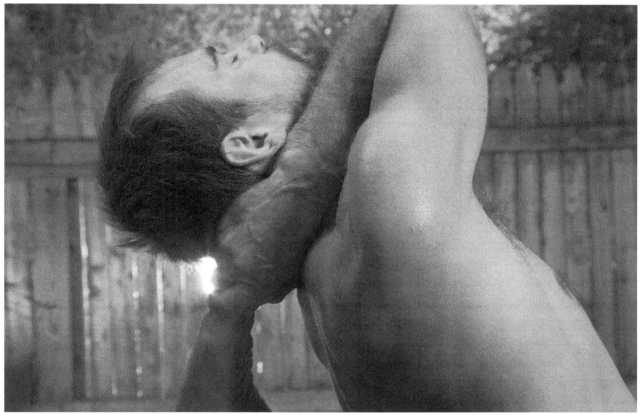

photo by Mauricio Velez

Backbends serve to activate the sympathetic nervous system, which stimulates the body. They open the front body while extending the spine. The cartilage of the vertebrae becomes lubricated and nourished with synovial fluid, which can promote healing and prevent injury. Backbends open the *chakras* and create more awareness the deeper you go. Backbends symbolically represent the unknown because it is impossible to see where we are going or what the potential is, but through practice, the mystery is revealed and the heart is awakened.

248. Sphinx pose

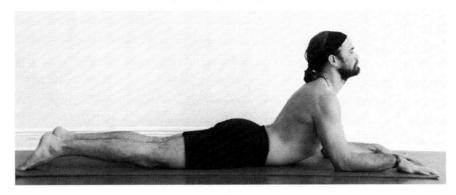

Come to lying flat on the stomach and bring the elbows under the shoulders. Pull the arms back toward the hips to engage the lower back muscles and extend the heart forward. Push the top of the toes down into the mat and pull the toes toward the hips. Scoop the tailbone under and then extend energy from the hips out through the heels.

Benefits: This is the best backbend for all back injuries. It gently extends the spine, and compresses lower back muscles, which releases tension and increases blood flow. When released into *apanavasana,* the muscles and vertebrae are saturated with healing fluids. The pose can be held up to 20 minutes, and during the hold, it is acceptable to rest intermittently. Holding the pose this long 2-3 times a day will slowly bring vertebrae into alignment if you have scoliosis, and relieve pain from disk herniation.
Contraindications: Avoid arching the neck with cervical herniation.
Modification: Place folded blankets under the floating ribs.
Chakra: root, sacral

249. Apanavasana (downward corpse pose)

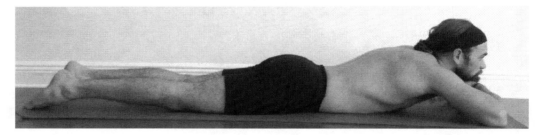

Stack one fist on top of the other, and then rest the chin down. Relax the body fully. The slight arch with the head elevated maintains the blood flow to the back muscles, which allows the muscles to absorb the fluid while relaxed.

Benefits: This is the best rest position when working backbends. It allows the back muscles to relax while they stay warm without dispersing blood by dropping the head. It calms the body and eases the mind.
Modification: Place folded blankets under the floating ribs.
Chakra: root

250. Majarasana (cat pose, "all fours position")

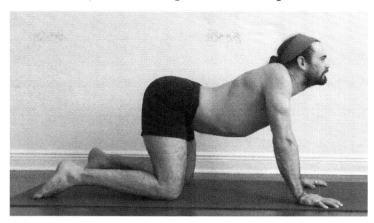

Place the hands slightly in front of the shoulders and the knees under the hips. Push the head up and curl in the upper back. Pull the shoulders down away from the ears and outer rotate the top of the arm bones. It can be held here or used as a transition into another pose. The pose can be used with breath movement to warm the back muscles by rounding the back on exhalation, and arching the back on inhalation.

Benefits: It prepares the body for more backbends.
Modification: Keep the neck neutral with cervical herniation.
Chakra: root

251. Bhujangasana (cobra pose preparation)

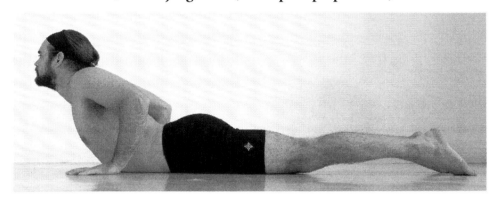

Lie flat down on the belly and bring hands beside the chest with the wrists under the elbows. Press down through the tops of the feet, squeeze the shins into the midline, and then scoop the tailbone under. Lengthen the shoulders toward the ears and then curl them onto the back body. Pull the hands back and extend the heart forward.

Benefits: This pose prepares the body for more backbends. It strengthens upper back integration.
Modification: Place a block between the legs to recruit more strength in the inner thighs.
Chakra: root, sacral

252. Bhujangasana (cobra pose)

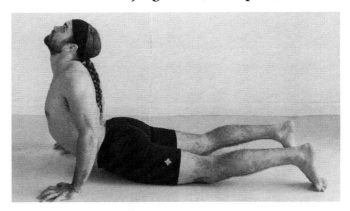

From *bhujangasana* prep, lift up higher by pulling the hands, arms, and shoulders back. Extend the heart forward, slide the palate back, and then push the head back. Keep the arms slightly bent, and the pelvis and thighs on the floor. Spiral the forearms in to root down through the index knuckles, and outer rotate the tops of the arms.

Benefits: This pose tones the spinal region and develops back strength. It opens the heart and lungs while stretching the abdomen. It stimulates the thyroid, kidneys, adrenals, and abdominal organs. It relieves sciatica and helps with stress and fatigue.
Contraindications: Avoid with carpal tunnel syndrome and during pregnancy.
Modification: Place a block between the legs to recruit more strength in the inner thighs.
Chakra: root, sacral

253. Prasarita Bhujangasana (extended wide cobra pose)

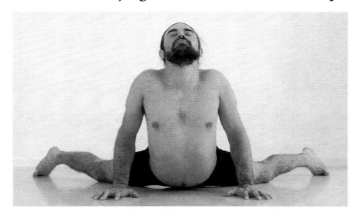

From *bhujangasana* prep, extend the legs out wide to the sides. Point the feet and inner rotate the top of the thighs. Keep the pinky toes pushing down and lengthen the shoulders toward the ears as you lift up higher. When you reach the peak, curl the shoulders back and extend the heart forward.

Benefits: This pose has the same benefits as *bhujangasana* but creates a stretch in the outer hip rotators.
Contraindications: Avoid with carpal tunnel syndrome and during pregnancy.
Chakra: root, sacral

254. Eka Pada Prasarita Bhujangasana (one leg stretched wide cobra pose)

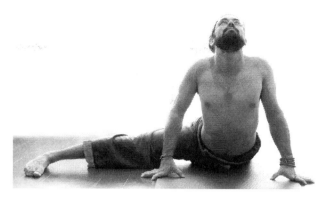

From *bhujangasana* prep, extend one leg directly out to the side with the bottom of the foot flush to the floor. Lengthen the shoulders toward the ears and lift up, as you push down through the extended foot and the back leg. When you reach the peak, curl the shoulders back and extend the heart forward.

Benefits: This pose has the same benefits as *bhujangasana* but creates strength in the ankles and inner thighs.
Contraindications: Avoid with carpal tunnel syndrome and during pregnancy.
Chakra: root, sacral

255. Utthita Eka Pada Prasarita Bhujangasana (extended one leg stretched wide cobra pose)

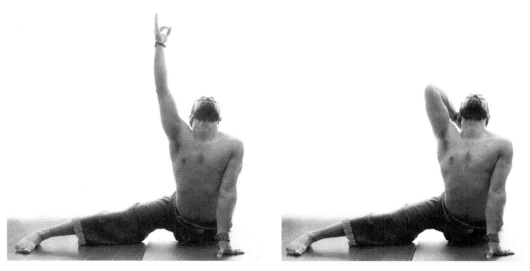

From *prasarita eka pada bhujangasana,* bring one hand under the face and place it in reverse ridgetop position. Outer rotate the arm, micro bend the elbow, and curl the shoulder back. Reach the same arm as the extended leg up toward the ceiling. Bend the arm and place the hand behind the head to take the pose deeper. Push the head back into the hand and curl more in the upper back.

Benefits: This pose has the same benefits as *bhujangasana* but creates strength in the ankles, inner thighs, and arms.
Contraindications: Avoid with carpal tunnel syndrome and during pregnancy.
Chakra: root, sacral

256. Urdhva Mukha Svanasana (upward facing dog)

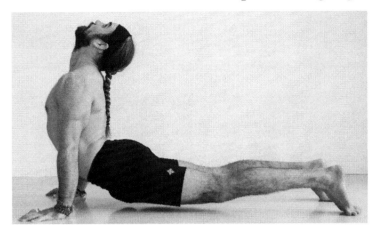

From *chaturanga dandasana,* lift the upper body up as the toes push down into the mat. Scoop the tailbone strong but relax the outer gluteal muscles. Pull the hands toward the feet and the feet toward the hands, as you lift up out of the hips and curl. Keep the arms completely straight, and the pelvis and thighs hovering off of the floor.

Benefits: This pose has the same benefits as *bhujangasana* but creates strength in the legs and arms.
Contraindications: Avoid with carpal tunnel syndrome and during pregnancy.
Modification: Use alternate hand positions.
Chakra: root, sacral

257. Uttana Shishosana (intense birthing pose, "puppy pose")

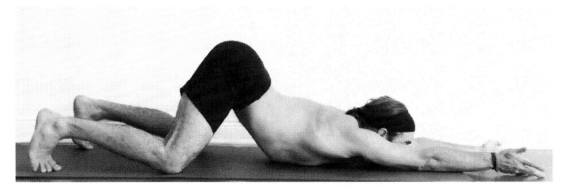

Set the knees just behind the hips and lean forward onto the chin and the chest. Reach the arms straight ahead with the palms facing up to outer rotate the shoulders. Relax in the upper back and let the heart and throat open. Placing palms face up allows the shoulders to safely open without hyperextending.

Benefits: This pose opens the spine and shoulders. It stretches the neck and tones the back muscles.
Contraindications: Avoid with knee injury or if there is too much weight on the chin.
Modification: Slide the knees back a few inches to lower the chest flat.
Chakra: heart, throat

258. Nirakunjasana I (heart opening pose I)

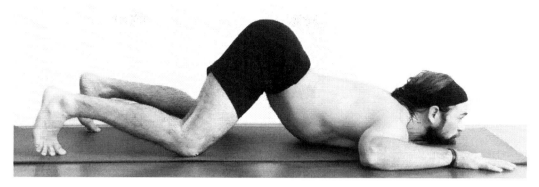

Set the knees just behind the hips and lean forward onto the chin and the chest with the arms bent out to the side and palms placed face-down. Relax in the upper back and let the heart and throat open.

Benefits: This pose opens the spine and shoulders. It stretches the chest and neck. It strengthens the diaphragm.
Contraindications: Avoid with knee injury.
Modification: Slide the knees back a few inches to lower the chest flat.
Chakra: heart, throat

259. Nirakunjasana II (heart opening pose II)

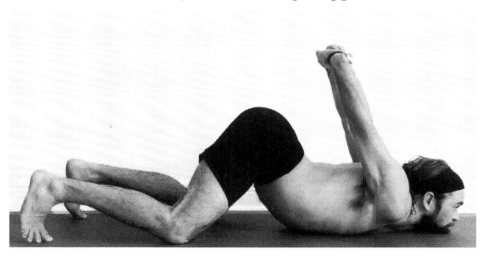

Assume *nirakunjasana I* position and clasp hands together behind the lower back and then extend the arms up. Squeeze the shoulder blades together and lengthen the chin forward to stretch the neck.

Benefits: This pose opens the spine and shoulders. It stretches the chest and neck. It creates strength in the upper back and diaphragm.
Contraindications: Avoid with knee injury.
Modification: Slide the knees back a few inches to lower the chest flat.
Chakra: heart, throat

260. Araniasana (dragon pose)

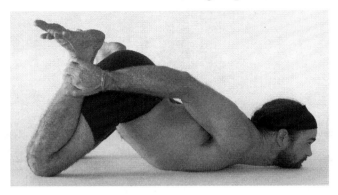

Assume *nirakunjasana I* position and elevate the feet then reach the hands back for the outside of the ankles. Bend the elbows up and squeeze the shoulder blades together. Kick the legs back and the pull forward with the arms. Use the strength recruited to lengthen and extend the spine.

Benefits: This pose opens the spine and shoulders and stretches the chest and neck. It creates strength in the upper back.
Contraindications: Avoid with knee injury.
Modification: Use straps to hold the ankles.
Chakra: heart, throat

261. Ardha Bhekasana (half frog pose)

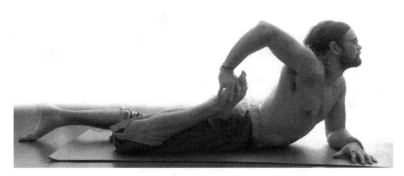

Lie flat on the belly and bring the legs together. Support the chest with the elbow under the shoulder and reach the other arm back for the inside edge of the foot with the thumb and index finger pinching the big toe. Kick back and resist first, then pull the foot in beside the hip, and pivot the hand on top of the foot. Push the foot down toward the floor and flex the toes back into the hand to keep the leg muscles around the knee engaged.

Benefits: This pose opens the spine and tones the back. It stretches the front of the shoulder and the quadriceps muscles. It strengthens the knees and relieves pain from rheumatism and gout.
Contraindications: Avoid with migraines. Avoid with lower back injuries or shoulder injuries.
Modification: If the hand cannot pivot on top of the foot due to shoulder tension, then hook the forearm over the foot.
Chakra: sacral, heart

262. Urdhva Ardha Bhekasana (upward half frog pose)

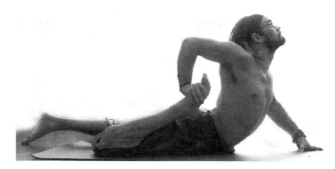

From *ardha bhekasana,* place the hand of the supporting arm at the top of the mat. Lift the upper body up, and keep the supporting arm slightly bent. Pull the stabilizing arm back toward the hip and push the foot down toward the floor. Flex the toes back into the hand to keep the leg muscles around the knee engaged.

Benefits: This pose has the same benefits as *ardha bhekasana* but creates a greater extension of the spine and a deeper stretch for the shoulder.
Contraindications: Avoid with migraines. Avoid with lower back injuries or shoulder injuries.
Modification: If the hand cannot pivot on top of the foot due to shoulder tension, then hook the forearm over the foot.
Chakra: sacral, heart

263. Urdhva Uttana Ardha Bhekasana (upward intense half frog pose)

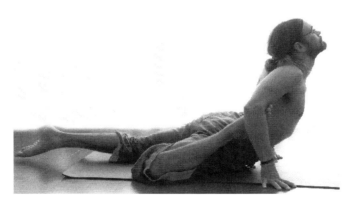

To deepen *urdhva ardha bhekasana,* hook the forearm over the foot and bring the foot into the elbow crease. Place both hands beside the hips and lift higher. Squeeze the elbows in and flex the toes back into the arm to hold the foot in position and to maintain the engagement of leg muscles.

Benefits: This pose has the same benefits as *ardha bhekasana* but creates a greater extension of the spine and a deeper stretch for the quadriceps.
Contraindications: Avoid with migraines. Avoid with lower back injuries or shoulder injuries.
Modification: If the hand cannot pivot on top of the foot due to shoulder tension, then hook the forearm over the foot.
Chakra: sacral, heart

264. Bhekasana (frog pose)

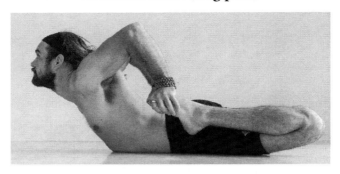

Reach both hands back for the inside of the feet with the thumb and index knuckles pinching the big toes. Pivot the hands on top of the feet while keeping the thumbs on the inside, and then push both feet down. Lift the upper body and extend the heart forward.

Benefits: This pose opens the spine and tones the back. It stretches the front of the shoulder and the quadriceps muscles. It strengthens the knees and relieves pain from rheumatism and gout. It stimulates the pancreas and abdominal organs.
Contraindications: Avoid with migraines. Avoid with lower back injuries or shoulder injuries.
Chakra: sacral, heart

265. Dhanurasana (bow pose)

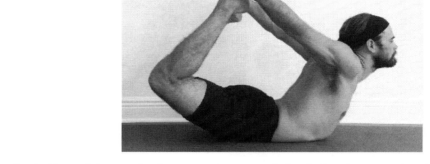

Lie flat on the belly and bring the legs together. Reach back for the outside edges of both feet. Push down through the knees first, lift the hips two inches, and then scoop the tailbone. Push the hips down, kick the legs back, and lift up as high as possible. Kick back more on the inhalation and extend the heart forward on exhalation. This creates a visceral massage and stimulates the pancreas.

Benefits: This pose opens the spine and tones the back. It stimulates the pancreas and massages the abdominal organs, kidneys, and liver. Activates the adrenals and the sympathetic nervous system. Relieves respiratory ailments.
Contraindications: Avoid with high blood pressure, hernia, colitis, or ulcers.
Chakra: sacral, heart

266. Baddha Dhanurasana (bound bow pose)

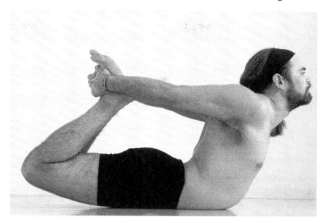

Lie flat on the belly and bring the legs together. Reach back for the outside edges of both feet and clasp hands over the feet. Squeeze the knees together and then scoop the tailbone. Kick the legs back and arch up. Keep the legs squeezing together and extend the heart forward.

Benefits: This pose has the same benefits as *dhanurasana* but creates a stretch for the shoulders and chest.
Contraindications: Avoid with high blood pressure, hernia, colitis, or ulcers.
Chakra: sacral, heart

267. Parsva Dhanurasana (side bow pose)

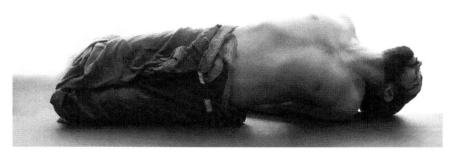

From *dhanurasana*, lift one knee higher and roll to the opposite side. Release the head, neck, jaw, and palate. Gaze up toward the ceiling.

Benefits: This pose tones the back and stretches the abdominals.
Contraindications: Avoid with high blood pressure, hernia, colitis, or ulcers.
Modification: Place a block under the head to keep it neutral if there is discomfort in the neck.
Chakra: sacral, heart

268. Purna Dhanurasana (full bow pose)

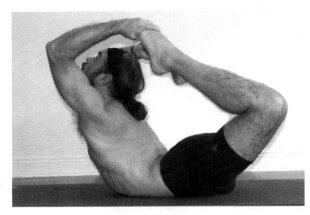

From sphinx pose, reach one hand back for the foot with the palm face-up. Grab the outside edge of the foot, and then grab the other foot the same way. Pivot the elbows forward and overhead, and then shift the hands to the top of the feet. Kick the feet back and lift the arms up. Extend the heart forward and hold the position or rock with the breath to come onto the chin.

Benefits: This pose creates strength in the back body. It stretches in the shoulders, abdominals, and hip flexors. It activates the adrenals and stimulates the sympathetic nervous system.
Contraindications: Avoid with high blood pressure, hernia, colitis, or ulcers.
Modification: Use straps to hold the feet.
Chakra: sacral, heart

269. Eka Pada Dhanurasana (one foot bow pose)

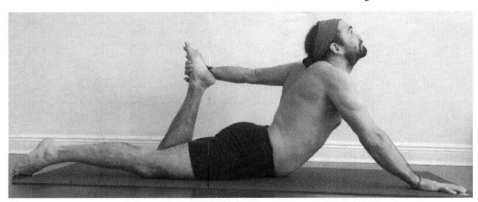

Lie flat on the stomach and bring the legs together. Bend one knee and reach back for the outside edge of the foot. Place the other hand in front of the shoulder and press up. Kick the leg back and straighten the arm. Twist away from the stretch to deepen the opening in the chest and abdomen.

Benefits: This pose strengthens the legs and stretches the chest and shoulders. It tones the back muscles and activates the adrenals.
Contraindications: Avoid with high blood pressure, hernia, colitis, or ulcers.
Chakra: sacral, heart

270. Baddha Eka Pada Dhanurasana (bound one foot bow pose)

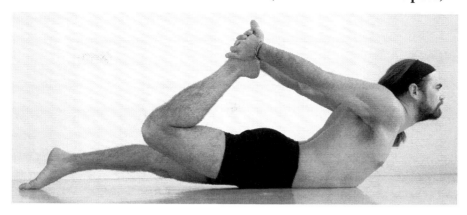

Lie flat on the stomach and bring the legs together. Bend one knee and clasp hands over the foot. Push down through the back foot and kick the bound leg back. Lift the chest and extend the heart forward.

Benefits: This pose strengthens the legs and stretches the chest and shoulders. It tones the back muscles and activates the adrenals.
Contraindications: Avoid with high blood pressure, hernia, colitis, or ulcers.
Chakra: sacral, heart

271. Purna Eka Pada Dhanurasana (full one foot bow pose)

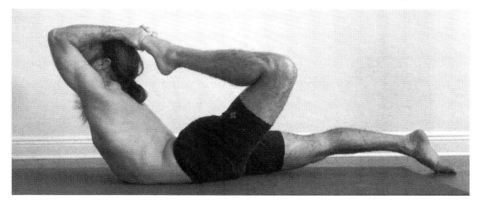

From sphinx pose, reach one hand back palm face-up, and grab the outside edge of the foot. Pivot the elbow forward and shift the hand on top of the foot. Reach the other arm overhead and grab the foot with both hands. Kick the leg up, and then bring it to the back of the head.

Benefits: This pose creates strength in the back body. It stretches in the shoulders, abdominals, and hip flexors. It activates the adrenals and stimulates the sympathetic nervous system.
Contraindications: Avoid with high blood pressure, hernia, colitis, or ulcers.
Modification: Use a strap to hold the foot.
Chakra: sacral, heart

272. Gherandasana (sage Gheranda's prep pose)

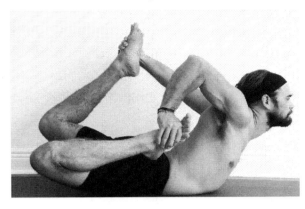

Bring one leg into *ardha bhekasana* and reach the other hand back for the outside of the foot. Push the foot down that is in in half frog position and kick the opposite foot back like in bow pose. Open the chest and extend the heart forward.

Benefits: This pose strengthens the legs and back. It stretches the shoulders and quadriceps. It massages the liver, kidneys, and abdominal organs. Stimulates the pancreas and sympathetic nervous system. Relieves pain in the knee joint from gout or rheumatism.

Contraindications: Avoid with high blood pressure, hernia, colitis, or ulcers.

Chakra: sacral, heart

273. Gherandasana I (sage Gheranda's pose I)

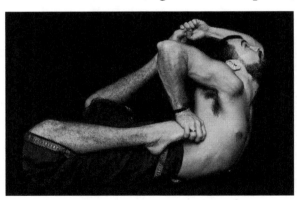

Bring one leg into *ardha bhekasana* and reach the other hand back with palm face up for the outside edge of the foot. Pivot the elbow up and grab the top of the foot. Push the foot in half frog position down and pull the elevated foot to the back of the head.

Benefits: This pose strengthens the back muscles. It stretches the shoulders, hip flexors, and quadriceps. It massages the liver, kidneys, and abdominal organs. Stimulates the pancreas and sympathetic nervous system. Relieves pain in the knee joint from gout or rheumatism.

Contraindications: Avoid with high blood pressure, hernia, colitis, or ulcers.

Modification: Use a strap to hold the foot overhead.

Chakra: sacral, heart

274. Gherandasana II (sage Gheranda's pose II)

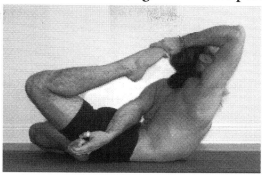

Bring one leg into half lotus position and then lie flat down on top of the leg, so the knee is pointing back behind you. Support the chest in sphinx pose. Reach the same arm as the leg in half lotus back and grab the foot. Reach the free hand back for the outside edge of the opposite foot. Pivot the elbow up and grab the top of the foot with the hand. Push the head up and extend the heart forward.

Benefits: This pose strengthens the back body. It stretches the shoulders, hip flexors, and quadriceps. It massages the liver, kidneys, and abdominal organs. Stimulates the pancreas and sympathetic nervous system. Relieves pain in the knee joint from gout or rheumatism.
Contraindications: Avoid with high blood pressure, hernia, colitis, or ulcers.
Modification: Use a strap to hold the foot overhead.
Chakra: sacral, heart

275. Ushtrasana (camel pose)

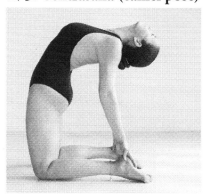

From a kneeling position, bow forward to the heart and widen the sitting bones back and apart. Draw the lower abdomen in and scoop the tailbone under. Lift the ribcage and shoulders up toward the ears, and then curl one arm back at a time placing the palms flat on the heels. Push down through the outside edges of the feet and extend energy forward through the hips and up through the heart. Keep the front of the neck engaged by extending the chin to the chest and then sliding the palate back.

Benefits: This pose strengthens the back muscles. It stretches the hip flexors and abdomen. It opens the heart and improves posture by lengthening the spine. It reduces fatigue, anxiety, menstrual discomfort, and respiratory ailments.
Contraindications: Avoid with high blood pressure or headache. Avoid taking the head back if have cervical herniation.
Modification: Place the feet in flexion with the toes curled under to elevate the heels.
Chakra: sacral, heart

276. Eka Pada Bheka Ushtrasana (one foot frog frog camel pose)

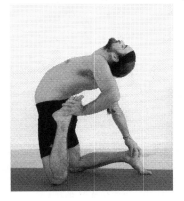

From a kneeling position, lift one foot up and grab the inside edge of the foot. Then pivot the elbow back behind you and shift the hand on top of the foot. Push the foot toward the outer edge of the hip, and then reach the opposite hand back for the foot on the floor. Extend the hips forward and the heart up.

Benefits: This pose strengthens the back muscles. It stretches the hip flexors, quadriceps, and abdomen. It opens the heart and expands the lungs.
Contraindications: Avoid with high blood pressure or headache. Avoid taking the head back if have cervical herniation.
Chakra: sacral, heart

277. Ardha Padma Ushtrasana (half lotus camel pose)

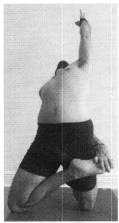

From a kneeling position, place one foot in flexion in front of the opposite knee. Then reach down, point the foot, and slide it up the thigh into half lotus position. Reach behind the back to clasp the foot. Reach the other hand overhead and curl into a backbend over the forearm.

Benefits: This pose opens the hips and the lower back. It stretches the hip flexors and shoulders.
Contraindications: Avoid with high blood pressure, headache, or knee injury. Avoid taking the head back if have cervical herniation.
Modifications: Use a strap to hold the foot. If the hips are tight, then keep the foot on the floor in flexion in front of the knee. One hand reaches back for the heel and the other is placed on the hip.
Chakra: sacral, heart

278. Laghuvajrasana (little thunderbolt pose)

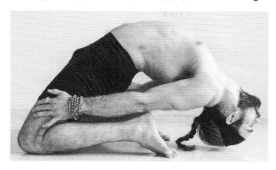

From camel pose, walk the fingers up the calves for the front of the thighs. Pull against the thighs with the fingers and lower the head toward the floor. Hold the pose with the head hovering off of the floor. Lowering the head to the floor with no hands and back up is a "pigeon dropping." The actions are repeated with the breath. Inhale down and exhale up. Pigeon droppings can be performed anytime *laghuvajrasana* appears in the sequencing or as an alternative after *ushtrasana*.

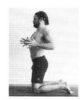 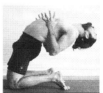 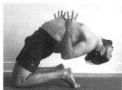 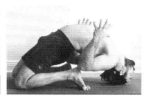 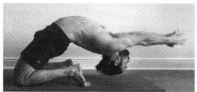

Benefits: This pose strengthens the back muscles, quadriceps, and abdominals.
Contraindications: Avoid with high blood pressure or headache.
Modification: Place the fingers on the lower abdomen or high on the thighs.
Chakra: sacral, heart

279. Kapotasana (pigeon pose)

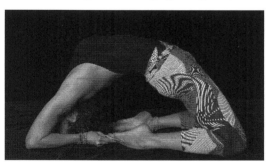

From *supta virasana* or *laghuvajrasana,* bring the hands beside the ears. Lift the hips, extend the arms straight, and push the hips forward. Rest the head down and walk the hands in to clasp the feet. When you reach your edge, relax the body but keep the feet and tailbone active.

Benefits: This pose strengthens the back muscles and opens the spine through extension. It stretches the abdomen and hip flexors. It opens the chest and expands the lungs.
Contraindications: Avoid with high blood pressure or headache.
Modification: Slide the head in as close as you can and keep the hands beside the head.
Chakra: sacral, heart

280. Eka Pada Kapotasana I (one foot pigeon pose I)

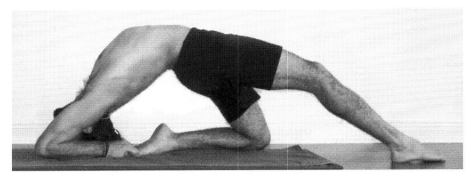

From *kapotasana,* clasp one foot with both hands and extend the other leg straight in front of you.

Benefits: This pose strengthens the back muscles and opens the shoulders and spine. It stretches the abdomen and hip flexors. It opens the chest and expands the lungs.
Contraindications: Avoid with high blood pressure or headache.
Modification: Use a strap to hold the foot.
Chakra: sacral, heart

281. Eka Pada Kapotasana II (one foot pigeon pose II)

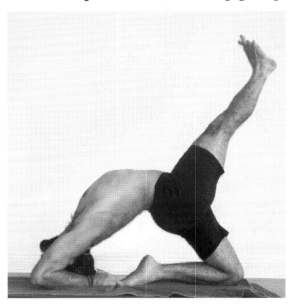

Assume *kapotasana I* position, holding the foot, and extend the leg straight up toward the ceiling.

Benefits: This pose strengthens the back muscles and hip flexors. It opens the shoulders and spine.
Contraindications: Avoid with high blood pressure or headache.
Modification: Slide the head in as close as you can and keep the hands beside the head.
Chakra: sacral, heart

282. Rajakapotasana (king pigeon pose)

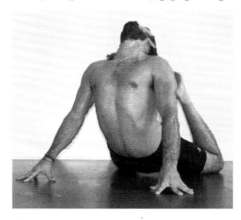

From *bhujangasana* prep position, elevate the hands and place them wider in front of you. Lift up, outer rotate the arms, and then straighten them all of the way. Slide the palate back and push the head back. Bend the knees and point the feet toward the back of the head.

Benefits: This pose strengthens the back muscles. It opens the chest and lungs. It stretches the thighs and hip flexors.
Contraindications: Avoid with sacroiliac injury.
Chakra: sacral, heart

283. Nasginyasana I (mermaid I pose)

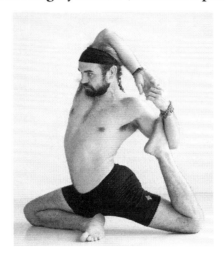

From *eka pada rajakapotasana* preparation, reach one hand back for the foot and trap it in the elbow crease. Push down through the knees and squeeze the legs together to lift the hips. Reach the other arm overhead and clasp hands. Push the head back into the top arm as you twist forward.

Benefits: This pose strengthens the back muscles. It opens the chest and lungs. It stretches the thighs and hip flexors.
Contraindications: Avoid with sacroiliac injury or knee injury.
Modification: Place a prop underneath the hip of the leading leg to maintain stability and to keep the hips level.
Chakra: sacral, heart

284. Nasginyasana II (mermaid II pose)

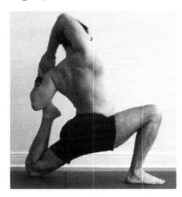

From a deep lunge position, reach back and grab the inside edge of the foot. Kick back into the hand to engage the thigh muscles and then pull the leg in and hook the arm over the foot. Clasp hands overhead and push the head up to deepen the opening.

Benefits: This pose strengthens the back muscles. It opens the chest and lungs. It stretches the thighs and hip flexors.
Contraindications: Avoid with sacroiliac injury or knee injury.
Chakra: root, heart

285. Eka Pada Rajakapotasana I (one leg king pigeon I)

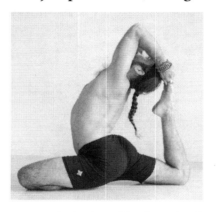

From *eka pada rajakapotasana* preparation, reach the hand back, palm face-up, to grab the outside of the foot of the back leg. Squeeze the legs together, lift up out of the hips, and then take the head back, as the elbow pivots up toward ceiling. The arm of the forward leg then reaches overhead to clasp the foot. The hips stay hovering off the floor and do not rest down. There are other techniques for clasping the foot, but the above method is the most accessible for practitioners.

Benefits: This pose strengthens the back muscles. It opens the chest and lungs. It stretches the thighs and hip flexors. It stimulates the thyroid, parathyroid, and adrenals.
Contraindications: Avoid with sacroiliac injury or knee injury.
Modification: Place a prop underneath the hip of the leading leg to maintain stability and to keep the hips level. Use a strap to hold the foot.
Chakra: sacral, heart

286. Baddha Eka Pada Rajakapotasana I (bound one leg king pigeon I)

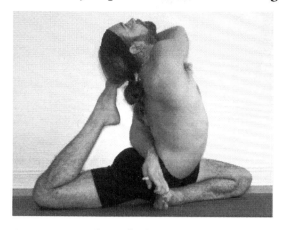

Assume *eka pada rajakapotasana I* position and reach the same hand as the forward leg behind the back and grab the foot. Then duck the head under the top arm as the elbow moves toward the opposite shoulder.

Benefits: This pose strengthens the back muscles. It opens the chest and lungs. It stretches the shoulders, thighs, and hip flexors. It stimulates the thyroid, parathyroid, and adrenals.
Contraindications: Avoid with sacroiliac injury or knee injury.
Chakra: sacral, heart

287. Eka Pada Rajakapotasana II (one foot king pigeon II prep)

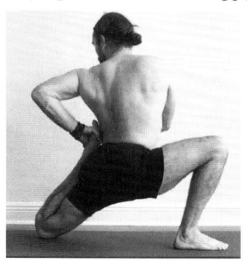

From a deep lunge position, reach back for the foot and pull it in beside the hip. Resist to engage the thigh muscles by pressing the foot back into the hands, and then deepen the opening by pushing the foot forward.

Benefits: This pose prepares the body for deep backbends. It stretches the shoulders, thighs, and hip flexors.
Contraindications: Avoid with sacroiliac injury or shoulder injury.
Chakra: root, sacral

288. Parivrtta Eka Pada Rajakapotasana II
(revolved one foot king pigeon II prep, "twisting thigh stretch")

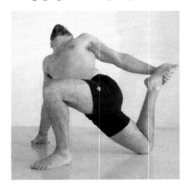

Step one foot up into a lunge and rest the back knee down. Twist and reach the opposite hand back for the outside edge of the opposite foot. Kick the foot back to engage the quadriceps, and then bring the heel in toward the hip. Deepen the twist and then move towards a backbend.

Benefits: This pose tones the back muscles and extends the spine. It opens the chest and lungs. It stretches the thighs and hip flexors. It stimulates the thyroid, parathyroid, and adrenals.
Contraindications: Avoid with knee injury.
Chakra: sacral, heart

289. Parivrtta Eka Pada Rajakapotasana II (revolved one foot king pigeon II prep variation)

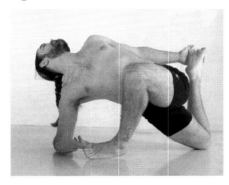

Step one foot into a lunge and rest the back knee on the mat. Twist and reach the opposite hand for the outside edge of the opposite foot. Lower down on the forearm and hook the big toe with the first two fingers, palm face-up. Rock over onto the outside edge of the forward foot and push down through the top edge to lift the heel. The ankle, shin, and knee should be aligned as the hips move forward and down. Keep the lower abdomen engaged and the thigh of the back leg moving back as the foot is drawn in. Work on creating strength in the pose to prevent over stretching of the hip flexors.

Benefits: This pose tones the back muscles. It opens the chest and lungs. It stretches the thighs and hip flexors. It stimulates the thyroid, parathyroid, and adrenals.
Contraindications: Avoid with knee or ankle injury.
Chakra: sacral, heart

290. Eka Pada Rajakapotasana II (one leg king pigeon II)

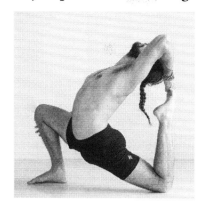

Step one foot into a lunge and rest the back knee on the mat. Reach one hand palm face up for the back foot. Grab the outside edge of the foot and pivot the elbow up as the hand shifts to the top of the foot. Place the free hand on the forward knee or the floor for stability. Grab the foot with both hands and kick the foot down toward the floor to deepen the pose. Extend the hips forward and down as the heart lifts up.

Benefits: This pose tones the back muscles and extends the spine. It opens the chest and lungs. It stretches the thighs and hip flexors. It stimulates the thyroid, parathyroid, and adrenals.
Contraindications: Avoid with high blood pressure or headaches.
Modification: Use a strap to hold the foot.
Chakra: sacral, heart

291. Eka Pada Rajakapotasana III (one leg king pigeon III)

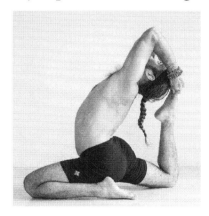

Bring one leg into *ardha virasana* and the other leg straight back behind you. Grab the outside edge of the back foot with palm face up. Push down through the back knee to keep the hips hovering off the floor. Pivot the elbow forward and up, as the hand grabs the top of the foot. Reach the other arm overhead and clasp the foot with both hands, or keep the hand on the floor for support.

Benefits: This pose tones the back muscles and extends the spine. It opens the chest and lungs. It stretches the thighs and hip flexors. It stimulates the thyroid, parathyroid, and adrenals.
Contraindications: Avoid with high blood pressure or headaches.
Modification: Use a strap to hold the foot.
Chakra: sacral, heart

292. Eka Pada Rajakapotasana IV (one leg king pigeon IV)

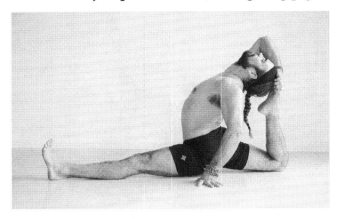

From *Hanumanasana,* reach one hand back, palm face-up, for the outside edge of the back foot. Squeeze the legs into the center to lift up out of the hips, and then pivot the elbow forward and up. Take the head back and lift the heart up. The free hand can reach overhead for the foot or remain on the floor for stability.

Benefits: This pose tones the back muscles and extends the spine. It opens the chest and lungs. It stretches the thighs and hip flexors, while lengthening the hamstrings. It stimulates the thyroid, parathyroid, and adrenals.
Contraindications: Avoid with high blood pressure or headaches.
Modification: Use a strap to hold the foot.
Chakra: sacral, heart

293. Eka Pada Rajakapotasana V (one leg king pigeon V)

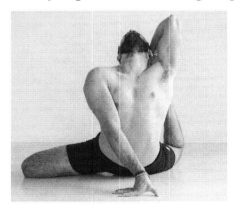

Place one leg in *ardha thavaliasana* position with the thigh parallel with the top edge of the mat, and the shin parallel with the outside edge. Reach the arm across the midline to stabilize and place the hand in ridgetop position. Grab the outside edge of the back foot and pivot the elbow up as the head moves back.

Benefits: This pose tones the back muscles and extends the spine. It opens the chest and lungs. It stretches the adductors, quadriceps, and hip flexors. It stimulates the thyroid, parathyroid, and adrenals.
Contraindications: Avoid with high blood pressure or headaches.
Modification: Use a strap to hold the foot.
Chakra: sacral, heart

294. Purvottanasana (east side stretch)

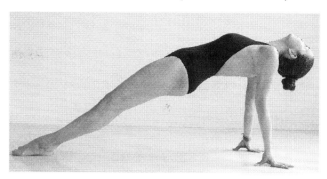

From sitting, reach the hands behind the hips with the arms in outer rotation. Place the hands flat with fingers pointing toward the feet, or elevate the wrists in fist or ridgetop position. If the wrists elevate in ridgetop, then outer rotate the hands with the arms, so the fingers point away. Extend the legs straight and point the feet as the hips lift. Take the head back and lift the heart as the throat opens.

Benefits: This pose tones the back muscles and extends the spine. It strengthens the triceps and legs. It stretches the abdomen and ankles.
Contraindications: Avoid with high blood pressure, heart disease, ulcers, or headaches.
Modification: Keep the knees bent and lift into a table position.
Chakra: sacral, heart

295. Setu Bandha Sarvangasana (half bound shoulder stand pose, "bridge pose")

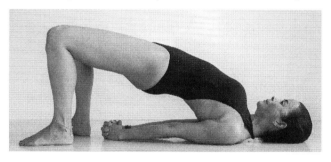

From a supine position, bring the feet under the knees hip distance apart. Lift the hips and bring the shoulder blades in toward the spine. Clasp hands underneath or place the hands on the floor palms face-up. Squeeze the legs in toward the midline to engage the inner thighs. Push down through the feet and pull them back to engage the hamstrings and gluteal muscles. Root down through the big toes as the heels widen apart. Draw the belly in and scoop the tailbone up. Push the head back to lift the chin away from the chest, and then lift the chest up toward the chin.

Benefits: This pose strengthens the legs and gluteal muscles. It tones the back muscles and stimulates the thyroid and parathyroid endocrine glands. It opens the shoulders and stretches the abdomen. It alleviates stress, fatigue, headache, and mild depression.
Contraindications: Avoid with neck injuries.
Modification: Place a block underneath the sacrum.
Chakra: root, throat

296. Eka Pada Setu Bandha Sarvangasana (one foot half bound shoulder stand pose)

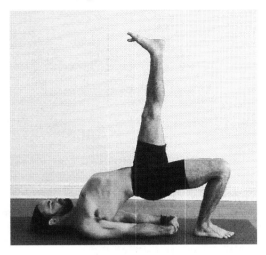

From *setu bandha sarvangasana,* bring one foot toward the center of the mat and extend the other leg straight up toward the ceiling. Press down through the arms, shoulders, and the back of the head.

Benefits: This pose strengthens the legs and gluteal muscles. It tones the back muscles and stimulates the thyroid and parathyroid endocrine glands. It opens the shoulders and stretches the abdomen. It alleviates stress, fatigue, headache, and mild depression.
Contraindications: Avoid with neck injuries.
Modification: Place a block underneath the sacrum.
Chakra: root, throat

297. Eka Pada Bheka Sarvangasana (one foot frog shoulder stand pose)

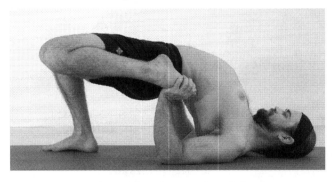

From *setu bandha sarvangasana,* reach one hand for the inside of the foot, pivot the hand, and push the foot up toward the outer edge of the hip. Place the elbow down and hold the hip with the other hand on the outside edge to stabilize.

Benefits: This pose strengthens the legs and gluteal muscles. It stretches the quadriceps and relieves stress in the knees.
Contraindications: Avoid with neck injury.
Chakra: sacral, throat

298. Bheka Sarvangasana (frog shoulder stand pose)

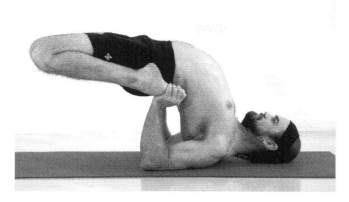

From *eka pada bheka sarvangasana,* reach the stabilizing hand for the inside edge of the foot. Rest the elbow down and pivot the hand on top of the foot. Push the feet up as the head pushes back.

Benefits: This pose strengthens the lower back, abdominals, and gluteal muscles. It stretches the quadriceps and relieves stress in the knees.
Contraindications: Avoid with neck injury.
Chakra: sacral, throat

299. Urdhva Dhanurasana (upward bow prep pose)

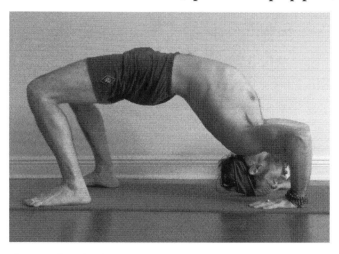

Lie flat on the back with the feet under the knees hip distance apart. Place the hands overhead beside the ears. Lift the hips and chest up, and then pause on top of the head. Draw the elbows in toward the armpits, and squeeze them toward each other. From here, straighten the arms to enter the pose.

Benefits: This pose prepares the body for the full backbend. It strengthens the neck, legs, and upper back. It helps in stabilizing the rotator cuff muscles.
Contraindications: Avoid with neck injury.
Chakra: root, crown

300. Urdhva Dhanurasana (upward bow pose)

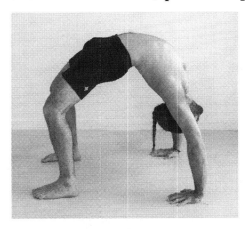

From *urdhva dhanurasana* prep, curl the chest forward and go all the way up straightening the arms. Squeeze the legs in toward the midline to engage the adductors. Push down through the feet and pull them back toward the hips to engage the hamstrings and gluteal muscles. Root down through the big toes and widen the heels apart. Scoop the tailbone strong without over gripping the gluteal muscles.

Benefits: This pose strengthens the legs, arms, and back muscles. It stretches the abdomen, chest, and lungs. It stimulates the nervous, digestive, respiratory, and cardiovascular systems. Increases vitality and alleviates depression.
Contraindications: Avoid with carpal tunnel syndrome, back injury, heart problems, and high or low blood pressure.
Modification: Place blocks at a 45-degree angle at the corner of the wall and floor. Rest on your back with the head between the blocks. Wrap the hands over the blocks with the fingers facing down or out to the side if tighter. From here, curl the chest toward the wall and push into the blocks to go up.
Chakra: sacral, heart

301. Dwi Pada Viparita Dandasana I (two foot inverted staff pose I)

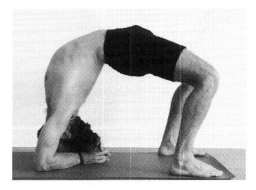

From *urdhva dhanurasana,* lower down onto the forearms and clasp hands behind the head. Push down through the arms and the wrists. Lift the head off the floor and curl the chest forward.

Benefits: This pose strengthens the shoulders and back muscles. It stretches the chest and abdomen. It helps with anxiety, fatigue, and depression.
Contraindications: Avoid with shoulder or lower back injury.
Chakra: sacral, heart

302. Dwi Pada Viparita Dandasana II (two foot inverted staff pose II)

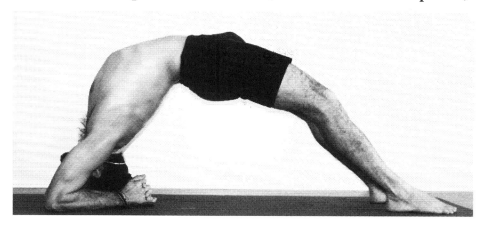

Assume *dwi pada viparita dandasana I* position and extend both legs straight. Squeeze the legs toward the midline and extend the chest forward.

Benefits: This pose strengthens the legs, shoulders, and back muscles. It stretches the chest and abdomen. It helps with anxiety, fatigue, and depression.
Contraindications: Avoid with shoulder or lower back injury.
Chakra: sacral, heart

303. Setu Bandhasana (bound lock pose)

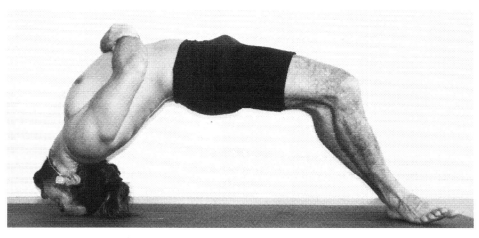

From *dwi pada viparita dandasana II,* outer rotate the legs, turning the heels in and toes out. Balance on the outside edges of the feet, extend forward, and come onto the forehead. Then reach the hands on top of the chest and grab opposing forearms.

Benefits: This pose strengthens the neck. It improves balance and concentration.
Contraindications: Avoid with neck injury.
Modification: Place the hands beside the head for stability.
Chakra: root, brow

304. Mandalasana (sacred circle pose)

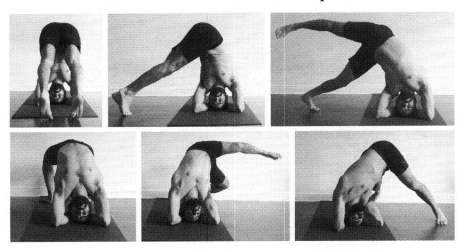

Clasp hands as in *sirsasana I* position and extend the legs straight. Walk, slide, or jump to one side. Lift the trailing leg up and rock onto the outside edge of the leading leg's foot. Outer rotate the lifting leg and pop the hips up toward the ceiling to flip over. Walk the feet over as in *dwi pada viparita dandasana*, and then lift the trailing leg again. Inner rotate the leg and turn the hips down. Return to the starting position. Repeat or switch directions.

Benefits: This pose strengthens the shoulders, back, and abdominal muscles. It opens the spine and expands the chest. It develops vigor and confidence.
Contraindications: Avoid with neck injury.
Chakra: heart, crown

305. Eka Pada Viparita Chakrasana (one foot inverted wheel pose)

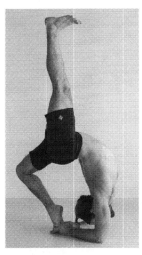

Assume *dwi pada viparita dandasana I* position and kick one foot in toward the head and then grab the foot with both hands. Curl the chest forward and then lift the other leg up toward the ceiling.

Benefits: This pose strengthens the shoulders and back muscles. It stretches the chest, abdomen, and lungs.
Contraindications: Avoid with shoulder injury.
Modification: Use a strap around the foot.
Chakra: sacral, heart

306. Makarasana (crocodile pose)

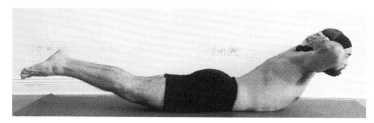

Lie flat on the stomach and bring the legs together. Clasp hands behind the head and lift up. Squeeze the legs and big toes together and push the head up strong into the hands.

Benefits: This pose strengthens the neck, back, and inner thigh muscles. It stimulates the appetite and digestive system. It tones the pancreas and autonomic nervous system.
Contraindications: Avoid with high blood pressure, heart disease, or peptic ulcer.
Chakra: root, throat

307. Shalabhasana I (locust pose I)

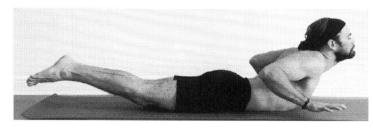

Lie flat on the stomach and bring the legs together with the hands beside the chest. Lift the feet and hands off the floor. Squeeze the legs and shoulder blades together. Hold the pose for five breaths and then rest in *apanavasana*.

The following benefits, contraindications, and *chakra* apply to all *shalabhasana* poses I-IV.

Benefits: This pose strengthens the back and inner thigh muscles. It stimulates the appetite and digestive system. It tones the pancreas and autonomic nervous system.
Contraindications: Avoid with high blood pressure, heart disease, or peptic ulcer.
Chakra: root, throat

308. Shalabhasana II (locust pose II)

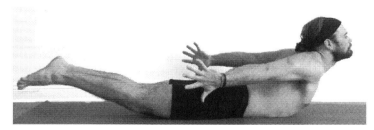

Lie flat on the stomach and bring the legs together with the hands beside the chest. Lift the legs and straighten the arms behind you with the palms facing in. Squeeze the legs and shoulder blades together as you hold the pose.

309. Shalabhasana III (locust pose III)

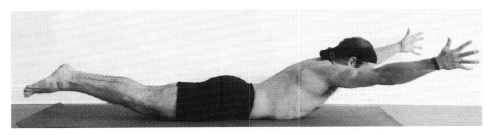

Lie flat on the stomach and bring the legs together with the hands beside the chest. Reach the arms straight ahead, lift the legs, and squeeze them together.

310. Shalabhasana IV (locust pose IV)

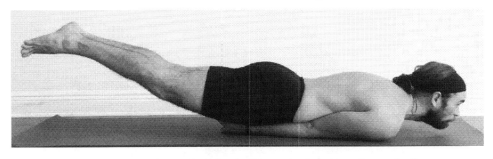

Lie flat on the stomach and clasp hands under the belly with the thumbs and elbow creases facing straight down. Lift the head and the legs. Push the belly into the arms to lift higher.

311. Baddha Hasta Shalbhasana (bound hand locust pose)

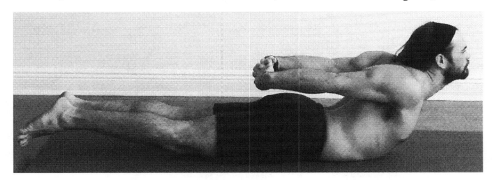

Lie flat on the stomach and clasp hands behind the back. Lift the shoulders toward the ears and then squeeze the shoulder blades together. Lift the feet and squeeze the legs together.

Benefits: This pose strengthens the back and inner thigh muscles. It stretches the chest and shoulders. It stimulates the appetite and digestive system. It tones the pancreas and autonomic nervous system.
Contraindications: Avoid with high blood pressure, heart disease, or peptic ulcer.
Chakra: root, throat

312. Viparita Shalabhasana (inverted locust pose)

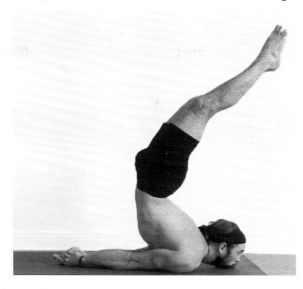

From *shalabhasana IV*, push down through the arms and lift the legs straight up toward the ceiling. The legs can widen and bend slightly to create an initial kick to lift vertical.

Benefits: This pose strengthens the arms, shoulders, and back muscles. It stretches the throat.
Contraindications: Avoid with high blood pressure or heart disease.
Chakra: root, throat

313. Purna Viparita Shalabhasana (full inverted locust pose)

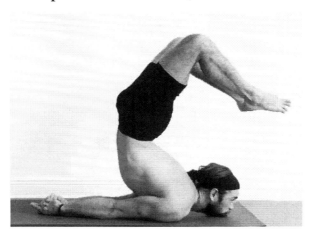

From *viparita shalabhasana*, bend the legs and squeeze the big toes together. Use the strength of the inner thighs to extend the feet toward the head.

Benefits: This pose strengthens the arms, shoulders, and back muscles. It stretches the throat and hip flexors.
Contraindications: Avoid with high blood pressure or heart disease.
Chakra: root, throat

314. Eka Pada Shalabhasana (one foot locust pose)

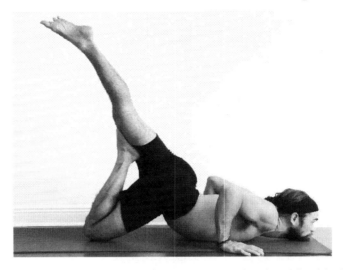

Lie flat on the stomach with the hands beside the chest. Squeeze the shoulder blades together, and then bend one leg up. Lift the opposite leg straight up and place the thigh on the arch of the foot of the bent leg. Curl in the upper back and extend the chin forward.

Benefits: This pose tones the back and stretches the throat. It relieves lower back stress.
Contraindications: Avoid with high blood pressure or heart disease.
Chakra: root, throat

315. Baddha Eka Pada Shalabhasana (bound one foot locust pose)

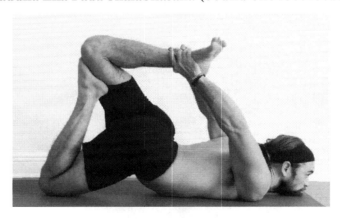

From *eka pada shalabhasana,* bend the top leg and grab the foot with both hands. Kick the leg up and lift the arms up. Curl in the upper back and extend the chin forward.

Benefits: This pose tones the back and stretches the throat. It improves balance and concentration.
Contraindications: Avoid with high blood pressure or heart disease.
Chakra: root, throat

316. Ghanda Bherundasana (formidable face pose)

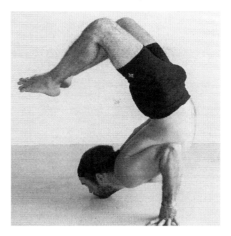

Lie flat on the stomach with the hands beside the chest. Place the chin on the floor and squeeze the shoulder blades on the back. Lift the hips and knees off the floor and walk the feet in toward the chest, while keeping the chin on the floor. Lift one leg toward the ceiling and kick up. Bend the legs and extend the feet toward the back of the head. Keep the shoulders lifting away from the floor. Curl in the upper back and release the heart down.

Benefits: This pose strengthens the shoulders and back muscles. It stretches the throat and hip flexors. It stimulates the nerve centers and glands in the pelvis plexus, hypo-gastric plexus and pharyngeal plexus.
Contraindications: Avoid with high blood pressure or heart disease.
Chakra: heart, throat

317. Simhasana (lion pose)

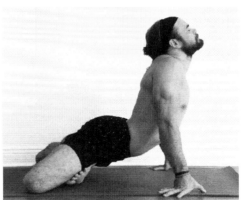

From *padmasana,* reach the hands forward and rock over the knees. Extend the hips down as you arch up. Exhale three times through the mouth, sticking the tongue out, and gaze up toward the third eye. This removes old air from the lungs, and releases negative energy, while stretching the muscles of the face.

Benefits: This pose tones the back and extends the spine. It opens the hips and relieves lower back stress. It stretches the hip flexors and muscles of the face.
Contraindications: Avoid with knee injury.
Chakra: sacral, throat

318. Parivrtta Simhasana (revolved lion)

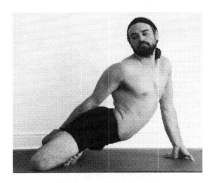

From *simhasana,* reach one hand back and grab the top shin. Pull up on the bound leg and twist. Gaze over the shoulder and stretch the side of the neck.

Benefits: This pose creates a greater opening for the hips and massages the abdominal organs. It relieves lower back stress and improves digestion.
Contraindications: Avoid with knee injury.
Chakra: sacral, solar plexus

319. Matsyasana (fish pose)

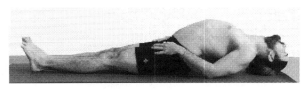

Lie flat on the back with the legs straight and the hands on top of the thighs. Push down through the elbows and the back of the head. Arch the spine and lift the heart space.

Benefits: This pose tones the back and strengthens the neck. It stimulates the abdominal organs and the thyroid. It alleviates constipation, respiratory ailments, mild backache, and fatigue.
Contraindications: Avoid with neck injury or pregnancy.
Chakra: root, throat

320. Padma Matsyasana (lotus fish pose)

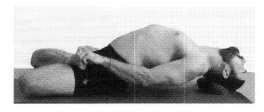

Lie flat on the back with the legs in lotus position with the hands holding the feet. Pull against the feet and push the head back into the floor. Arch the spine and expand the heart.

Benefits: This pose tones the back and strengthens the neck. It opens the hips and expands the lungs.
Contraindications: Avoid with neck injury or pregnancy.
Chakra: sacral, throat

321. Uttana Padasana (intense foot pose)

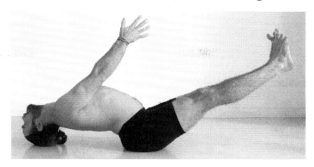

From *matsyasana,* lift the legs and arms at forty-degree angles, while maintaining the arch of the spine.

Benefits: This pose tones the back and strengthens the neck.
Contraindications: Avoid with neck or lower back injury. Avoid during pregnancy.
Chakra: sacral, throat

322. "Drop-back"

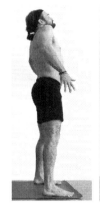 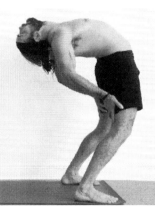 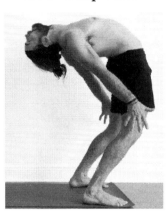 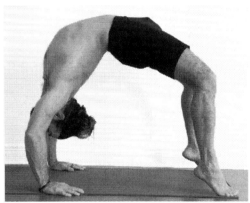

From *tadasana,* squeeze the legs into the midline, draw the belly in, and scoop the tailbone. Lift the ribcage and shoulders up to lengthen the sides of the body. Curl the shoulders back and open the heart. Place the hands on the hamstrings and extend the hips forward. Take the head back and look for the back of the mat. Outer rotate the arms as they straighten, and then reach both hands for the floor. The heels can lift to transfer the energy to the front body. This reduces impact for the wrists and strengthens the quadriceps, hip flexors and lower abdominals. If the feet remain flat, then they should not turn out to the sides during the descent with outer rotation of the thighs. This will narrow the lower back and compress the vertebrae. The feet should stay parallel with heels up or down.

Benefits: This pose sequence strengthens the legs, abdominals, and back muscles. It expands the lungs and tones the diaphragm. It increases vitality and removes mild depression.
Contraindications: Avoid with wrist injury.
Modification: Lower down with the hands in fingertips or fists. The drop-back can also be performed with one hand by placing one hand on the front of the thigh and reaching the other arm overhead.
Chakra: sacral, heart

323. Viparita Chakrasana (inverted wheel)

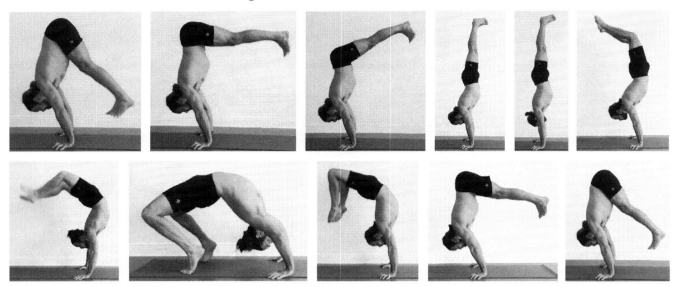

Jump or press into a handstand with legs straight. Bend the legs and drop over into *urdhva dhanurasana*. Lean the weight over the feet then jump up into a scorpion position. Extend the chest forward and push the head up to bring the legs back up and over. Lower into a forward bend or *adho mukha svanasana*. Repeat as many times as possible. The Skanda Yoga record is 72 in nine minutes.

Benefits: This pose sequence strengthens the legs, abdominals, neck, and back muscles. It expands the lungs and tones the diaphragm. It increases vitality and removes mild depression.

Contraindications: Avoid with shoulder and wrist injury.

Chakra: sacral, heart

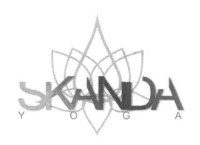

CHAPTER 13

Shoulders, Wrists, and Core

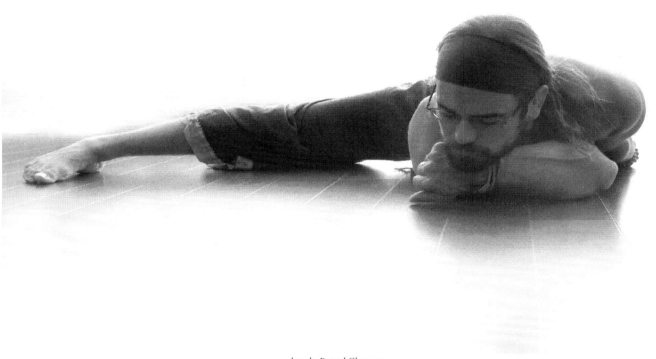

photo by Raquel Glottman

Shoulder openers are important to practice in order to keep the rotator cuff injury-free. Arm balances and *vinyasas* create a lot of strength, which can lead to tension. The following poses in this section will keep the shoulders open and healthy. The wrist exercises are also therapeutic in application, as they promote healing and prevent injury. The exercises for the core are practiced to strengthen the connection to the lower and upper body. Additionally, it is important to have a strong core to be able to maintain the *shakti*. The spiritual power can dissipate if we don't have physical integrity. Practice the following exercises with the intention of retaining personal power.

324. Skanda Chakrasana (Skanda's wheel)

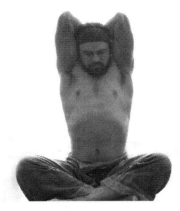 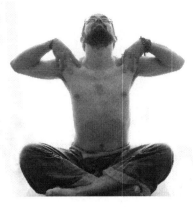 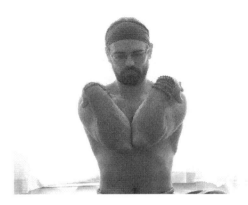

From sitting in *sukhasana,* place the fingers on top of the shoulders and lift the elbows straight up. Squeeze in strong with the arms pinching the head and hold for a few seconds. Lower the arms down parallel with the floor and pull the elbows apart. Squeeze the shoulder blades together on the back and open the heart. Hold the engagement for a few seconds, and then bring the elbows together in front of the chest. Pinch the elbows together and pull the shoulders back for a few seconds holding the engagement. Repeat the cycle many times holding a strong engagement in each position before transitioning to the next one.

Benefits: This exercise is good for strengthening and stabilizing the rotator cuff.
Chakra: heart

325. Uttana Garuda Bhujasana I, II, III (intense eagle arm pose I, II, III)

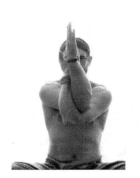 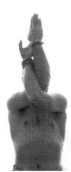 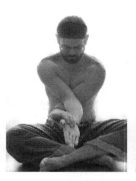 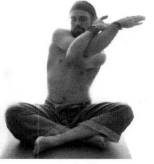 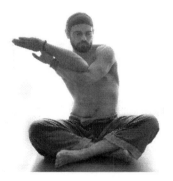

Start in a comfortable seated position and wrap the arms into eagle position. Lift the arms straight up toward the ceiling and hold for at least five seconds. For the second position bring the arms back down and point them toward the floor. Hold the stretch for at least five seconds. For the third position, bring the hands back up, so the underarm is parallel with the floor, and then point the hands to one side and lift the elbows. Stretch toward one side, hold, and then the other.

Benefits: This exercise stretches the infraspinatus and supraspinatus rotator cuff muscles.
Modification: Hold a towel between the hands if the bottom hand doesn't wrap around the top wrist.
Chakra: heart

326. Eka Bhuja Swastikasana I (one arm auspicious pose I)

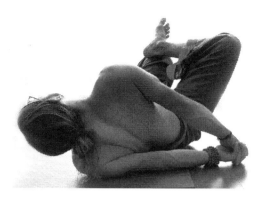

From lying face down, extend one arm out to the side perpendicular with the body. Turn the palm face up with the thumb pointing toward the feet. Roll over onto the hip and shoulder. Step one foot on the floor behind you, and then reach back and clasp hands. Twist both knees up toward the ceiling, and place one ankle on top of the thigh to deepen the twist in the lower body. The bottom hand can then turn down toward the floor to deepen the opening, but be careful not to hyperextend the elbow. If the hand is placed palm face down in the beginning, it will place more pressure in the elbow joint before the shoulder can open.

Benefits: This exercise stretches the deltoid and relieves lower back stress.
Modification: Use a strap to hold the hands or just rest the top hand on the hip.
Chakra: solar plexus, heart

327. Eka Bhuja Swastikasana II (one arm auspicious pose II)

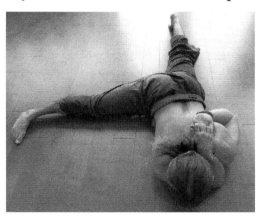

From *eka bhuja padmasana*, slide the chin off of the wrist and reach the hand over the shoulder onto the back. Then reach the arm that was beside the hip behind the back and clasp hands.

Benefits: This exercise stretches the triceps, infraspinatus, and supraspinatus. It opens the hips and calms the nervous system.
Contraindication: Avoid with shoulder injury.
Modification: Use a strap to hold the hands.
Chakra: heart, throat

328. Supta Vira Eka Bhuja Swastikasana (supine hero one arm auspicious pose)

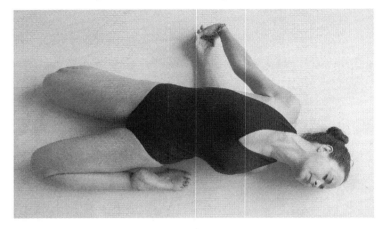

Start from a *supta vira prep* position with the ankles on the outside of the hips. Use the hands for support, lean back, and then begin to twist and reach one arm behind you with the palm face up. Lower straight down on top of the shoulder, then reach the other arm back and clasp hands.

Benefits: This exercise stretches the thighs, shoulders and neck.
Contraindication: Avoid with shoulder or lower back injury.
Modification: Use the top hand on the floor in front of the chest for support instead of clasping.
Chakra: sacral, heart

329. Supta Agnistambha Eka Bhuja Swastikasana (supine fire log one arm auspicious pose)

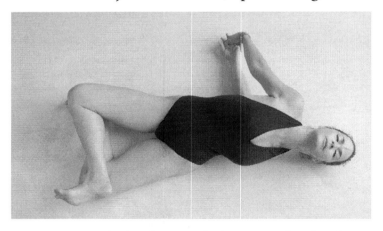

Start from *agnistambhasana* position with the shins stacked on top of each other. Reach one arm back with the palm face up, rest down onto the shoulder, then reach back and clasp hands. Arch the lower back and lower the top knee down over the ankle.

Benefits: This exercise stretches the hip flexors and shoulders.
Contraindication: Avoid with shoulder or lower back injury.
Modification: Use a partner to stabilize the legs and to push the top knee down if it is lifting. Practice *supta agnistambhasana* first to open the hips, and then add in the shoulder opening later when it is accessible.
Chakra: sacral, heart

330. Eka Bhuja Padmasana (one arm lotus pose)

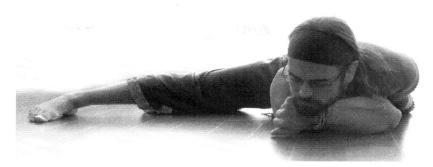

From lying face down on the stomach, extend one leg directly out to the side with the foot flat on the floor. Bend the same arm and place the elbow under the opposite shoulder with the thumb pointing down in fist position. Hook the chin over the wrist and push it flat into the floor. Extend the free arm straight back beside the hip in fist position palm up toward ceiling. Press the back of the hand into the floor to shift the energy forward into the upper body.

Benefits: This exercise stretches the arms and shoulders. It opens the hips and calms the nervous system.
Contraindication: Avoid with shoulder injury.
Chakra: sacral, heart

331. Eka Bhuja Virasana (one arm hero prep pose)

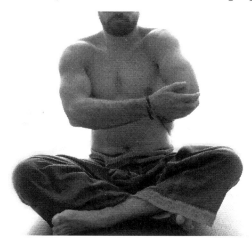

From sitting in *sukhasana,* bring one hand palm face out on the outer edge of the ribcage. Reach across with the other hand and grab the elbow. Slowly pull the elbow forward toward the center.

The following benefits and contraindications apply to poses 332 & 333.

Benefits: The *buja virasana* series releases tension in the front of the shoulder and stretches the teres major and teres minor muscles.
Contraindication: Avoid if the infraspinatus or supraspinatus muscles are injured.
Chakra: heart

332. Dwi Bhuja Virasana I (two arm hero pose I)

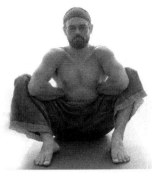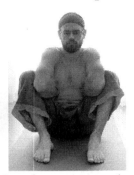

From sitting with the knees bent up, bring both hands palms facing out to the sides of the ribcage. Separate the knees then twist and hook one elbow in at a time. Slowly squeeze the elbows together using the knees.

333. Dwi Bhuja Virasana II (two arm hero pose II)

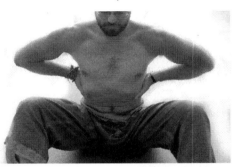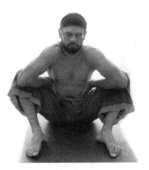

From sitting with the knees bent up, bring both hands with palms facing in to the sides of the ribcage. The hands are over the lower floating ribs with the thumbs pointing straight ahead. Separate the knees then twist and hook one elbow in at a time. Slowly squeeze the elbows in and let the shoulders release.

334. Dwi Bhuja Virasana III (two arm hero pose III)

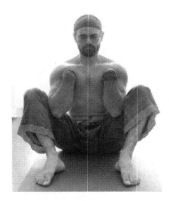

From sitting with the knees bent up, cup the hands and then bring the root knuckles on the inside edge of the pectoral muscles. Bring the elbows down and squeeze the knees into the arms. Then push the wrists up into the chest.

Benefits: This pose stretches the top of the hands and relieves stress in the wrists.
Chakra: heart

335. Supta Eka Bhuja Virasana
(supine one arm hero pose)

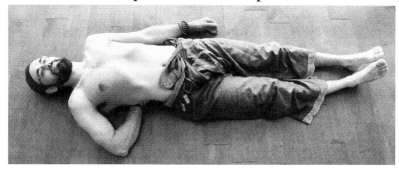

From lying in a supine position, bring one hand palm face down under the back. The edge of the wrist should be directly under the outer edge of the rib cage. Roll over onto the arm and grab the triceps. Lightly pull up on the bent arm to deepen the twist.

Benefits: This pose releases tension in the front of the shoulder and stretches the teres major and teres minor muscles.
Contraindication: Avoid if the infraspinatus or supraspinatus muscles are injured.
Chakra: heart

336. Supta Eka Bhuja Vira Padangusthasana
(supine one arm hero hand to big toe pose)

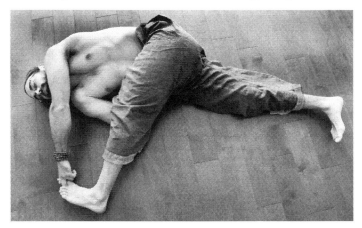

From *supta eka bhuja virasana* position, reach the free hand up and clasp the big toe. Then slowly twist over the bent arm and lower the foot to the floor.

Benefits: This pose releases tension in the front of the shoulder, lower back, and IT band. It stretches the teres major and teres minor muscles.
Contraindication: Avoid if the infraspinatus or supraspinatus muscles are injured.
Chakra: solar plexus, heart

337. Eka Bhuja Anahata Chapasana (one arm heart sugarcane pose, "heartbreaker")

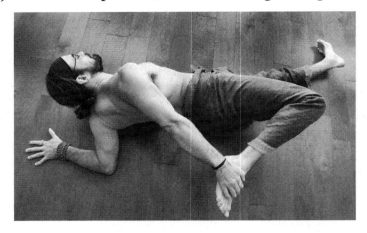

From lying face down, bend one arm out to the side at a 90-degree angle and place the palm face down. The bottom of the elbow should be aligned with the bottom edge of the shoulder. Roll over toward the bent arm and swing the bottom foot in front of you to stabilize. Reach the top arm back for the top foot. Kick the leg back behind you then curl the heart forward and down.

Benefits: This pose stretches the front of the shoulders and the pectoral muscles. It tones the back and opens the thighs.
Contraindication: Avoid if have a shoulder injury.
Modification: Place the top hand on the floor in front of the chest for support instead of reaching for the foot.
Chakra: sacral, heart

338. Dwi Bhuja Visvajrasana (two arm double diamond pose)

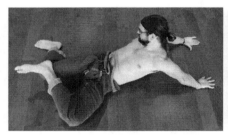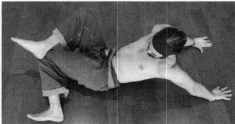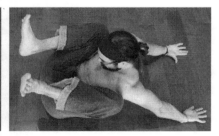

From sitting, reach the hands behind you with the palms face up. When you cannot go any further, push down through the wrists, lift the hips, and slide them away from the hands. Cross one ankle on top and twist to one side. Extend energy from the hip out through the knee. To exit the pose, bring both knees to the chest and then kick out into a forward bend.

Benefits: This pose stretches the front of the shoulders and the pectoral muscles. It relieves lower back tension.
Contraindication: Avoid if have a shoulder injury.
Modification: Place the hands palms face up on a desk or table then squat down to stretch the shoulders.
Chakra: sacral, heart

339. Supta Bhuja Vinyasa (supine arm transitions, "arm raises with block")

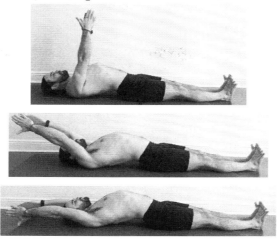

Lie flat on your back and place a block between the hands. Press into the block with the palms of the hands. Avoid gripping the block with your fingertips. Straighten the arms and draw them down into the shoulder sockets. Push the shoulder blades down into the floor and arch the lower back. Keep squeezing into the block and pulling the arms down, and then slowly lower the arms overhead to touch the floor with the thumbs. Bring the arms back up, repeating the same actions of squeezing in and pulling down. Go slow to focus on the alignment and build more strength in the arms. Repeat up to 13.

Benefits: This exercise strengthens and stabilizes the rotator cuff muscles. It improves posture and increases concentration.
Modification: Place a blanket or a pillow between the hands to build more strength in the arms, or use a small weight to focus on the shoulders and upper back integration.
Chakra: sacral, heart

340. Adho Baddha Mustiasana (downward bound fists, "thumb breaker")

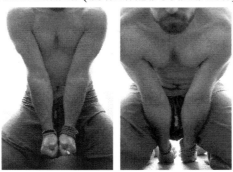

Start from sitting in *virasana* with the knees separated. Clasp the fingers over the thumbs to make a fist. Lift the hips and reach the fists back under the hips. Place the inside edge of the hands on the floor, so the thumb joint is pressing straight down. The hands should be aligned with the ankles. Slowly lower the hips down onto the forearms, while lifting the arms and shoulders pull up.

Benefits: This stretches the tendon of the thumb. It relieves forearm stress and prevents injury from text messaging.
Contraindication: Avoid if have a thumb injury.
Modification: From sitting or standing, wrap the fingers over one thumb and wrap the other hand on top. Keep the arms straight and strong, and then pull the hand down without moving the wrist.
Chakra: root

341. Parivrtta Eka Hastasana I (revolved one hand pose)

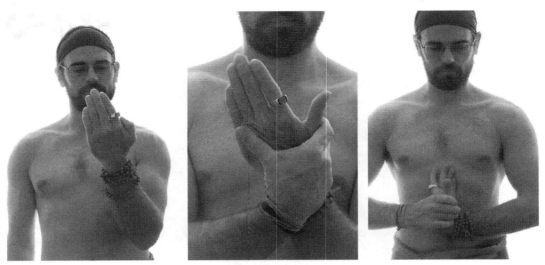

Look at the palm of one hand. Place the thumb of the other hand between the two outer metacarpal bones. Wrap the fingers over and grab the inside edge of the hand below the thumb joint. Push with the thumb, and pull with the fingers to twist the hand. Then lower the wrist toward the navel with both elbows bent out to the side. Lightly push the palm of the hand toward the forearm as the hand twists. Hold for 30 seconds, release, and then give the wrist a gentle squeeze.

Benefits: This pose and *parivrtta eka hastasana II* relieve stress in the wrists and increases the flow of synovial fluid to the articular cartilage when the positions are released.

342. Parivrtta Eka Hastasana II (revolved one hand pose II)

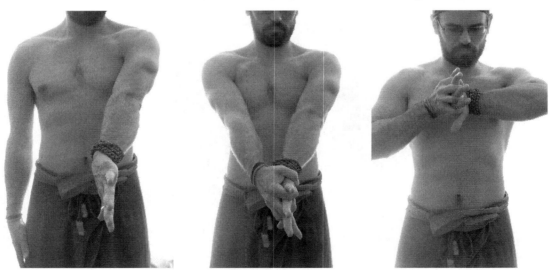

Extend one hand in front and turn the thumb down. Clasp on the back of the hand and push the palm toward the forearm then bring the wrist toward the chest. Lightly twist the fingers up and hold for 30 seconds, and then release and give the wrist a gentle squeeze.

343. Parivrtta Baddha Hastasana (revolved bound hand pose)

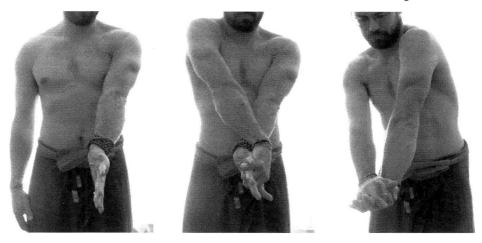

Extend one hand in front and turn the thumb down. Cross wrists and clasp hands palm to palm. Roll the bottom arm in and pull up with the top hand then push the wrist down.

Benefits: This pose stretches the top of the forearms and relieves stress in the wrists.
Modification: Extend the arms overhead while holding the clasp and twisting the arm.

CORE

344. Ardha Chaturanga Dandasana (half four limb staff pose)

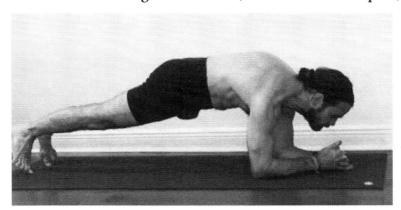

Place the elbows under the shoulders and clasp hands. Come onto the tips of the toes and strengthen the core. Draw the belly in and scoop the tailbone under. Hold the pose here or lean forward on inhalation and push back toward a dolphin pose on exhalation. This can be repeated to warm the body or as an alternative to inversions.

Benefits: This pose is a good substitute for plank pose if working with a wrist injury. It also can be used to strengthen the core and prepare for forearm stand.
Chakra: solar plexus

345. Vayu Vinyasa (wind flow)

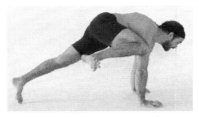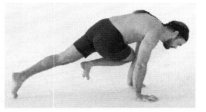

From plank position with the inhalation, bring one knee to the outside of one elbow and then twist and touch the opposite elbow on exhalation. Repeat several times or repeat the number found on the Dreamspell calendar for the tone of the day. From here, enter *trianga dandasana, chaturanga dandasan*a, or an arm balance.

Benefits: This core strengthening exercise also builds power in the arms and legs. It prepares the body for arm balances.
Contraindications: Avoid with high blood pressure or wrist injuries.
Modification: Use alternate hand positions to prevent stressing the wrists.
Chakra: sacral, solar plexus

346. Navasana (boat pose)

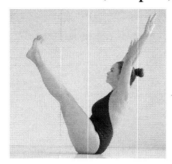

From sitting, lift the legs at a 45-degree angle and reach the arms parallel with the floor or straight up toward the ceiling. Flex the feet or activate *pada bandha.* Engage the quadriceps muscles and extend energy from the hips out through the heels.

Benefits: This pose strengthens the thighs, hip flexors, abdomen, and lower back. It stimulates abdominal organs, kidneys, prostate, and thyroid. It is beneficial for inguinal hernias. It aids in stress relief and improves balance.
Contraindications: Avoid with lumbar herniation.
Modification: Bend the knees and hold the back of the legs for support.
Chakra: sacral, throat

347. Ardha Navasana (half boat pose)

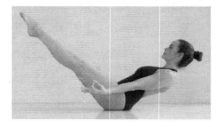

From *navasana,* lower halfway down. Point the feet and reach the arms straight ahead parallel with the floor.
Benefits: This pose strengthens the abdominals and lower back. It is beneficial for inguinal hernias.
Chakra: sacral, solar plexus

348. Parsva Navasana (side boat pose)

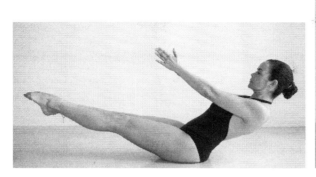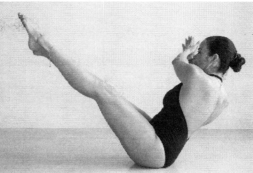

From *ardha navasana* position, lean over onto one hip and lift the legs up in that direction and reach the hands in the opposite direction. Deepen the twist at the end of the exhalation and then lower back down. Stay on the same hip and repeat up to 13 times, then switch sides.

Benefits: This pose strengthens the abdominals, obliques, and intercostal muscles.

Chakra: sacral, solar plexus

349. Supta Garudasana (supine eagle pose, "eagle crunches")

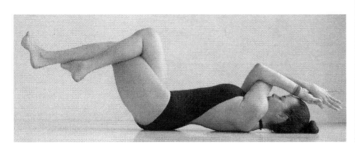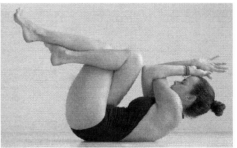

From a supine position, wrap one leg over the other and hook the ankle under if possible. The same arm as the top leg wraps under the opposite arm. Stretch yourself apart, taking the arms and legs away from each other, and then curl in, pushing the elbow into the top of the thigh. Squeeze the arms and legs together strong at the end of the exhalation. Open back up on inhalation, stretching apart, and then curl back in on the next exhalation. Repeat up to 13 times, then switch sides.

Benefits: This pose strengthens the abdominals.

Contraindication: Avoid with lumbar herniation.

Modification: Clasp hands behind head instead of wrapping arms if shoulders are tight.

Chakra: sacral, solar plexus

350. Urdhva Eka Padasana (upward one foot pose)

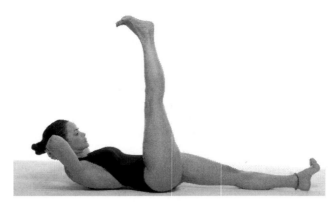

From a supine position, lift one leg straight up toward ceiling. Keep both legs straight and clasp hands behind the head. Lift the upper body on exhalation and hold the breath out for a few seconds. Rest the head back down on the inhalation. Switch legs and repeat up to 13 times.

Benefits: This pose strengthens the abdominals and the legs. It is beneficial for inguinal hernias.
Chakra: root, solar plexus

351. Urdhva Dwi Padasana (upward two foot pose)

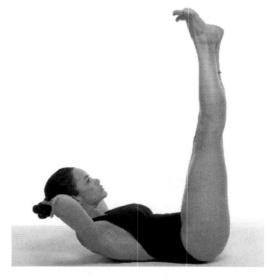

From a supine position, lift both legs straight up toward ceiling. Keep both legs straight, and then clasp hands behind the head. The upper body curls up on inhalation, and then the lower body curls up on exhalation. The shoulder blades and hips should be off of the floor at the end of exhalation. Hold the breath out for a few seconds, then inhale, and rest the head back down. Repeat up to 13 times.

Benefits: This pose strengthens the abdominals and inner thigh muscles. It is beneficial for inguinal hernias.
Modification: Place a block or blanket between the legs to recruit more strength.
Chakra: sacral, solar plexus

352. Supta Krishnasana (supine Krishna pose, "Krishna crunches")

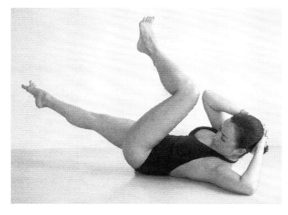 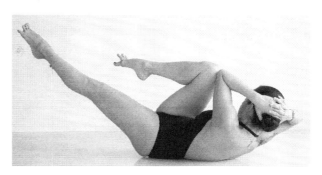

From a supine position, clasp hands behind the head and lift both feet off of the floor. Twist up on exhalation and bring the opposite knee to the opposite elbow. Hold the breath out and create a strong contraction. Switch sides on inhalation, and curl in on exhalation. Repeat up to 13 times.

Benefits: This pose strengthens the abdominals and hip flexors. It is beneficial for inguinal hernias.

Chakra: solar plexus

353. Pincha Araniasana (dragon tail pose, "dragon flags")

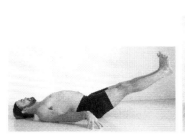 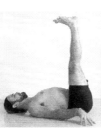 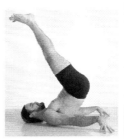 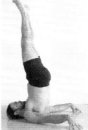 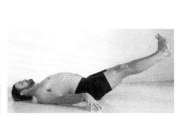

From a supine position with the legs together on the floor, extend the arms out to the side of the body on fingertips. Lift the legs perpendicular, then press down through the fingers and lift the hips. The legs can come overhead, but then straighten the body out, and extend the legs straight up toward the ceiling. Engage the core and hold the body upright at the end of the inhalation. On exhalation, slowly lower the hips down and then the legs, but the feet don't touch the floor. Lift the legs back up on inhalation and repeat up to 13 times.

Benefits: This pose strengthens the abdominals and lower back muscles.

Contraindications: Avoid with neck injury and during menstruation.

Chakra: solar plexus, throat

354. Supta Vayu Vinyasa (supine wind transition, "windshield wipers")

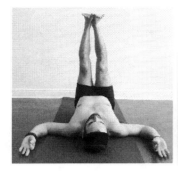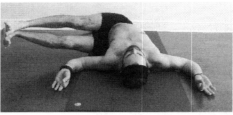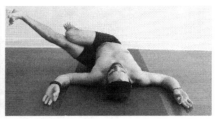

Lie flat on your back and bend the arms at 90-degree angles. Bring the shoulder blades in close toward the spine and extend the legs straight up toward the ceiling. Keep the shoulder blades flush to the floor and slowly lower the legs to one side. Don't let the legs touch the floor or the shoulders lift off of the floor. Stay focused on keeping the arms and shoulders pushing down strong. If it is too difficult with the legs straight, then bend the top leg or both legs if needed. Link the actions with the breath. Exhale over, and inhale up.

Benefits: This pose strengthens the abdominals, obliques, anterior serratus, and upper back muscles. It stabilizes the rotator cuff.
Contraindications: Avoid with lumbar herniation.
Modification: Place a blanket between the legs to develop inner thigh strength.
Chakra: solar plexus, heart

355. Supta Kali Vinyasa (supine Kali transitions, "Kali crunches")

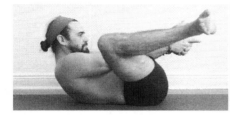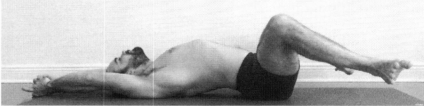

From a supine position, open the knees wide to the sides with the legs bent at 90-degree angles. Reach the arms overhead with hands clasped in *Kali mudra*. Arch the lower back and take a deep inhalation. On exhalation, curl in reaching the arms straight ahead, and bring the knees toward the shoulders. Hold the breath out, then inhale and repeat up to 13 times.

Benefits: This pose strengthens the abdominals, obliques, anterior serratus, and hip flexors.
Contraindications: Avoid with lumbar herniation.
Chakra: root, sacral

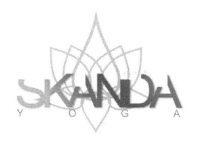

CHAPTER 14

Forward Folds, Twists, and Hip Openers

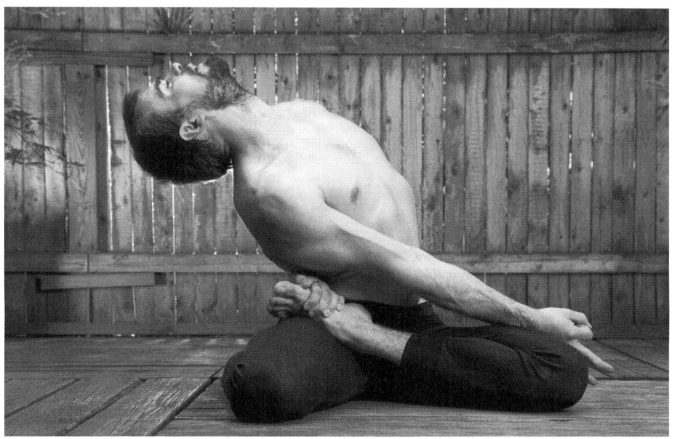

photo by Mauricio Velez

Forward folds and hip openers have a calming effect on the body as the parasympathetic nervous system is stimulated. Twists have a neutralizing effect energetically. They lengthen and extend the spine. Twists also have detoxifying effects for the internal organs. Hip openers are used to prepare for backbends, while forward folds and twists counterbalance backbends. Forward folds should be avoided if working with a spinal injury or back pain.

356. Dandasana (staff pose)

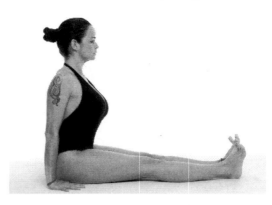

Extend both legs straight and place the hands beside the hips. Lengthen the spine and draw the navel in firming the lower abdomen. Curl the shoulders back and lift the heart up. Slide the lower jawbone back and release the palate. Activate the feet in *pada bandha*. Maintain core alignment with the pelvic floor toned and lower abdomen firm.

Benefits: This pose tones the legs, abdomen, and back muscles. It improves posture and stabilizes the pelvis. It activates the kidneys and removes bloating sensation.
Contraindications: Modify the pose if the hamstrings are tight and the lower back is rounding.
Modification: Place a folded blanket under the sitting bones. Increase blankets until the pelvis can return to neutral and the lower back can arch.
Chakra: root, sacral

357. Paschimottanasana I (west side stretch I, "forward bend")

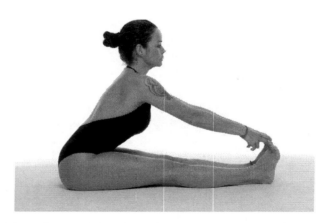

Extend both legs straight and bow forward, hooking the big toes with the first two fingers. Lengthen the spine and arch up. Bow forward, bending the elbows out to the side and squeeze the shoulder blades on the back. Keep the arms and shoulders pulling back. Curl in the upper back and extend the heart forward. Create a strong engagement in the quadriceps as you deepen the pose.

All of the following benefits, contraindications, modifications, and chakra innervation apply to all paschimottanasana poses I-IV.

Benefits: This pose tones the legs and stretches the back muscles. It improves posture and stabilizes the pelvis. It tones the kidneys, liver, spleen, and adrenal glands. It can be beneficial for managing prolapse, menstrual disorders, diabetes, colitis, and bronchitis. It activates the parasympathetic nervous system and increases relaxation.

Contraindications: Avoid rounding the lower back in this pose. Avoid with asthma, slipped disks, or sciatica.

Modification: Use a belt to hold the feet to keep the legs straight and strong. Place a blanket under the sitting bones if the lower back rounds to create more tilt in the pelvis.

Chakra: root, sacral

358. Paschimottanasana II (west side stretch II)

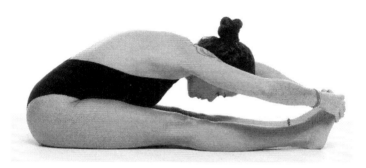

Assume *paschimottansana I* position and reach the hands for the outside edges of the feet. Pull back on the outside edges and extend the mounds of the feet forward. Bend the elbows out to the side and lift them up to engage the back body. Pull the shoulders down the back and sweep the heart forward. Keep the shoulders lifting above the ears as the pose is deepened.

Benefits: This pose strengthens the upper back integration.

359. Paschimottanasana III (west side stretch III)

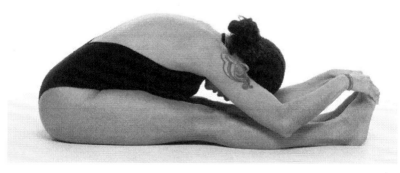

From *paschimottanasana II,* shift the hands to the tops of the feet and bend the elbows down toward the floor. Keep the arms active pulling against the feet and push the feet out into the hands. Create more strength in the legs and arms as you deepen the opening.

Benefits: This pose strengthens the stretches the upper back.

360. Paschimottanasana IV (west side stretch IV)

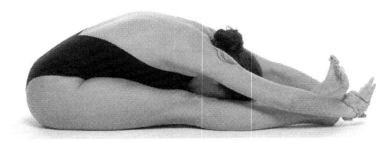

From *paschimottansana III,* clasp one wrist over the arches of the feet. Keep the arms and shoulders actively lifting above the ears as you deepen the pose. Hold a strong engagement in the legs and push the thighbones into the floor.

Benefits: This pose creates a deeper stretch for the lower back and more length for the hamstrings.

361. Parivrtta Paschimottanasana (revolved forward bend)

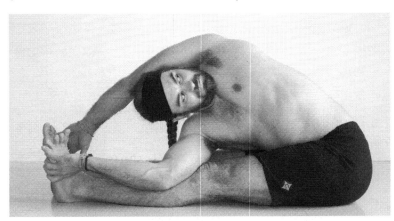

Assume *paschimottansana I* position and reach one arm across with the palm face up to the opposite leg. Hook the elbow over the outside of the shin, and grab the outside edge of the foot with the hand. Grab the outside edge of the opposite foot with the other hand. Duck the head under the top arm, and push it back to deepen the twist. Pull the hands against the feet and push the feet out to create a stronger engagement in the body to deepen the opening.

Benefits: This pose stretches the back and side body. It lengthens the latissimus dorsi muscles and hamstrings. It massages the abdominal organs and improves digestion.
Contraindications: Avoid with lumbar herniation.
Modification: Use a belt to hold the feet to keep the legs straight and strong.
Chakra: sacral, solar plexus

362. Uttana Paschimottanasana (intense forward bend)

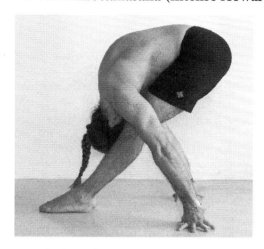

Assume *paschimottansana I* position and place the hands in front of the hips. Push down through the hands and lift the hips, and then slide the feet back toward the hips. Bow forward and rest the head on the legs. Engage the core strong to hold the pose.

Benefits: This pose strengthens the arms and abdominals. It stretches the back and neck.
Contraindications: Avoid with lumbar herniation.
Modification: Place blocks under the hands if you need more height to slide the legs back.
Chakra: sacral, brow

363. Ardha Baddha Padma Paschimottanasana (half bound lotus west side stretch)

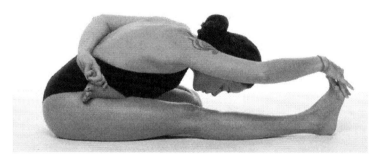

Assume *paschimottansana I* position and bring one leg into half lotus position. Reach the same arm behind the back and grab the foot. Bow forward and grab the foot of the straight leg. Bend the arm out to the side and pull the shoulder down the back.

Benefits: This pose opens the hips and lengthens the hamstrings. It relieves lower back stress and stretches the shoulders.
Contraindications: Avoid with lumbar herniation or medial collateral ligament injury in the knee.
Modification: Place a block or blanket under the knee of the bent leg to support the opening. Use a strap to hold the foot.
Chakra: sacral, brow

364. Trianga Mukhaikapada Pashimottanasana (three limbs face to one leg west side stretch)

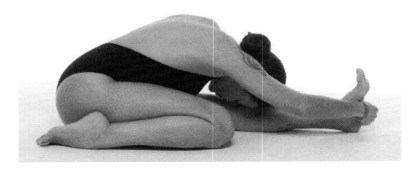

From *paschimottanasana,* bring one leg into *ardha vira* position. Both sitting bones should be evenly rooted. If the body tilts off to the side of the straight leg, then support the outer hip with a rolled towel so the hips are level. If there is discomfort in the knee, then sit on a block or blanket. Bow forward and reach both hands for the foot while keeping the arm bones lifting above the ears.

Benefits: This pose opens the thighs and lengthens the hamstrings. It relieves lower back stress and calms the nervous system.
Contraindications: Avoid with lumbar herniation or knee injury.
Modification: Place a blanket underneath the hip of the straight leg if the pelvis tilts over to that side.
Chakra: sacral, brow

365. Eka Pada Gomukha Paschimottanasana (one foot cow west side stretch)

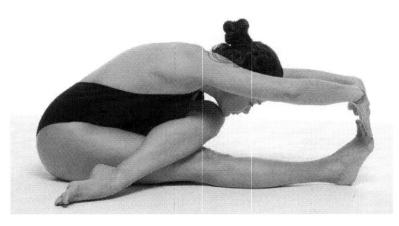

From *paschimottanasana,* cross one leg on top of the other and place the foot beside the opposite hip. Bow forward and grab the foot of the straight leg. Rest the chest on top of the leg, and hook the chin over the knee.

Benefits: This pose opens the outer hip rotators and lengthens the hamstrings. It relieves lower back stress and calms the nervous system.
Contraindications: Avoid with lumbar herniation.
Chakra: sacral, brow

366. Janu Sirsasana I (head to knee pose I)

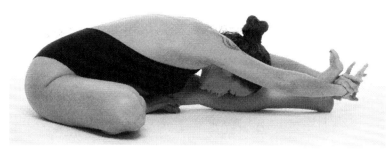

Extend one leg straight and bend the other out to the side. Place the foot against the inner thigh of the straight leg for a standard alignment and to build strength. For dynamic alignment, open the knee wider out to the side and turn the foot, sole face up, so it points toward the inner thigh of the straight leg. This allows the hips to open and decreases stress in the knee. Bow forward and clasp the foot. Lift the arms and shoulders up and extend the heart forward.

Benefits: This pose opens the hips and lengthens the hamstrings. It relieves lower back stress and calms the nervous system. It tones the liver, kidneys, and spleen.
Contraindications: Avoid with lumbar herniation or knee injury.
Modification: Place a blanket or block under the bent leg to support the knee.
Chakra: sacral, brow

367. Janu Sirsasana II (head to knee pose II)

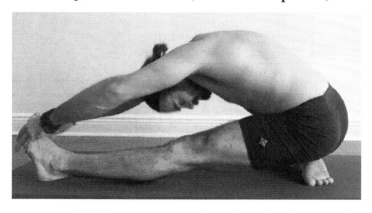

Assume *janu sirsasana I* position and lift the hips up to place the pelvic floor on the heel of the foot. The toes can point straight ahead or out to the side. This serves to awaken the *muladhara chakra*. Lift up from the hips and bow forward for the foot of the straight leg.

Benefits: This pose opens the hips and lengthens the hamstrings. It relieves lower back stress and calms the nervous system.
Contraindications: Avoid with lumbar herniation or knee injury.
Modification: Place a blanket underneath the hips.
Chakra: sacral, brow

368. Janu Sirsasana III (head to knee pose III)

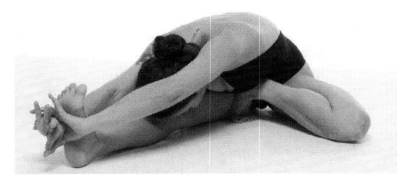

Assume *janu sirsasana I* position and turn the foot of the bent leg under with the foot flexed. The ball of the foot is flush with the floor, and the heel is pointing straight up. Bow forward for the foot. Keep the arm bones lifting and *uddiyana* engaged as the heel presses into the navel.

Benefits: This pose opens the hips and lengthens the hamstrings. It relieves lower back stress and calms the nervous system.
Contraindications: Avoid with lumbar herniation or knee injury.
Modification: Place a blanket under the hip to work the inner rotation of the thigh and placement of the foot.
Chakra: sacral, brow

369. Parivrtta Janu Sirsasana I (revolved head to knee pose I)

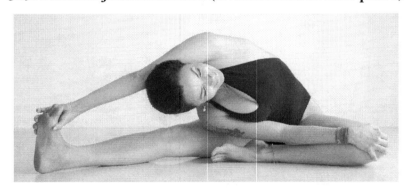

Assume *janu sirsasana I* position and reach the arm of the straight leg across and grab the opposite knee. The other arm reaches overhead for the big toe or outside edge of the foot. Pull with the hands and deepen the twist as the head ducks under the top arm.

Benefits: This pose opens the hips and lengthens the hamstrings. It stretches the obliques, intercostals, anterior serratus, and latissimus dorsi muscles. It massages the abdominal organs and improves digestion.
Contraindications: Avoid with lumbar herniation or knee injury.
Modification: Use a strap to hold the foot.
Chakra: sacral, solar plexus

370. Parivrtta Janu Sirsasana II (revolved head to knee pose II)

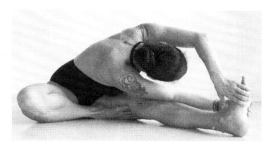

From *parivrtta janu sirsasana,* twist the opposite way for position II. Reach the arm of the bent leg across to the outside of the straight leg with palm face up. Grab the outside edge of the foot and reach the other arm overhead to grab the inside edge of the foot. Pull against the foot and push it forward to deepen the twist.

Benefits: This pose opens the hips and lengthens the hamstrings. It stretches the obliques, intercostals, anterior serratus, and latissimus dorsi muscles. It massages the abdominal organs and improves digestion.
Contraindications: Avoid with lumbar herniation or knee injury.
Modification: Place a blanket underneath the knee of the bent leg if it lifts and hold the foot of the straight leg with a strap.
Chakra: sacral, solar plexus

371. Bharadvajasana I (sage Bhardva's pose I)

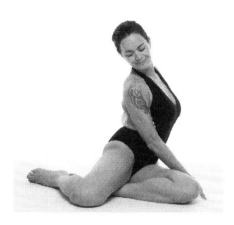

From sitting, bend the knees to one side and point the feet in the opposite direction. Place one hand behind the hips for support, and reach the other arm across to the outside of the thigh to initiate the twist. The head can stay twisting back over the leading shoulder or gaze down toward the feet to stretch the neck. To deepen the pose reach behind the back and grab the twisting arm.

Benefits: This pose opens the hips, lengthens the spine, and stretches the neck. Alleviates sciatica, backache, and stress. It improves digestion.
Contraindications: Avoid with lumbar herniation, headache, or insomnia.
Modification: Elevate the hips with blankets if the hips are tight.
Chakra: sacral, solar plexus

372. Bharadvajasana II (sage Bhardva's pose II)

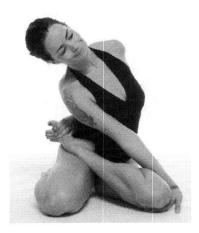

Bring one foot into *ardha virasana* position and the other into half lotus. Reach behind the back and grab the big toe. The opposite hand presses on the outside of the thigh to deepen the twist. Twist back over the leading shoulder for standard alignment or reach the ear toward the forward shoulder to stretch the neck.

Benefits: This pose opens the hips and stimulates the abdominal organs. It lengthens the spine in the dorsal and lumbar regions. It relieves tension in the neck and jaw. It alleviates sciatica, backache, and stress. It improves digestion.
Contraindications: Avoid with lumbar herniation, headache, or insomnia. Avoid with knee injury.
Modification: Elevate the hips with blankets or a block if the hips are tight. Place a towel under the ankle if experience discomfort. Hold the foot with a strap.
Chakra: sacral, solar plexus

373. Bharadvajasana III (sage Bhardva's pose III)

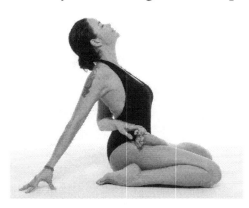

From *Bharadvajasana II,* hold onto the bound foot and reach the twisting arm behind you for position III. Arch up and curl back over the forearm. Unhinge the jaw and stretch the neck up.

Benefits: This pose tones the back muscles and spinal nerves. It opens the shoulders and hips. It stretches the abdomen and neck.
Contraindications: Avoid with headache or insomnia. Avoid with knee injury.
Modification: Elevate the hips with blankets or a block if the hips are tight, and use a block for the supporting hand. Hold the foot with a strap.
Chakra: sacral, heart

374. Ardha Matsyendrasana (lord of the fish pose prep)

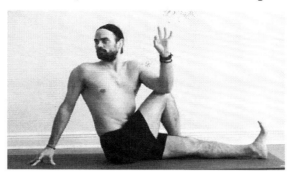

From sitting, extend one leg straight and cross the leg over with the knee pointing straight up. Extend the opposite arm up and arch the spine. Then twist and hook the arm over the opposite side of the leg.

Benefits: This pose tones the back muscles and spinal nerves. It stimulates the liver and kidneys. It alleviates sciatica, lumbago, fatigue, and menstrual discomfort.
Contraindications: Avoid with lumbar herniation or slipped disks.
Modification: Elevate the hips with blankets if the hips are tight. Place a block under the supporting hand to increase spinal extension.
Chakra: solar plexus

375. Ardha Matsyendrasana I (lord of the fish pose I)

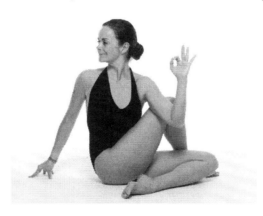

Bend one leg in and rest it on the floor. Cross the other leg over with the knee pointing straight up. Reach the arm of the top leg back in an elevated position for support. The opposite arm reaches across the outside of the elevated leg. Arch the lower back, lift the heart, and then push into the leg to deepen the twist. Outer rotate the hip to keep both sitting bones rooted.

Benefits: This pose tones the back muscles and spinal nerves. It stretches the outer hip rotators. It stimulates the liver and kidneys. It alleviates sciatica, lumbago, fatigue, and menstrual discomfort.
Contraindications: Avoid with lumbar herniation or slipped disks. Place a block under the supporting hand to increase spinal extension.
Modification: Elevate the hips with blankets if the hips are tight.
Chakra: solar plexus

376. Baddha Ardha Matsyendrasana (bound lord of the fish pose)

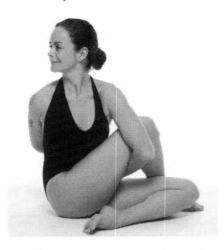

From *ardha Matsyendrasana,* inner rotate the twisting arm, and pass the wrist under the knee. The supporting hand then reaches behind the back to clasp. Keep the hip of the twisting leg outer rotating, so both sitting bones stay evenly weighted.

Benefits: This pose tones the back muscles and spinal nerves. It stretches the outer hip rotators and shoulders.
Contraindications: Avoid with shoulder injury, lumbar herniation, or slipped disks.
Modification: Elevate the hips with blankets if the hips are tight.
Chakra: solar plexus

377. Baddha Uttana Ardha Matsyendrasana (bound intense lord of the fish pose)

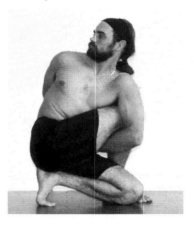

Curl the toes under of one foot and sit on the heel with the perineum resting directly on top. Cross the opposite leg over. Twist and wrap the arm under the elevated leg and clasp hands behind the back. Squeeze the arms together to deepen the twist.

Benefits: This pose tones the back muscles and spinal nerves. It stretches the outer hip rotators, shoulders, and toes. It develops balance and concentration.
Contraindications: Avoid with shoulder injury, knee, or ankle injury. Avoid with lumbar herniation.
Chakra: root, solar plexus

378. Ardha Matsyendrasana II (lord of the fish pose II)

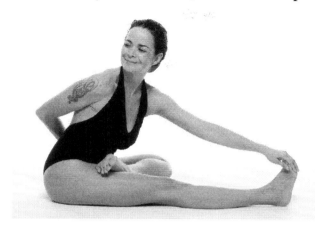

Extend one leg straight and bring the other foot on top of the thigh in half lotus position. Twist away from the bent leg and reach the opposite hand across for the outside edge of the foot of the straight leg. Reach the other hand behind the back for the thigh. Pull against the foot to deepen the twist.

Benefits: This pose opens the hips and relieves lower back tension.
Contraindications: Avoid with lumbar herniation or slipped disks.
Modification: Elevate the hips with blankets if the hips are tight. Use a strap to hold the foot.
Chakra: sacral, solar plexus

379. Ardha Matsyendrasana III (lord of the fish pose III)

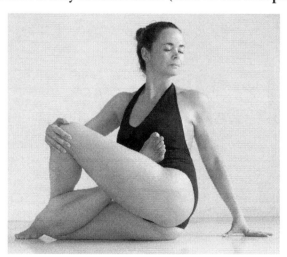

From *ardha Matsyendrasana II,* lean to the side of the bent leg and cross the opposite foot over the knee. Place one hand back for support, and hold the knee with the other hand. Arch up and lengthen the spine. Pull against the knee, outer rotate the elevated hip and deepen the twist.

Benefits: This pose opens the hips and relieves lower back tension.
Contraindications: Avoid with lumbar herniation or knee injury.
Chakra: sacral, solar plexus

380. Bhunamananasana (saluting mother earth pose)

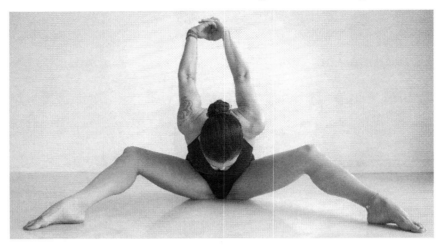

From sitting, bend both knees up and widen the legs apart. Place the feet flat on the floor. Clasp hands behind the back and arch up. Bow forward and take the head toward the floor.

Benefits: This pose opens the hips and relieves lower back tension. It stretches the shoulders and the upper back.
Contraindications: Avoid with lumbar herniation.
Modification: Elevate the hips with blankets if the hips are tight. Use a strap to hold the hands.
Chakra: root, sacral

381. Upavishta Konasana (seated wide angle pose)

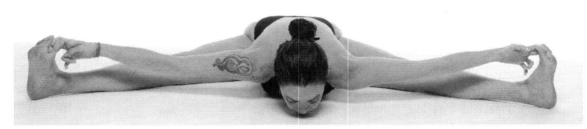

From sitting with the legs wide apart, clear the sitting bones first, and then manually inner rotate each thigh to clear the hamstrings. Flex or floint the feet and activate the leg muscles. Arch the lower back and tilt the top of the pelvis forward. Maintain the extension of the spine as you bow forward. Lift the arms and pull the shoulders down the back, as the heart moves forward. Reach out and grab the big toes with the first two fingers.

Benefits: This pose opens the hips and relieves lower back tension. It lengthens the hamstrings and stretches the adductor muscles. It calms the nervous system and stimulates the ovaries.
Contraindications: Avoid with lumbar herniation.
Modification: Elevate the hips with blankets if the hips are tight. Use straps to hold the feet.
Chakra: sacral

382. Parivrtta Upavishta Konasana (revolved seated wide angle pose)

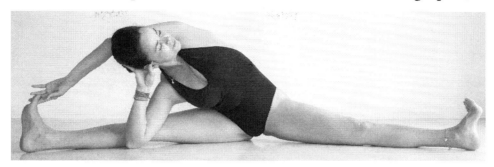

From *upavishta konasana,* reach one arm overhead for the opposite foot. Place the elbow on the floor on the inside of the leg to support the head with the other hand. Push the hand up into the head and then push the head back into the top arm to deepen the twist.

Benefits: This pose stretches the side body muscles of the obliques, anterior serratus, and intercostals. It also stretches the back muscles of the latissimus dorsi and quadratus lumborum. It lengthens the hamstrings and opens the shoulders.
Contraindications: Avoid with lumbar herniation.
Modification: Elevate the hips with blankets if the hips are tight. Use a strap to hold the foot.
Chakra: solar plexus

383. Samakonasana (even angle pose)

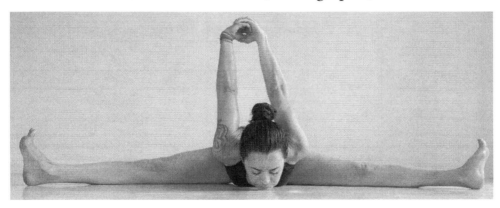

From *upavishta konasana,* take the feet wider apart, so the legs are at a 180-degree angle. Bow forward and rest the chin on the floor. Clasp hands behind the back or bring the hands into reverse prayer position. Push the middle of the back down as you stretch the chin forward.

Benefits: This pose opens the hips, shoulders, and throat. It stretches the adductors and lengthens the hamstrings. It releases lower back tension and stimulates the kidneys. It increases circulation to reproductive organs.
Contraindications: Avoid with lumbar herniation or knee injury.
Modification: Elevate the hips with blankets if the hips are tight. Use a strap to hold the hands.
Chakra: sacral, throat

384. Rajasamakonasana (royal even angle pose)

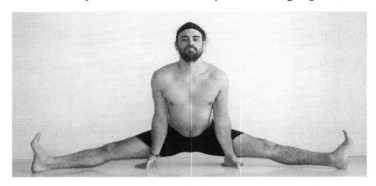

From *prasarita padottanasana V* position, lift the torso upright and bring the hands in front of the inner thighs. Place the hands in reverse ridgetop or fist position and outer rotate the arms. Outer rotate the legs, lifting the toes, and press down through the heels. Move the hips forward and bring the legs into a 180-degree opening. Bend the elbows and press the forearms into the inner thighs and press the legs into the arms. Tilt the pelvis forward and slowly let the hips sink down to increase the opening.

Benefits: This pose creates strength in the legs and arms. It opens the hips and releases lower back tension. It stretches the adductors and lengthens the hamstrings.
Contraindications: Avoid with knee injury.
Modification: Use blocks or blankets under the feet to work the scientific stretching technique of shutdown threshold isometrics.
Chakra: root, sacral

385. Eka Hasta Raja Samakonasana (one hand royal even angle pose)

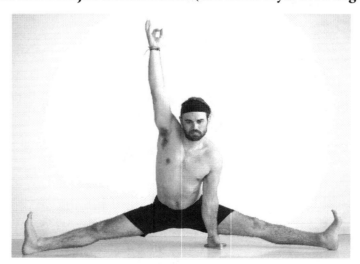

From *raja samakonasana,* reach one hand for the ceiling and hold, and then switch arms.

Benefits: This pose has the same benefits as *rajasamakonasana* but recruits more strength from the arms and legs.
Contraindications: Avoid with knee injury.
Chakra: root, sacral

386. Kurmasana (tortoise pose)

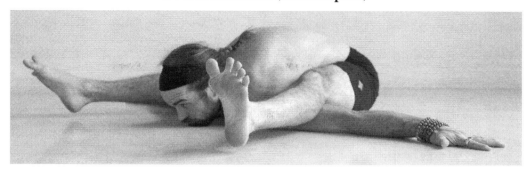

From *upavishta konasana,* bend the knees and slide the arms underneath. The arms are completely flat with palms face down. Engage the thigh muscles and straighten the legs. Lift the heels off of the floor and squeeze the shins into the center.

Benefits: This pose creates strength in the legs and opens the hips. It increases circulation in the spine and calms the nervous system. It tones the abdominal organs and stimulates the pancreas.
Contraindications: Avoid with knee or hamstring injury. Avoid placing pressure on the elbows.
Modification: Keep the legs bent until the arms are over the shoulders and the chest is flat.
Chakra: sacral, throat

387. Supta Kurmasana (sleeping tortoise pose)

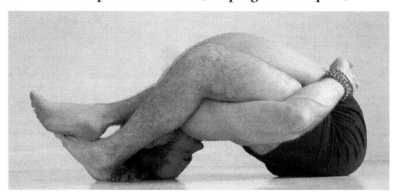

From *kurmasana,* bend the legs and slide the ankles toward each other. Lift the head, cross ankles, and then duck the head under. Clasp hands behind the back.

Benefits: This pose opens the hips and stretches the back muscles. It calms the nervous system and initiates *pratyahara.*
Contraindications: Avoid with lower back injury.
Modification: Bring one leg behind the head at a time or use a strap to hold hands.
Chakra: sacral, crown

388. Balasana (child's pose)

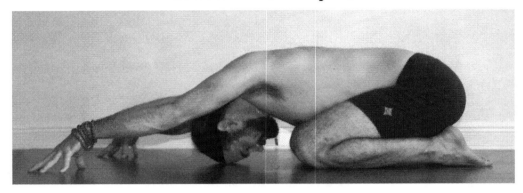

Sit back on the heels and take the knees wide apart. Reach the arms in front of you with the hands in fingertip position. Lift the arms and shoulders away from the floor. Release the neck and the heart.

Benefits: This pose tones the upper back and expands the lungs. It releases lower back tension and calms the nervous system. It reduces stress and fatigue.
Contraindications: Avoid with knee or hip flexor injury.
Modification: Rest the hips on a bolster or block to reduce pressure in the knees. Place blankets over the thighs to prevent resting down all of the way, which can irritate the hip flexors if strained.
Chakra: sacral, brow

389. Salamba Balasana (supported child's pose)

Sit back on the heels and take the knees wide apart. Stack the fists up in front of you and rest the forehead down. This allows the neck muscles to relax but keeps the spine neutral, which is more beneficial after a long headstand or several backbends.

Benefits: This pose releases tension in the upper and lower back.
Contraindications: Avoid with knee or hip flexor injury.
Modification: Rest the hips on a bolster or block to reduce pressure in the knees. Place blankets over the thighs to prevent resting down all of the way, which can irritate the hip flexors if strained.
Chakra: sacral, brow

390. Virasana (hero's pose)

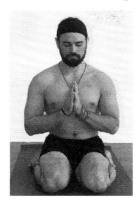

Come to kneeling on the mat and spread the calves evenly by sliding the thumbs down the head of the muscles as you sit back between the feet. Push down through the pinky toes and squeeze the heels in toward the outer hips. Sit on a block or blanket if necessary to relieve pressure in the knees.

Benefits: This pose stretches the quadriceps. It opens the knees and the ankles. It increases synovial fluid to the cartilage and connective tissue. It relieves pressure on the heart and improves digestion. It alleviates varicose veins, rheumatic pains in the knee, and gout.
Contraindications: Avoid sitting all of the way down if there is stress in the knees or ankles. Avoid turning the feet out to the sides.
Modification: Sit on a bolster or block to reduce pressure in the knees. Place a towel or blanket under the ankles to reduce pressure. A small rolled towel can be placed tightly in the knee pits to increase space in the joint.
Chakra: root, sacral

391. Vajrasana (diamond pose)

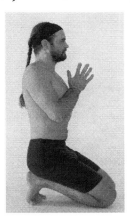

Curl the toes under and sit on the heels to stretch the toes and open the *nadis* of the feet. Transition between *vajrasana* and *virasana* to lubricate and open the knee joint. This pose is also good for creating more *tapas* and inner heat for meditation.

Benefits: This pose stretches the quadriceps and toes. It increases the arches of the feet and opens the knees.
Contraindications: Avoid sitting all of the way down if there is stress in the knees or feet.
Modification: Sit on a bolster or on stacked blocks to reduce pressure in the knees.
Chakra: root, sacral

392. Sukhasana (sweet pose)

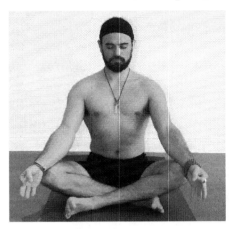

From sitting, cross the legs in front of you so the shins are supported by the opposite heel. Activate the feet and push the outside edges into the floor, so the ankles stay aligned with the shins. The tops of the knees are aligned with the top of the pelvis. If the knees are higher than the pelvis, then elevate the hips by sitting on a prop.

Benefits: This pose increases physical relaxation and mental alertness. It is beneficial for meditation and *pranayama*.
Contraindications: Avoid sitting with the knees higher than the top of the pelvis. Avoid rounding the lower back or excessive arching.
Modification: Sit on a bolster, blanket, or block to lift the hips and bring the pelvis into a neutral position.
Chakra: root, sacral

393. Siddhasana (spiritual power pose)

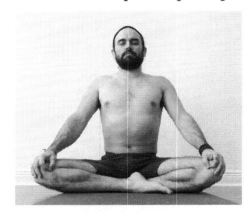

From sitting, place one heel under the perineum and cross the other leg in front. Maintain an internal lift from the pelvic floor during meditation.

Benefits: This pose increases physical relaxation and mental alertness. It is beneficial for meditation and *pranayama*. It tones the lower back and the abdominals.
Contraindications: Avoid with knee injury.
Modification: Sit on a bolster, blanket, or block to lift the hips and bring the pelvis into a neutral position.
Chakra: root, sacral

394. Siddhasana II (spiritual power pose II)

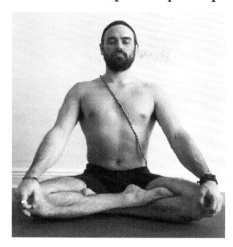

From sitting, place the top of one foot in the knee pit of the opposite leg. Reach underneath that leg and grab the top of the opposite foot. Pull it up and over the bottom calf.

Benefits: This pose balances the pelvic floor and synergistically engages *mula bandha*. It is beneficial for meditation and *pranayama*. It tones the lower back and the abdominals.
Contraindications: Avoid with knee injury.
Chakra: root, sacral

395. Gomukhasana (cow face prep pose)

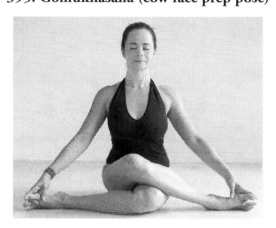

Cross one leg over the other with one knee on top of the other, and the feet beside the opposite hip. Shift the hips off to the side of the bottom leg an inch or two, so that both sitting bones are evenly weighted. Hook the big toes with the first two fingers, arch up, and lengthen the spine.

Benefits: This pose opens the outer hip rotators. It increases circulation to the reproductive organs.
Contraindications: Avoid with hip replacement.
Modification: Sit on a bolster, blanket, or block to lift the hips and remove stress from the knees or ankles.
Chakra: root, sacral

396. Gomukhasana I (cow face pose I)

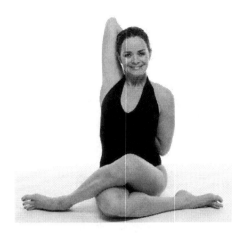

From *gomukhasana* prep, bring the same arm as the top leg behind the back with the pinky finger side of the hand turned in. Reach the other arm in front of you then draw the arm bone back into the shoulder socket. Bend the arm overhead and clasp hands.

Benefits: This pose opens the outer hip rotators. It stretches the triceps, supraspinatus and infraspinatus rotator cuff muscles.
Contraindications: Avoid with hip replacement.
Modification: Sit on a bolster, blanket, or block to lift the hips and remove stress from the knees or ankles. Use a strap to clasp the hands.
Chakra: root, sacral

397. Gomukhasana II (cow face pose II)

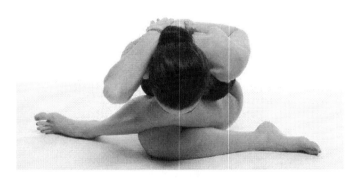

Assume *gomukhasana I* position and fold forward while pulling up on the hands. Push down through the pinky toes and release tension in the hips.

Benefits: This pose releases outer hip tension. It stretches the triceps, supraspinatus and infraspinatus rotator cuff muscles.
Contraindications: Avoid with hip replacement or shoulder injury. Do not fold forward if you have to sit on props for *gomukhasana I* position.
Modification: Use a strap to clasp hands.
Chakra: sacral, throat

398. Garuda Gomukhasana (eagle cow face pose)

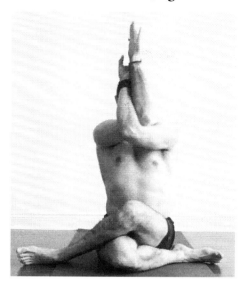

From *gomukhasana* prep position, wrap the same arm as the top leg under the opposite arm, and reach the arms up toward the ceiling. From here, perform the *uttana garuda bhujasana* series by extending the arms to the right, left, and down.

Benefits: This pose opens the outer hip rotators and releases IT band tension. It stretches the rotator cuff muscles.
Contraindications: Avoid with hip replacement or shoulder injury.
Chakra: root, heart

399. Swastikasana (auspicious pose)

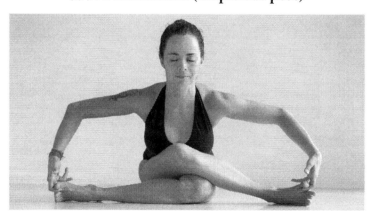

From *gomukhasana* prep, slide the feet forward and bring the shins into a single line. Pull up on the big toes and push the pinky toes down into the floor. Bow forward while keeping the arms and shoulders lifting up.

Benefits: This pose opens the outer hip rotators and releases IT band tension.
Contraindications: Avoid with hip replacement.
Chakra: root, sacral

400. Eka Pada Rajakapotasana (one leg king pigeon prep pose)

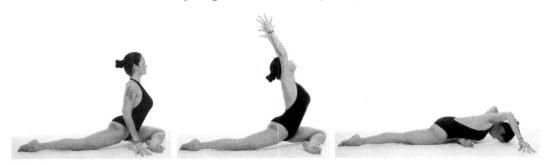

Bring one leg forward with the thigh parallel with the outer edge of the mat, or take the knee wider to deepen the opening. Inner rotate the back leg, bring it in toward the midline, and then slide it back. The back leg should be straight and parallel with the outer edge of the mat. Point the foot to increase flexibility, or curl the toes under to increase strength in the pose. Place the hands beside the hips and push down through the knees, squeeze the legs toward each other, and lift up out of the hips as they square forward. Reach the arms overhead to increase muscle energy in the legs. Then bow forward and push the hips down. Place the hands in fingertip position in front of you and lift the elbows and shoulders up.

Benefits: This pose strengthens the thighs and ankles. It stretches the outer hips and the hip flexors. It stimulates the adrenals, thyroid and parathyroid. It alleviates disorders of the urinary system and enhances *bramacharya*.

Contraindications: Avoid with knee injury.

Modification: Place a blanket or block under the hip of the forward leg to keep the pelvis level and to relieve pressure in the knee.

Chakra: sacral, heart

401. Parivrtta Eka Pada Kapotasana (revolved one leg pigeon pose)

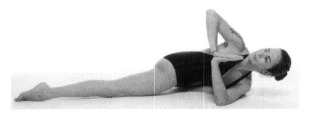

From pigeon preparation, lean off to the side of the expanding leg and pull the foot up with the shin parallel with the top edge of the mat. Grab the foot and pull yourself across to hook the elbow or the shoulder into the arch of the foot. Place the hands in prayer position. Push down through the hands and deepen the twist. Push down through the grounding leg and keep the thigh inner rotating.

Benefits: This pose stretches the outer hips and relieves lower back tension. It massages the abdominal organs and improves digestion.

Contraindications: Avoid with knee injury.

Modification: Place the top hand on the pelvis to deepen the pose instead of having the hands in prayer position. Push in on the hip and roll it down toward the floor to increase the stretch in the opposite hip.

Chakra: sacral, heart

402. Eka Bhuja Padma Eka Pada Kapotasana (one arm lotus one leg pigeon pose)

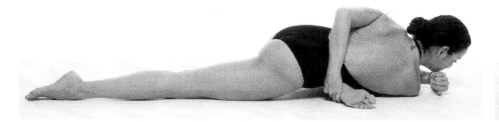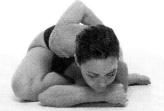

From pigeon preparation, reach behind the back and grab the heel. Pull up on the heel and push the pinky toe down. Bend the other arm and place the elbow under the opposite shoulder. Make a fist and hook the chin over the wrist with the thumb pointing straight down. Lean the shoulders forward and push the wrist into the floor.

Benefits: This pose stretches the outer hips and opens the shoulders.
Contraindications: Avoid with knee or shoulder injury.
Modification: If the heel is unavailable, then grab the big toe or use a strap to hold the foot.
Chakra: sacral, throat

403. Vamadevasana I (sage Vamadeva's pose I)

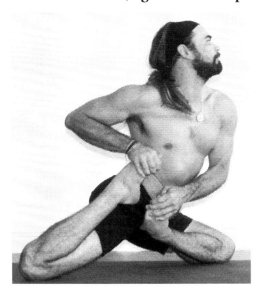

From *eka pada rajakapotasana* prep, reach for the inside edge of the back foot and bring it into a quad stretch with the foot beside the hip. Reach down and grab the foot of the front leg. Squeeze the legs toward each other, lift the hips, and then bring the feet toward each other.

Benefits: This pose stretches the thighs. It tones the spine and gluteal muscles. It prevents impotence.
Contraindications: Avoid with knee injury.
Chakra: root, sacral

404. Vamadevasana II (sage Vamadeva's pose II)

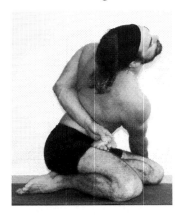

Bring one leg into *ardha mulabandhasana*. Inner rotate the leg and sit on the heel with the toes pointing behind you. Bring the other leg into *ardha padma* position and clasp the big toe behind the back. Reach the opposite arm across and deepen the twist.

Benefits: This pose opens the hips and stretches the shoulders. It massages the abdominal organs and improves digestion. It relieves neck and jaw tension.
Contraindications: Avoid with knee injury.
Chakra: root, solar plexus

405. Agnistambhasana I (fire log pose I)

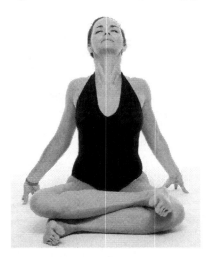

From sitting, stack one shin on top of the other with the opposite ankle aligned with the opposite knee. Flex the top foot and lock it off on the outside edge of the bottom thigh. Push energy out from the mound of the big toe and pull the pinky toes back. Take the hands behind the hips and arch up. If the top knee lifts, push it down with one hand, and then twist slightly and lean back away from that leg.

Benefits: This pose stretches the outer hip rotators and the hip flexors. It reduces mental tension and calms the mind.
Contraindications: Avoid with knee injury.
Modification: Elevate the hips with a blanket if the lower back rounds.
Chakra: root, sacral

406. Agnistambhasana II (fire log pose II)

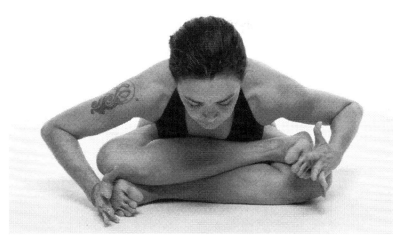

Assume *agnistambhasana I* position and place the hands on the balls of the feet. Push in with the hands and out through the balls of the feet. If the top knee is still elevated, then cross-grab the feet with the hands. Pull into the center as the feet push out. This increases muscle energy and brings the thighbones deeper into the hip sockets, which allows the hips to open and release tension.

Benefits: This pose stretches the outer hip rotators. It reduces mental tension and calms the mind.
Contraindications: Avoid with knee injury.
Chakra: root, sacral

407. Agnistambhasana III (fire log pose III)

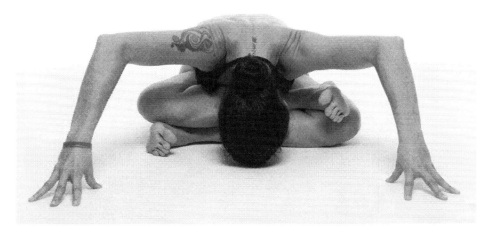

From *agni stambhasana II,* reach the arms straight ahead and rest the chest over the legs. Maintain the engagement in the feet to keep the ankles, shins, and knees aligned. Lift the elbows up to engage the upper back and open the heart.

408. Parivrtta Agnistambhasana I (revolved fire log I pose)

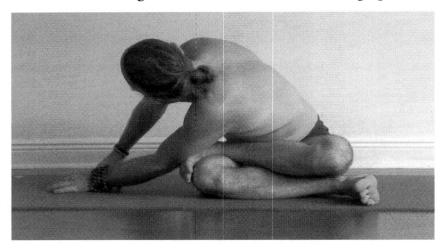

From *agni stambhasana III,* reach the arm across and hook it over the sole of the foot. Place the forearm on the floor and the other hand on fingertips out wide. Push the arm into the foot and then press down through the fingers to deepen the twist.

Benefits: This pose stretches the outer hip rotators and the quadratus lumborum. It releases lower back tension and stimulates the internal organs.
Contraindications: Avoid with knee injury. Avoid deepening the twist if the knee lifts up off of the bottom ankle.
Chakra: sacral, solar plexus

409. Parivrtta Agnistambhasana II (revolved fire log II pose)

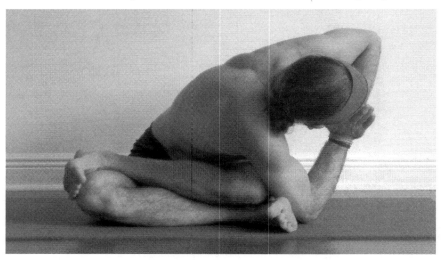

From *parivrtta agni stambhasana* position, lift up and twist in the opposite direction. Bring the hands into prayer position and press down to deeper the twist.

410. Baddha Konasana I (bound angle pose I)

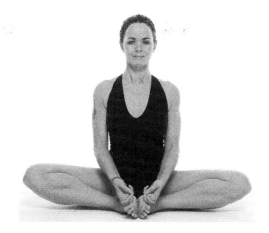

Bring both feet together in front of you and open the knees out to the side. Push the heels and balls of the feet together, and then clasp the big toes with the first two fingers. Arch the spine and tilt the pelvis forward. Press the outer edges of the feet together to lift the heels and create more external rotation.

Benefits: This pose stretches the outer hip rotators and the adductors. It stabilizes the pelvis and balances the brain hemispheres. It relieves tension from sciatica and tones the reproductive organs. It stimulates the kidneys and prostate.
Contraindications: Avoid with knee injury.
Modification: Elevate the hips with a blanket if the lower back rounds and the knees are elevated.
Chakra: root, sacral

411. Baddha Konasana II (bound angle pose II)

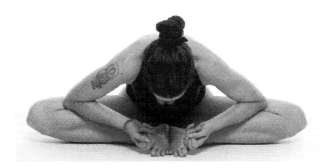

Assume *baddha konasana I* position and then bow forward over the feet. Push the elbows down into the thighs. Pull up on the feet as the feet push down into the floor. Squeeze the outer edges of the feet together and let the heels lift and widen apart.

Benefits: This pose stretches the outer hip rotators and the adductors. It strengthens the feet and the ankles. It relieves lower back tension.
Contraindications: Avoid with knee injury. Avoid if the knees are lifting.
Modification: If the knees are lifting, then slide the feet forward and perform *tarasana* (star pose).
Chakra: root, sacral

412. Baddha Konasana III (bound angle pose III)

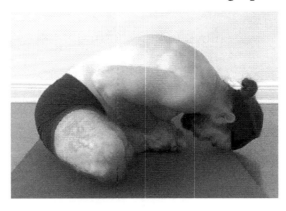

From *baddha konasana II* position, continue bowing forward over the feet. Pull up strongly on the feet and take the head to the floor. From here, squeeze the elbows into the ribcage.

Benefits: This pose stretches the outer hip rotators and the adductors. It strengthens the abdominals, feet, and the ankles. It relieves lower back tension.
Contraindications: Avoid with knee or ankle injury.
***Chakra*:** root, sacral

413. Ardha Mulabandhasana (half root lock pose)

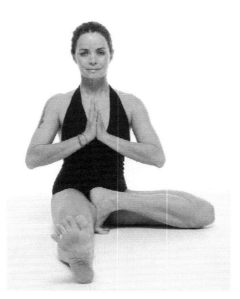

From *baddha konasana,* extend one leg straight and inner rotate the opposite leg. Flex the foot and place the ball of the foot flat on the floor. Bring the hands in prayer position or bow forward for *janu sirsasana III.*

Benefits: This pose opens the hips and ankles. It stretches the feet.
Contraindications: Avoid with knee or ankle injury.
***Chakra*:** root, sacral

414. Mulabandhasana I (root lock pose I)

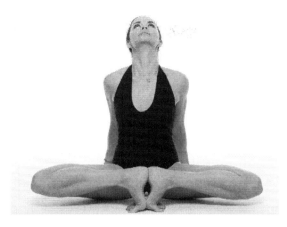

From *baddha konasana,* press the feet together, inner rotate the thighs, and lift the heels straight up. Place the hands behind the back to support the opening of the hips moving forward and down. To deepen the opening, the hands can come forward into prayer position, or clasp hands behind the back and extend the arms up.

Benefits: This pose opens the hips and ankles. It stretches the feet.
Contraindications: Avoid with knee or ankle injury.
Chakra: root, sacral

415. Mulabandhasana II (root lock pose II)

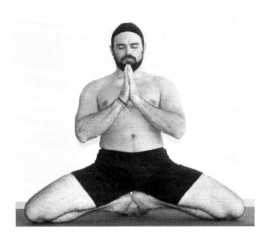

Assume *mulabandhasana I* position and turn the feet under. Arch up and tilt the pelvis forward. Lift the hips and increase the inner rotation of the thighs. Sit on the outside edges of the heels and maintain an internal lift with the *mula bandha.*

Benefits: This pose opens the hips and ankles. It tones the reproductive organs. It induces *mula bandha* and is used to awaken the *muladhara chakra.*
Contraindications: Avoid with knee or ankle injury.
Chakra: root, sacral

416. Tarasana (star pose)

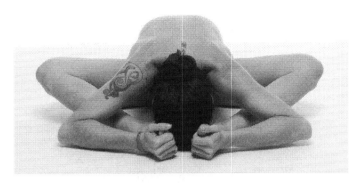

From *baddha konasana,* slide the feet forward and hold onto the feet. Pull yourself forward from the waistline. Rest the head in the arches of the feet or keep the head pushing up to deepen the opening. Hook the elbows over the legs and bend them out to the sides on the floor. The body is in the form of a 6-pointed star.

Benefits: This pose opens the hips and relieves lower back tension. It calms the nervous system and induces relaxation.
Contraindications: Avoid with lower back injury.
Chakra: root, sacral

417. Parivrtta Tarasana (revolved star pose, "stargazer")

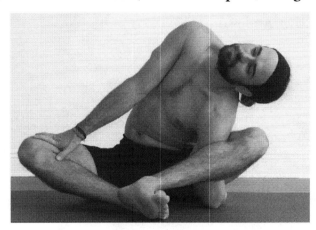

From *tarasana,* hook one foot on top of the other, and wrap the same arm under the leg. Rest the forearm on the floor and push the opposite knee down with the free hand. Lean away from the leg to stretch the adductors, and lengthen up out of the hip to stretch the side body. Release the ear toward the shoulder, and unhinge the jaw to stretch the neck.

Benefits: This pose opens the hips. It stretches the neck and the sides of the body. It releases tension from the quadratus lumborum, obliques, and anterior serratus muscles.
Contraindications: Avoid with lumbar herniation.
Chakra: root, sacral

418. Parivrtta Baddha Tarasana (revolved bound star pose)

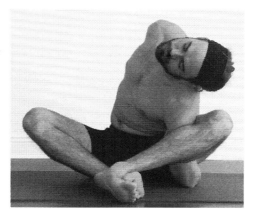

From *parvritta tarasana,* reach the free arm back and clasp hands. Lean onto the grounding forearm and release the head toward the shoulder. Unhinge the jaw and stretch the neck.

Benefits: This pose opens the shoulders and hips. It stretches the neck and the sides of the body. It releases tension from the quadratus lumborum, obliques, and anterior serratus muscles.
Contraindications: Avoid with lumbar herniation.
Modification: Use a strap for the hands to clasp.
Chakra: root, sacral

419. Surya Yantrasana I (sun dial pose I)

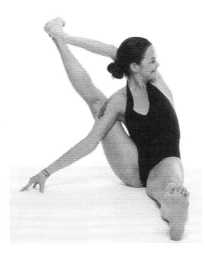

Bring one leg over the arm and extend the hand out to the side for support. Grab the outside edge of the foot with the opposite hand. Bow forward, inner rotate the thigh, and straighten the leg. Then outer rotate the thigh and push out through the heel. Duck the head under the expanding arm and twist away from the expanding leg.

Benefits: This pose opens the hips. It stretches the hamstrings, intercostals, and shoulders.
Contraindications: Avoid with hamstring injury.
Modification: Use blankets under the hips and a strap to hold the foot.
Chakra: root, throat

420. Surya Yantrasana II (sun dial pose II)

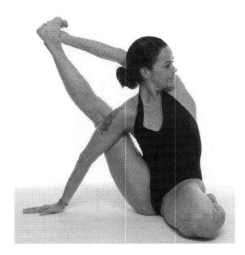

Fold one leg back with the foot beside the hip in *ardha vira* position. Grab the outside edge of the foot with the opposite hand. Bow forward, lift the hips off of the floor, and inner rotate the expanding leg. Then straighten the leg fully, rest the hips back down, and push out through the foot.

Benefits: This pose opens the hips. It stretches the hamstrings, intercostals, and shoulders.
Contraindications: Avoid with hamstring injury.
Modification: Use blankets under the hips and a strap to hold the foot.
Chakra: root, throat

421. Krounchasana I (heron pose I)

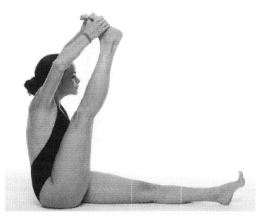

Extend one leg straight up and grab the ankle or the ball of the foot with both hands. Resist the stretch initially to engage the leg muscles. Push the thighbone away from the hip and then bring the leg closer to the chest. Pull down on the leg with the hands to lift and open the heart.

Benefits: This pose stretches the hamstrings. It stimulates the abdominal organs and the heart.
Contraindications: Avoid with hamstring injury.
Modification: Use blankets under the hips and a strap to hold the foot.
Chakra: root, heart

422. Krounchasana II (heron pose II)

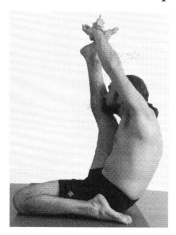

Fold one leg back with the foot beside the hip in *ardha vira* position. Grab the foot of the expanding leg on the outside edges or clasp hands over the foot in *jnana mudra*. Pull the leg and arm bones down. Extend the spine and lift the heart up.

Benefits: This pose stretches the thighs and the hamstrings. It stimulates the abdominal organs and the heart. It opens the knees and the ankles.
Contraindications: Avoid with hamstring or knee injury.
Modification: Use blankets under the hips and a strap to hold the foot.
Chakra: root, heart

423. Parivrtta Krounchasana (revolved heron pose)

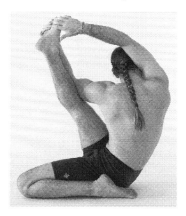

From *krounchasana,* grab the outside of the elevated foot with the opposite hand. The other hand can be placed behind the back for support if needed. If not, then hook the elbow on the outside of the shin with the palm face up. Grab the foot overhead with the other hand and duck the head under to deepen the twist.

Benefits: This pose stretches the thighs and the outer hip rotators. It releases tension in the IT band. It stimulates the abdominal organs and the heart. It opens the knees and the ankles.
Contraindications: Avoid with hamstring or knee injury.
Modification: Use blankets under the hips and a strap to hold the foot.
Chakra: root, heart

424. Marichiasana I (sage Marichi's pose I)

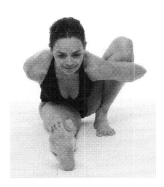

From sitting, extend one leg straight and bend the other leg in with the foot placed in line with the outer edge of the hip. Bow forward and wrap the arm around the leg to clasp hands behind the back. Use a strap to maintain the bind if necessary. Push the head up, fold forward, and then release the head to the knee. The sitting bone of bound leg will be off of the floor. To deepen all clasps, the wrapping arm can grab the extending arm's wrist, and then pull the arm straight. Marichi was a son of Brahma.

Benefits: This pose opens the hips and tones the thighs. It stretches the shoulders and the dorsal region of the spine. It lengthens the hamstrings and improves circulation to the abdominal organs. It stimulates the kidneys and the liver.
Contraindications: Avoid clasping with shoulder injury. Avoid bowing forward with lumbar herniation.
Modification: Elevate the hips with blankets if the extended leg wants to bend or turn out to the side.
Chakra: root, sacral

425. Marichiasana II (sage Marichi's pose II)

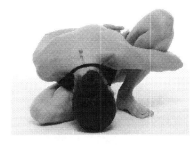

Place one foot on top of the opposite thigh in *ardha padma* position. Bend the other knee up with the foot aligned with the outer edge of the hip. If the knee of the leg in half lotus is on the floor, then bow forward, wrap, and clasp. If the knee hovers off the floor, then lift the hips and angle the knee down. Rest the hip back down, bow over the knee, and slowly move towards the center using the hands in front for support and let the hip release. You should never feel any pressure or stress in the knee in any pose.

Benefits: This pose opens the hips and releases neck tension. It stretches the shoulders and the dorsal region of the spine. It stimulates the kidneys, liver, spleen, and the abdominal organs. It activates parasympathetic nervous system and releases mental tension.
Contraindications: Avoid clasping with shoulder injury. Avoid with knee or ankle injury.
Modification: If the knee wants to lift off the floor, then bow over the bent leg instead of forward. If there is stress in the knee or the ankle, then place the foot on the floor underneath the opposite leg.
Chakra: root, brow

426. Marichiasana III (sage Marichi's pose III)

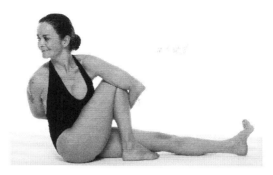

Assume *Marichiasana I* position and place the hand of the bent leg back for support on fingertips or ridgetop position. Arch the lower back up and in, then take the opposite arm across to the outside of the leg. Push the knee across the midline and outer rotate the hip. Wrap the arm around the leg and clasp hands behind the back.

Benefits: This pose lengthens the spine. It stretches the outer hip rotators, shoulders, and the obliques. It stretches the shoulders, lower back, and abductor muscles. It improves circulation to the back muscles and abdominal organs. It stimulates the kidneys, liver, pancreas, and spleen. It relieves backaches, lumbago, sciatica, and digestive disorders.
Contraindications: Avoid clasping with shoulder injury. Avoid with lumbar herniation.
Modification: If the lower back wants to round, then elevate the hips with blankets and avoid clasping.
Chakra: sacral, solar plexus

427. Marichiasana IV (sage Marichi's pose IV)

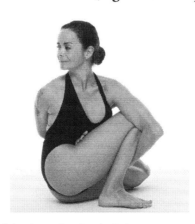

From *Marichiasana II,* reach the hand of the bent leg back for support on fingertips or ridgetop position. Arch the lower back up and in, then take the opposite arm across to the outside of the leg. Wrap the arm around the leg and grab the shin that is in half lotus, then reach the other hand back and clasp.

Benefits: This pose opens the hips and releases lower back tension. It stretches the shoulders, lower back, and abductor muscles. It stimulates the kidneys, liver, pancreas, and spleen. It rejuvenates nerves around the navel.
Contraindications: Avoid clasping with shoulder injury, lumbar herniation, or knee injury.
Modification: If the knee wants to lift off the floor, then lean back to keep it rooted down, and avoid twisting further to clasp. If there is stress in the knee, then slide the foot out of half lotus and place it on the floor.
Chakra: sacral, solar plexus

428. Marichiasana V (sage Marichi's pose V)

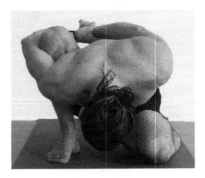

Bend one leg in with the foot beside the outer hip in *ardha vira* position. Fold the other leg in with the knee pointing up and the foot aligned with outside edge of the hip. Bow forward and place the hands on the floor. Push the head up then wrap the arm around and clasp. Both sitting bones should hover off of the floor in this pose. Take the head down first, and then extend energy down through the sitting bones.

Benefits: This pose opens the hips, ankles, and the knees. It stretches the shoulders and the dorsal region of the spine. It stimulates the kidneys, liver, and abdominal organs. It activates the parasympathetic nervous system and releases mental tension.

Contraindications: Avoid clasping with shoulder injury. Avoid with knee injury.

Modification: Sit on a block if there is stress in the knee or ankle.

Chakra: sacral, throat

429. Marichiasana VI (sage Marichi's pose VI)

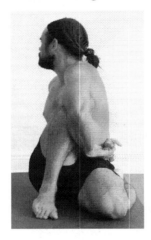

From *Marichiasana V,* reach one arm back for support with the hand in an elevated position. Inner rotate the opposite arm and wrap it around the elevated knee. Clasp hands behind the back, rest the hips down, and deepen the twist.

Benefits: This pose opens the hips, ankles, and the knees. It stretches the shoulders, lower back, and abductor muscles. It alleviates lower back tension and promotes healing for stomach disorders. It stimulates the kidneys, liver, pancreas, and abdominal organs.

Contraindications: Avoid clasping with shoulder injury. Avoid with knee injury.

Modification: Sit on a block if there is stress in the knee or ankle.

Chakra: sacral, solar plexus

430. Marichiasana VII (sage Marichi's pose VII)

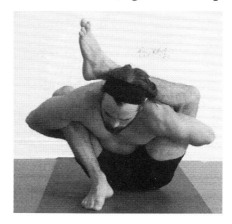

Bring one leg behind the head and bend the other leg in with the foot under the knee and aligned with the outside edge of hip. Push the head up strong, bow forward, wrap, and clasp hands behind the back.

Benefits: This pose opens the hips and strengthens the neck. It stretches the shoulders, lower back, and the outer hip rotators. It stimulates the kidneys, liver, abdominal organs, thyroid and parathyroid.
Contraindications: Avoid clasping with shoulder injury. Avoid with neck, lower back, or hamstring injury.
Modification: Use one hand to hold the foot behind the head or place the hands in front of you on the floor for support.
Chakra: sacral, throat

431. Marichiasana VIII (sage Marichi's pose VIII)

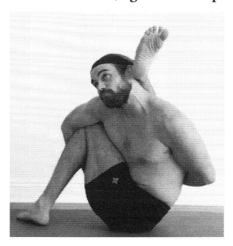

From *Marichiasana VII,* wrap the opposite arm around the outside of the bent leg, and clasp hands behind the back.

Benefits: This pose opens the hips and strengthens the neck. It stretches the shoulders, lower back, and abductor muscles. It stimulates the kidneys, liver, pancreas, abdominal organs, thyroid and parathyroid.
Contraindications: Avoid clasping with shoulder injury. Avoid with neck, lower back, or hamstring injury.
Modification: Use one hand to hold the foot behind the head or place the hands in front of you on the floor for support.
Chakra: solar plexus, throat

432. Marichiasana IX (sage Marichi's pose IX)

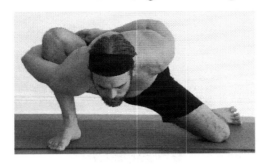

Place one knee on the edge of the mat with the thigh parallel with the top edge of the mat and the shin parallel with the outer edge. Turn the foot out to the side. Bend the other knee up with the foot underneath. The knee on the floor should be aligned with the arch of the opposite foot. The wider the stance, the deeper the hip opening. Push the head up, bow forward, and clasp hands behind the back. Keep the head pushing up so the hips stay moving forward and down.

Benefits: This pose opens the hips. It stretches the shoulders and adductor muscles.
Contraindications: Avoid clasping with shoulder injury. Avoid with inner thigh injury.
Modification: Use the hands on the floor for support. Place a blanket under the knee if experience discomfort.
Chakra: sacral, throat

433. Marichiasana X (sage Marichi's pose X)

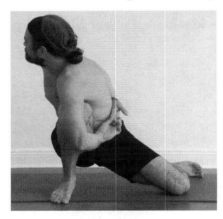

From *Marichiasana IX,* twist and take the opposite arm around the elevated leg. Clasp hands behind the back, and then move the hips forward and down. The knee and ankle press down lightly to maintain the engagement of the targeted muscles.

Benefits: This pose opens the hips. It stretches the shoulders, adductors, and abductor muscles. It stimulates the kidneys, liver, pancreas, and abdominal organs.
Contraindications: Avoid clasping with shoulder injury. Avoid with inner thigh injury.
Modification: Hold onto the elevated knee for support and focus on moving the hips forward and down. Place a blanket under the knee if experience discomfort.
Chakra: sacral, solar plexus

434. Thavaliasana (monkey frog pose)

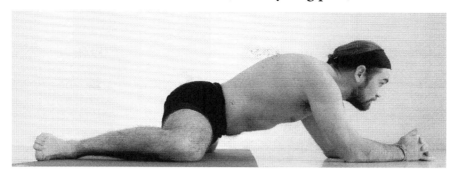

Come onto the forearms and take the legs as wide apart as possible with the thighs aligned and the shins parallel. Engage the lower abdomen and scoop the tailbone. Press the knees and the ankles down into the floor, and then push the hips back.

Benefits: This pose opens the hips and stretches the adductor muscles. It strengthens the lower abdominals.
Contraindications: Avoid with inner thigh injury.
Modification: Place a blanket under the knees if experience discomfort.
Chakra: root, sacral

435. Urdhva Mukha Thavaliasana (upward facing monkey frog pose)

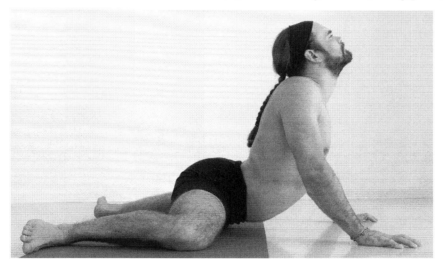

From *thavaliasana,* place the hands under the shoulders, and lift up into a backbend. Let the hips relax and get heavy. Pull the hands and shoulders back and extend the spine forward.

Benefits: This pose opens the hips and stretches the adductor muscles. It tones the spinal nerves and the sympathetic nervous system.
Contraindications: Avoid with inner thigh injury.
Modification: Place a blanket under the knees if experience discomfort.
Chakra: root, sacral

436. Hanumanasana (Hanuman prep pose)

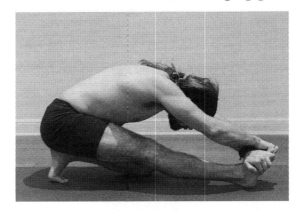

From a lunge position, rest the back knee down and curl the toes under. Sit back on the heel and straighten the other leg. Bow forward and cross wrists and grab the foot with both hands. Pull back on the inner and outer edges of the foot and push the foot forward. Lift the arms above the ears and pull the shoulders down the back.

Benefits: This pose opens the thighs and knees. It stretches the feet and lengthens the hamstrings. Alleviates pain from sciatica.
Contraindications: Avoid with knee injury.
Modification: Sit on a block or bolster instead of the heel if experience discomfort in the foot.
Chakra: root, sacral

437. Parivrtta Hanumanasana (revolved Hanuman prep pose)

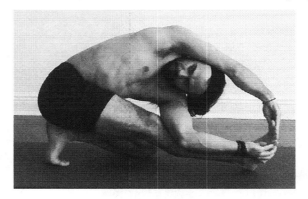

From *Hanuman* prep pose, lift up and reach the opposite arm across the straight leg with the palm face up. Grab the outside edge of the foot then reach overhead with the other arm. Pull against the foot with both hands to deepen the twist.

Benefits: This pose opens the thighs and knees. It stretches the feet and back muscles. It lengthens the hamstrings and stimulates the abdominal organs.
Contraindications: Avoid with knee injury or lumbar herniation.
Modification: Sit on a block or bolster instead of the heel if experience discomfort in the foot.
Chakra: sacral, solar plexus

438. Hanumanasana I (Hanuman's pose I)

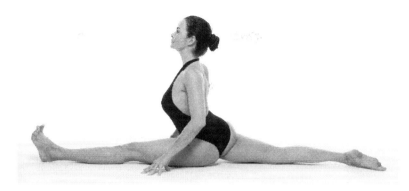

Extend one leg straight in front and one directly behind you. Flex the forward foot and point the back one. Squeeze the legs in toward the hips and square them forward. Arch the spine and tilt the top of the pelvis forward.

Benefits: This pose stretches the thighs and hip flexors. It lengthens the hamstrings and tones the abdominal organs. It relieves sciatica and is beneficial for treating pulled hamstring muscles when performed with PNF technique.
Contraindications: Avoid straightening the back leg if the pelvis opens up asymmetrically. Avoid with psoas injury and hamstring strains.
Modification: Use blocks under the hands for support and to keep the pelvis squared forward.
Chakra: root, sacral

439. Hanumanasana II (Hanuman's pose II)

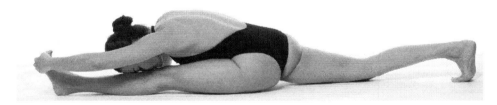

For position II, flex the back foot and bow forward. Clasp hands over the forward foot and rest the head on the leg.

Benefits: This pose stretches the thighs and hip flexors. It lengthens the hamstrings and releases lower back tension. It tones the liver, kidneys, spleen, and adrenal glands.
Contraindications: Avoid bowing forward if the hips are not on the floor. Avoid with hamstring strains.
Modification: Place blocks under the feet to deepen the pose.
Chakra: root, sacral

440. Hanumanasana III (Hanuman's pose III)

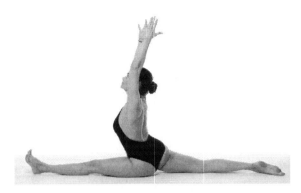

For position III, lift back up and reach the arms overhead. The back foot can be pointed or flexed.

Benefits: This pose creates strength in the legs. It stretches the thighs and hip flexors. It lengthens the hamstrings and tones the back muscles.
Contraindications: Avoid with psoas injury or hamstring strains.
Modification: Place blocks under the feet to deepen the pose.
Chakra: root, sacral

441. Hindolasana (baby cradle)

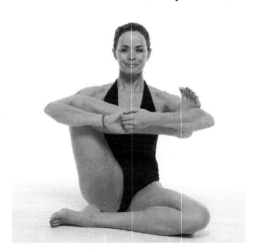

From sitting, bring one leg up and place the foot and knee in the elbow creases. Clasp hands in *Ganesha mudra* in front of the shins. Activate the foot by pushing out through the big toe and pull the outer edge of the foot back. Arch up and bring the leg in tight to the upper body.

Benefits: This pose opens the hips and stretches the abductors. It prepares the body for deeper hip openers.
Contraindications: Avoid disengaging the foot and letting the ankle sickle.
Modification: Hold the knee and foot with the hands instead of clasping in front of the shin.
Chakra: root, sacral

442. Salamba Hindolasana (supported baby cradle)

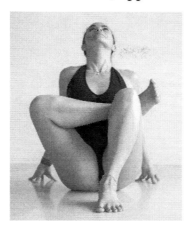

From sitting, bend both knees straight up, and then bring one ankle on top of the thigh with the foot flexed. Reach the hands back in an elevated position behind you to support the arch and extension of the spine. Lift the hips and bring the torso toward the bent leg to deepen the opening.

Benefits: This pose is preparation for *yoga dandasana*. It releases tension in the hip and stretches the front of the neck.
Chakra: heart, throat

443. Yoga Dandasana (yogi's staff pose prep)

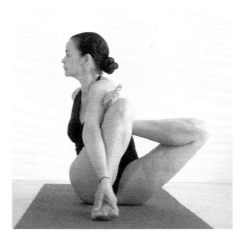

From *salamba hindolasana,* reach one arm across and place it in the arch of the foot. Push the arm into the top foot and twist. Reach the hand down for the supporting foot to deepen the opening.

Benefits: This pose opens the hips. It stretches the lower back and abductors. It prepares the body for *yoga dandasana*. It massages the abdominal organs.
Contraindications: Avoid with lumbar herniation or ankle injury.
Modification: Keep the arm bent and pressing into the sole of the foot instead of reaching down for the stabilizing foot.
Chakra: sacral, solar plexus

444. Yoga Dandasana (yogi's staff pose)

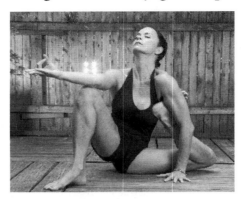

From *yoga dandasana* preparation, inner rotate the top arm and bend the elbow to trap the foot in the armpit. Lean back and take the knee to the floor. Turn the stabilizing leg out to the side for balance. Reach the hand down for the knee or for the floor. Extend the free arm over the elevated knee with the palm face up in *jnana mudra*.

Benefits: This pose opens the hips and stretches the abductors, ankles, and feet.
Contraindications: Avoid with lumbar herniation or ankle injury.
Modification: Use both hands to hold the foot until the knee reaches the floor.
Chakra: sacral, solar plexus

445. Baddha Yoga Dandasana (bound yogi's staff pose)

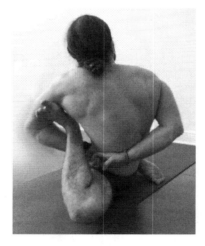

Start with one leg in *ardha vira* position. Take the other foot with both hands and push the knee down toward the floor behind you. Hold the heel with the opposite hand and reach the other arm over the foot. Hook the foot into the armpit and wrap the arm around the leg to clasp behind the back.

Benefits: This pose opens the hips and thighs. It stretches the abductors, ankles, and feet.
Contraindications: Avoid with lumbar herniation, ankle or shoulder injury.
Modification: Use a strap to bind.
Chakra: sacral, solar plexus

446. Padmasana (lotus pose)

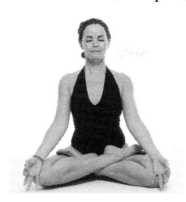

From sitting, grab the inside of one knee and bring the heel toward the navel. Point the foot and rest it on top of the opposite thigh. Bend the other leg up, point the foot, and bring it on top of the opposite leg. Flex both feet to hold the engagement in the legs. Rest the hands over the knees in *jnana* or *chin mudra*. In order to avoid an imbalance in the pelvis, make sure to work both sides evenly with the right foot on top first and then the left.

Benefits: This pose opens the hips and relaxes the nervous system. It tones the coccygeal and sacral nerves. It stimulates the pelvis, spine, abdomen, and bladder. It relieves menstrual discomfort and purifies the *nadis* when held for 20 minutes.

Contraindications: Avoid with knee injury or hip replacement.

Modification: Place one foot in half lotus and the other foot rests on the floor. Place a block under the knee if it lifts, or place a sandbag on top of the thigh and work on releasing the knee to the floor. There should be no stress in the knees at any point.

Chakra: root, crown

447. Parivrtta Padmasana (revolved lotus pose)

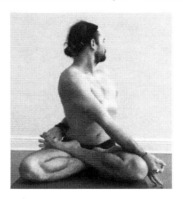

From lotus pose, reach one arm across with palm face out and press against the outside of the opposite thigh. Reach the other arm behind the back and hold the foot. Twist over the leading shoulder.

Benefits: This pose opens and massages the internal organs and improves digestion. It relieves lower back tension and balances life force energy.

Contraindications: Avoid with knee injury or hip replacement.

Modification: Use a strap to hold the foot.

Chakra: sacral, solar plexus

448. Goraknathasana (sage Goraknath's pose)

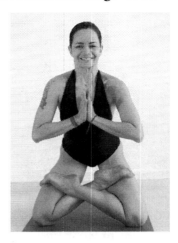

From *padmasana,* rock forward and stand up on the knees. Bring the hands together into prayer position. Bow forward slightly to hold the balance.

Benefits: This pose opens the hips and tones the muscles of the pelvic floor. It improves balance and concentration.
Contraindications: Avoid with knee injury or hip replacement.
Chakra: root, sacral

449. Garbha Pindasana (baby in the womb pose)

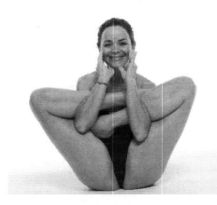

From *padmasana,* thread the arms through the legs under the calves. Lean back and bring the knees to the chest and the hands to the chin.

Benefits: This pose opens the hips and regulates the adrenal glands. It massages and tones the abdominal organs. It stimulates digestion and improves balance.
Contraindications: Avoid with knee injury or hip replacement.
Modification: Place the hands in prayer instead of bringing them to the face. If it is not possible to thread the arms through, then wrap the arms around the legs and clasp in *Ganesha mudra*. Squeeze the legs together and bring them to the chest.
Chakra: sacral, solar plexus

450. Yoga Mudrasana I (yoga seal pose)

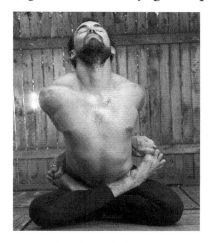

From *padmasana,* reach behind the back and hook both big toes. Grab the foot that is on top first and then the one that is underneath. Arch up and extend the spine.

Benefits: This pose opens the hips and stretches the shoulders. It opens the chest and expands the lungs. It increases digestive power.
Contraindications: Avoid with knee injury or hip replacement.
Modification: Use straps around the feet to clasp.
Chakra: root, crown

451. Yoga Mudrasana II (yoga seal pose II)

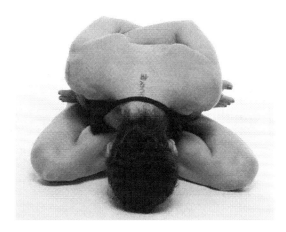

Assume *yoga mudrasana I* position and bow forward. Rest the forehead on the floor and pull up on the feet.

Benefits: This pose opens the hips and calms the nervous system. It stimulates the abdominal organs and kidneys.
Contraindications: Avoid with knee injury or hip replacement.
Modification: Use straps around the feet to clasp.
Chakra: root, brow

452. Akarna Dhanurasana I (archer's pose I)

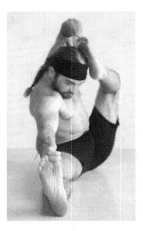

Grab both big toes with the legs stretched forward. Push down through one heel, and lift the other leg up. Bend the knee, and bring the foot beside the head. Switch sides and repeat several times.

Benefits: This pose opens the hips and strengthens the abdominal muscles. It stretches the shoulders and hamstrings.
Contraindications: Avoid with lumbar herniation.
Modification: Use straps around the foot of the straight leg.
Chakra: root, solar plexus

453. Akarna Dhanurasana II (archer's pose II)

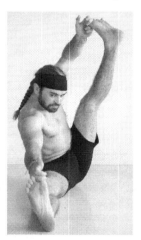

Grab both big toes with the legs stretched forward. Push down through one heel and lift the other leg up. Keep the expanding leg straight. Outer rotate the hip, inner rotate the thighbone, and then bring the leg toward the head. Use the strength of the arm to pull the leg back as it lifts.

Benefits: This pose opens the hips and strengthens the abdominal muscles. It stretches hamstrings.
Contraindications: Avoid with lumbar herniation or hamstring injury.
Modification: Use straps around the feet.
Chakra: root, solar plexus

454. Arjunasana (Arjuna's pose)

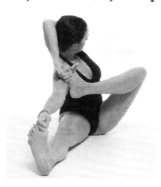

From *hindolasana* position, pull the leg in tight and hold it close with the opposite arm. Wrap the other arm behind the head and grab the foot. Push the head up into the top arm then bow forward and clasp the big toe of the straight leg. Twist and gaze behind you. Alternatively, the pose can be entered from *akarna dhanurasana* by ducking the head under the arm and pulling the foot across to the opposite shoulder.

Benefits: This pose opens the abductors and strengthens the neck. It prepares the body for bringing the foot behind the head.
Contraindications: Avoid with lumbar herniation or neck injury.
Modification: Use straps around the feet.
Chakra: root, throat

455. Eka Pada Sirsasana I (one leg over the head pose I)

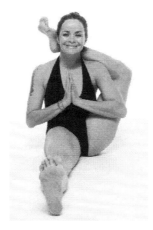

Grab one foot with both hands and bring the knee over the shoulder. Then hold onto the foot with the opposite hand and duck the head under the leg. Push the head back into the leg with the strength of the neck, and bring the hands together in *anjali mudra*.

Benefits: This pose opens the abductors and strengthens the neck. It stretches the lower back and tones the reproductive organs.
Contraindications: Avoid with lumbar herniation or strain.
Modification: Perform *hindolasana* until the hip is open enough to duck the head under.
Chakra: sacral, throat

456. Eka Pada Sirsasana II (one leg over the head pose II)

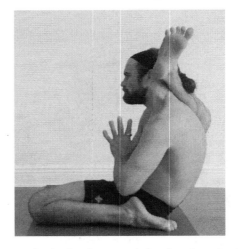

Bring one foot into *ardha vira* position with the leg bent and the foot beside the hip. Grab the other foot and bring the knee over the shoulder. Bring the leg behind the head and lean back to stretch the thigh and open the hip.

Benefits: This pose opens the abductors and strengthens the neck. It stretches the lower back and thighs. It tones the reproductive organs.
Contraindications: Avoid with lumbar herniation or strain.
Chakra: sacral, throat

457. Skandasana (warrior Skanda's pose)

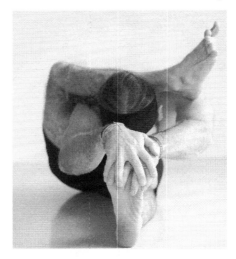

Assume *eka pada sirsasana I* position and bow forward. Reach both hands for the foot or place them on the floor for support. Push the head up strong and keep both feet active.

Benefits: This pose opens the abductors and strengthens the neck. It stretches the lower back and lengthens the hamstrings. It stimulates the liver, kidneys, spleen, and abdominal organs. It tones the reproductive organs.
Contraindications: Avoid with lumbar herniation or strain. Avoid overstretching the lower back.
Modification: Hold the foot with the opposite hand and lift it beside the ear, and then bow forward.
Chakra: sacral, throat

458. Viranchyasana I (Viranchi's pose I)

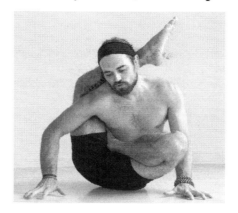

Bring one foot into half lotus position and the other leg behind the head. Use the hands for support or bring the hands into *anjali mudra*.

Benefits: This pose opens the hips and strengthens the neck. It stretches the lower back and tones the reproductive organs.
Contraindications: Avoid with lumbar herniation or knee injury.
Modification: Place the hands on the floor for support.
Chakra: sacral, throat

459. Dwi Pada Sirsasana I (two feet behind head pose I)

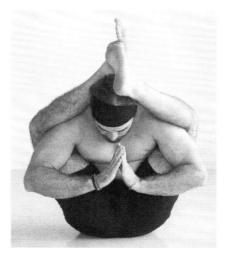

Bring both knees over the shoulders and clasp ankles. Duck the head under, and push it up. Use the hands for support or bring them into *anjali mudra*.

Benefits: This pose opens the hips and strengthens the neck. It stretches the lower back and tones the reproductive organs.
Contraindications: Avoid with lumbar herniation or neck injury.
Modification: Cross ankles in front of the chest and bring the arms under.
Chakra: sacral, throat

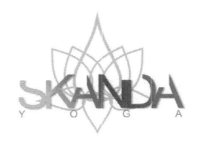

CHAPTER 15

Supine poses

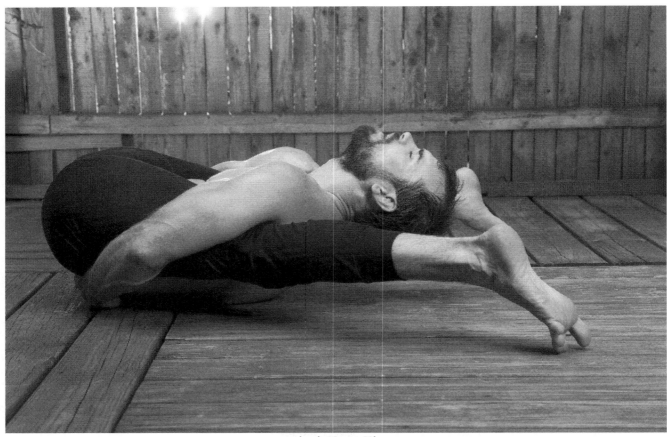

photo by Mauricio Velez

460. Supta Bhairavasana I (reclined formidable pose I)

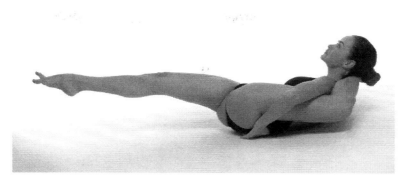

Bring one leg behind the head and lean back. Extend the free leg straight and activate *pada bandha*. Bring the hands into *anjali mudra* or wrap the arm over the leg to deepen the opening.

Benefits: This pose opens the hips and strengthens the neck. It stretches the abductors and hamstrings. It tones the reproductive organs.
Contraindications: Avoid with lumbar herniation or neck injury.
Modification: Grab one foot with both hands and push the knee into the floor while lifting the ankle straight over the knee.
Chakra: sacral, throat

461. Supta Bhairavasana II (reclined formidable pose II)

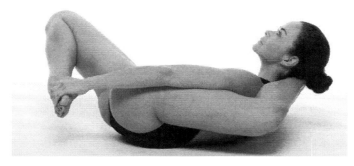

Assume *supta bhairavasana I* position and then grab the extended foot with the opposite hand. Pull the heel in toward the hip and then extend the knee away.

Benefits: This pose opens the hips and strengthens the neck. It stretches the hip flexors, abductors, and hamstrings. It tones the reproductive organs.
Contraindications: Avoid with lumbar herniation or neck injury.
Chakra: sacral, throat

462. Supta Valgulasana (sleeping bat pose)

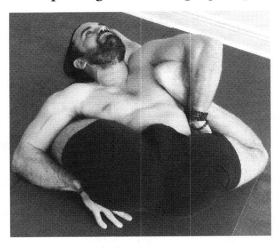

From *supta bhairavasana I* position, bring the extended foot into the armpit by wrapping the arm over the foot. Reach the hands down to clasp for a bound variation, or reach the hand down to hold the thigh or knee.

Benefits: This pose opens the hips and strengthens the neck. It stretches the outer hip rotators and tones the reproductive organs.
Contraindications: Avoid with lumbar herniation or neck injury.
***Chakra*:** sacral, throat

463. Yoganidrasana (sleeping yogi's pose)

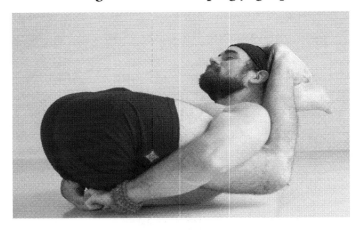

From a supine position, grab both feet and hook the arms over the legs. Bring both feet behind the head and cross ankles. Clasp the hands under the hips.

Benefits: This pose opens the hips and strengthens the neck. It stretches the shoulders, abductors, and hamstrings. It tones the reproductive organs and calms the nervous system.
Contraindications: Avoid with lumbar herniation or neck injury.
Modification: Hold both feet with the hands and work on pushing both knees down into the floor in happy baby pose.
***Chakra*:** sacral, throat

464. Eka Pada Sirsa Shayanasana (one leg over head resting pose)

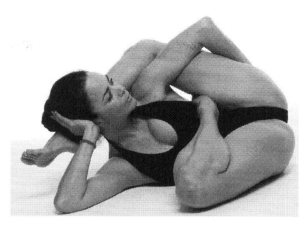

From a reclined position, bring one leg into half lotus and the other leg behind the head. Lean over to the side of the leg in half lotus and reach the opposite arm around the top leg. Support the head with the hand and push the head back into the leg.

Benefits: This pose opens the hips and strengthens the neck. It stretches the abductors and hamstrings. It tones the reproductive organs and calms the nervous system.
Contraindications: Avoid with lumbar herniation, knee or neck injury.
Chakra: sacral, throat

465. Supta Konasana (reclined angle pose)

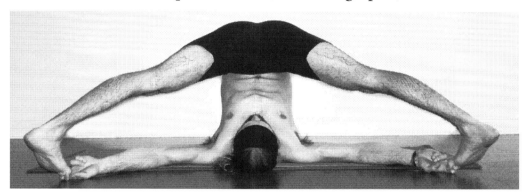

From a supine position, roll onto the shoulders, lift the hips, and then place the feet overhead on the floor. Hook both big toes and extend the feet out to the sides. Pull the arms back in toward the shoulders and push the head down into the floor.

Benefits: This pose opens the inner thighs and releases lower back tension. It tones the reproductive organs and calms the nervous system.
Contraindications: Avoid with a flat neck.
Modification: Hold both feet with straps.
Chakra: sacral, throat

466. Supta Baddha Konasana (supine bound angle pose)

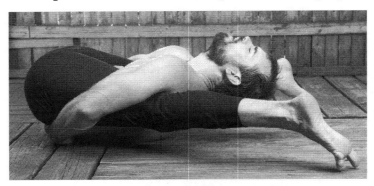

From *supta konasana,* lower the hips back down and hook the arms over the legs to clasp hands under the hips. Engage the quadriceps and hamstrings to straighten the legs and touch the floor with the toes.

Benefits: This pose opens the hips and releases lower back tension. It stretches the shoulders and hamstrings. It tones the reproductive organs and calms the nervous system.
Contraindications: Avoid with lumbar strain or herniation.
Chakra: sacral, throat

467. Supta Virasana (supine hero's prep pose)

From kneeling, spread the head of the calves evenly, and then rest the hips down between the ankles. Place the hands behind you for support as you lean back. Rest onto the forearms or lay back over bolsters.

Benefits: This pose opens the knees and ankles. It stretches the thighs and prepares the body to enter *supta virasana*.
Contraindications: Use props for support with knee, ankle, or back injury.
Modification: If there is discomfort in the knees, then place a prop underneath the hips. A small towel roll can be placed in the knee pits to increase space in the joint. If there is discomfort in the top of the feet, then a blanket can be placed under them.
Chakra: sacral, throat

468. Supta Virasana (supine hero's pose)

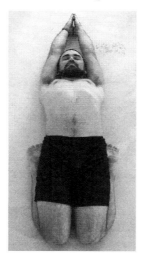

From kneeling, spread the head of the calves evenly, and then rest the hips down between the ankles. Rest the shoulders down then reach the arms overhead. Press the outside edges of the feet down and squeeze the heels in toward the hips. Maintain the natural curve of the lumbar spine. Don't over-arch or over-scoop the tailbone. The tailbone scoops but does not override the action of the pubic bone descending. If the tops of the thighs lift up, then the tailbone is scooping too hard.

Benefits: This pose opens the knees and ankles. It stretches the thighs and lengthens the hip flexors. It relieves leg aches and menstrual discomfort. It is beneficial for healing pulled back muscles and knee injuries.
Contraindications: Use props for support with knee, ankle, or back injury.
Modification: If there is discomfort in the knees then lift the hips and place a prop underneath. A small towel roll can be placed in the knee pits to increase space in the joint. If there is discomfort in the top of the feet, then a blanket can be placed under them. The upper body can rest on a bolster to decrease pressure in the back.
Chakra: sacral, throat

469. Supta Uttana Virasana (supine intense hero pose)

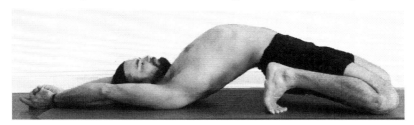

From kneeling, curl the toes under and rest the hips down between the hips. Reach the arms back for support, and then rest the shoulders down.

Benefits: This pose opens the knees and lengthens the hip flexors. It stretches the toes and increases the arch of the feet.
Contraindications: Use props for support with knee, ankle, or back injury.
Chakra: sacral, throat

470. Supta Baddha Virasana (supine bound hero pose)

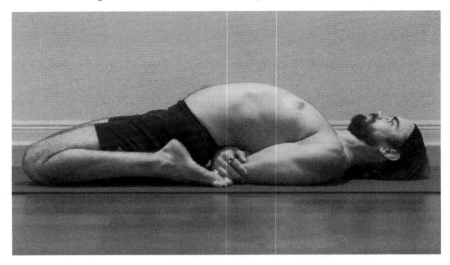

From *virasana,* clasp elbows behind the back and slowly lower down over the arms. Push the elbows into the floor and the wrists up into the back. Scoop the tailbone without lifting the pubic bone. Pull the shoulders down into the floor and lightly press the head back.

Benefits: This pose opens the knees and lengthens the hip flexors. It stretches the toes and increases the arch of the feet. It supports the spine as the body opens. It is beneficial for meditation and lucid dreaming.
Contraindications: Use props for support with knee, ankle, or back injury.
Chakra: sacral, throat

471. Eka Pada Supta Virasana I (one foot supine hero pose I)

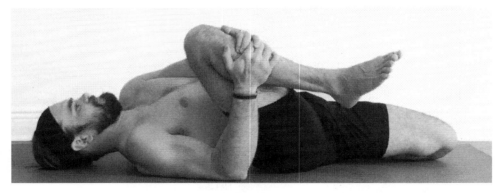

Bring one foot into *ardha vira* position with the foot beside the hip. Rest back and grab the shin of the other leg. Bring the knee toward the armpit to stretch the quadriceps and release tension in the hip flexors.

Benefits: This pose opens the knees and ankles. It stretches the thighs and releases tension in the hip flexors.
Contraindications: Use props for support with knee, ankle, or back injury.
Chakra: sacral, throat

472. Eka Pada Supta Virasana II (one foot supine hero pose II)

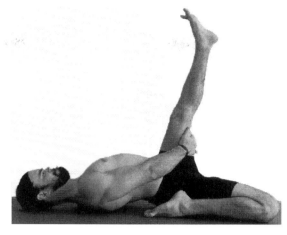

Bring one foot into *ardha vira* position with the foot beside the hip. Rest back and clasp hands behind the hamstrings. Kick the leg into the hands and engage the leg muscles fully. Arch the lower back, lift and open the heart, and then bring the leg closer to the chest. Use a strap to deepen the pose.

Benefits: This pose opens the knees and ankles. It stretches the thighs, hamstrings, and the hip flexors.
Contraindications: Use props for support with knee, ankle, or back injury.
Chakra: sacral, throat

473. Eka Pada Supta Virasana III (one foot supine hero pose III)

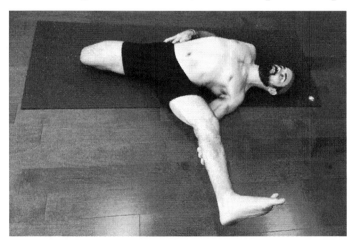

From *eka pada supta virasana II* position, extend the leg out to the side. Support the leg with the hand or reach the opposite hand overhead to hold the foot, but don't let the bent knee lift off of the floor.

Benefits: This pose opens the knees and ankles. It stretches the thighs, adductors, hamstrings, and the hip flexors.
Contraindications: Use props for support with knee, ankle, or back injury.
Modification: Use a strap to hold the foot.
Chakra: sacral, throat

474. Supta Padangusthasana I (supine single leg stretch prep pose I)

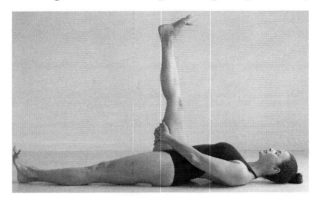

From a reclined position, extend one leg up and clasp hands behind the hamstrings. Kick the leg back into the hands to engage the leg muscles. Arch the lower back up and bring the leg closer to the chest.

Benefits: This pose prepares the body to deepen the pose. It relieves stress in the lower back and aligns the hamstrings on the thighbone. It alleviates sciatica and menstrual pain. It improves posture.
Contraindications: Avoid lying flat if pregnant after first trimester. Use props under the hips and back.
Modification: If the hamstring is injured, then cross the wrists in front of the thigh and grab the hamstrings. Pull with the hands and root the thighbone away to re-attach the muscle on the bone.
Chakra: root, sacral

475. Supta Padangusthasana I (supine single leg stretch pose I)

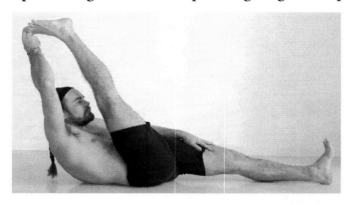

Assume *supta padangusthasana* prep and engage the leg muscles by resisting the stretch. Arch the lower back to clear the hip flexors, and then reach up and hook the big toe with one hand. Round the lower back and push down on the grounding leg with the other hand. Lift the face to the knee using the strength of the abdominals.

Benefits: This pose strengthens the abdominals and stretches the hamstrings.
Contraindications: Avoid lying flat if pregnant after first trimester. Use props under the hips and back. Avoid with lumbar herniation or hamstring injury.
Modification: Use a strap to hold the foot.
Chakra: sacral, solar plexus

476. Supta Padangusthasana II (supine single leg stretch II)

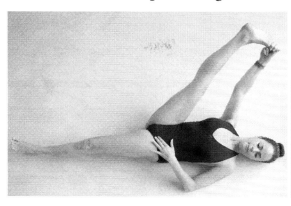
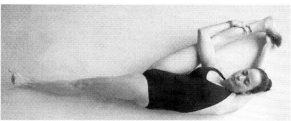

Assume *supta padangusthasana I* position and outer rotate the leg and extend it out to the side. Place the other hand on the hip and push the thigh of the grounding leg down. Reach the free arm overhead and grab the foot with both hands to deepen the opening.

Benefits: This pose opens the hips and lengthens the hamstrings.
Contraindications: Avoid lying flat if pregnant after first trimester. Use props under the hips and back.
Modification: Use a strap to hold the foot.
Chakra: root, sacral

477. Supta Padangusthasana III (supine single leg stretch III)

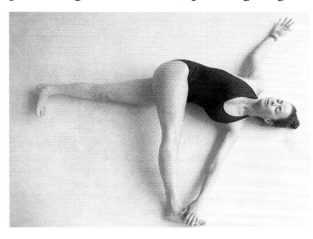

From *supta padangusthasana II,* roll over onto the opposite hip and take the leg over into a twist. Outer rotate the thigh and hip of the expanding leg. Flex the foot of the stabilizing leg and pull it in toward the hip. The free hand can reach out to the side if both shoulders are down; if not, then place the hand on the ribcage.

Benefits: This pose opens the hips. It stretches the abductors and releases tension in the IT band.
Contraindications: Avoid twisting if pregnant. Use props under the hips and back.
Modification: Use a strap to hold the foot. Bend the stabilizing leg and grab the inside edge of the foot to deepen the stretch and open the thighs.
Chakra: sacral, solar plexus

478. Supta Urdhva Eka Pada Vajrasana (supine one foot upward diamond pose prep)

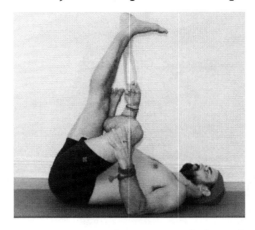

From *sucinrandrasana,* extend the bottom leg straight up toward the ceiling. Clasp hands around the calf or use a strap to hold the foot. Use one hand to pull the leg in closer to the chest, while the opposite arm pushes the bent leg away from you.

Benefits: This pose opens the hips and lengthens the hamstrings. It relieves lower back tension and reduces stress.
Contraindications: Avoid lying flat if pregnant after first trimester. Use props under the hips and back.
Modification: Use a strap to hold the foot.
Chakra: sacral

479. Anantasana (infinity pose)

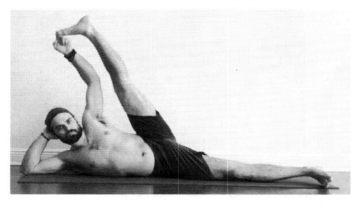

From lying in a supine position, roll over to one side and support the head with one hand. The elbow, hip, and foot should all be in a single line. Extend the top leg up toward the ceiling and hook the big toe with the first two fingers. Resist the stretch by pushing the thighbone away and engaging the quadriceps. Then deepen the opening by lifting the leg higher. This pose is dedicated to *Adi-Ananta-Sesha,* the serpent with an infinity of heads, who serves as the couch for Vishnu when he sleeps.

Benefits: This pose opens the hips and lengthens the hamstrings. It develops balance and concentration.
Contraindications: Avoid with hamstring injury.
Modification: Use a strap to hold the foot. The bottom elbow can be placed a few inches forward to increase balance.
Chakra: sacral

480. Supta Visvajrasana (supine double diamond)

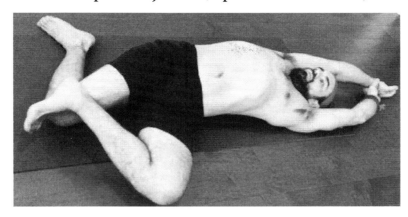

From a supine position, bend both knees up and place the feet underneath hip distance apart. Cross one ankle on top of the thigh. Extend the knees over to the side of the top leg and wiggle the foot of the bottom leg behind you a few inches. Push down through the top leg to lower the bottom leg to the floor. Extend energy from the hip out through the bottom knee. Clasp the wrist of the leg that is stretching overhead and pull the arm straight. Stretch the side body while attempting to bring the knee and shoulder flush to the floor.

Benefits: This pose stretches the thighs, hip flexors, intercostals, and obliques. It releases abdominal tension and prepares the body for backbends.
Contraindications: Avoid with knee injury.
Chakra: sacral

481. Supta Swastikasana (supine auspicious pose)

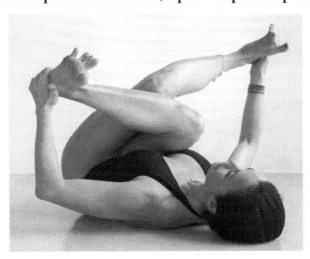

From a supine position, cross the knees and grab the outside edges of the feet. Lift the ankles up and bring the shins in a straight line, and then pull the feet down. The feet stay flexed or flointed to keep the ankles, shins, and knees aligned.

Benefits: This pose stretches the abductors and relieves lower back tension.
Contraindications: Avoid with lumbar herniation or during pregnancy after first trimester.
Chakra: root, sacral

482. Supta Swastikasana II (supine auspicious pose II)

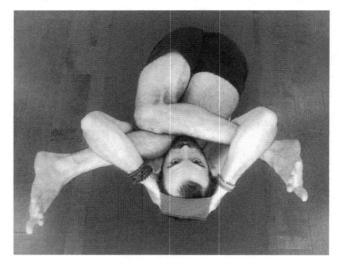

From *supta swastikasana,* hook the arms over the legs. Pull the legs down and clasp hands behind the head. Widen the elbows apart and lift the ankles higher, as you lift the head with the hands.

Benefits: This pose deepens the stretch in the outer hip rotators.
Contraindications: Avoid with lumbar herniation or knee injury.
Chakra: sacral, throat

483. Supta Ganeshasana (supine Ganesha's pose)

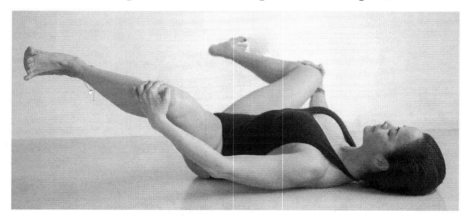

From a supine position, reach up and grab the knees. Bring the thighs in a single line parallel with the top edges of the mat, and the shins parallel with outer edges of the mat. Arch the lower back and bring the shoulder blades flat on the back. Pull the knees directly down toward the floor.

Benefits: This pose stretches the adductors and relieves lower back tension. It increases awareness of *mula bandha.*
Chakra: root, sacral

484. Supta Hindolasana I (supine baby cradle pose I)

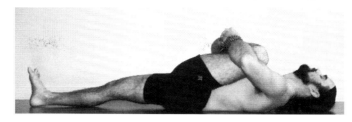

From a supine position, bring one leg up and clasp hands over the shin with the knee and foot in the elbow creases. Flex the foot to keep the ankle, shin, and knee aligned. Push the head and shoulders down to increase the hip opening.

Benefits: This pose stretches the abductors and relieves lower back tension.
Contraindications: Avoid with lumbar herniation or during pregnancy after first trimester.
Chakra: sacral, throat

485. Supta Hindolasana II (supine baby cradle pose II)

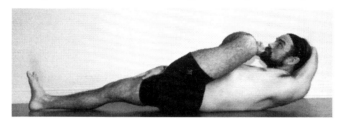

Assume *supta hindolasana I* position and reach the same arm as the expanding leg behind the head and grab the foot. Place the other hand on top of the grounding leg. Push the head back into the top elbow to open the hip.

Benefits: This pose stretches the abductors and shoulders. It strengthens the neck and relieves lower back tension.
Contraindications: Avoid with lumbar herniation or during pregnancy after first trimester.
Chakra: sacral, throat

486. Sucinrandrasana (eye of the needle pose)

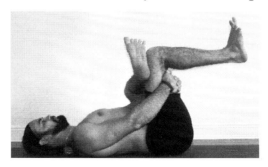

From a supine position, bend both knees up with the feet underneath and hip distance apart. Cross one ankle on top and flex the foot. Reach one arm through the center and clasp hands behind the hamstrings. Arch the lower back and resist the stretch. Push the leg into the hands, and then bring both legs toward the chest to deepen the hip opening.

Benefits: This pose stretches the abductors and releases hip flexor tension.
Contraindications: Avoid with lumbar herniation or during pregnancy after first trimester.
Chakra: sacral, throat

487. Supta Balasana (supine child's pose)

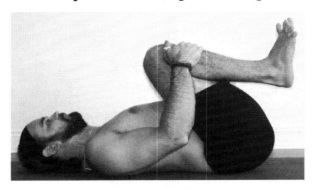

From a supine position, bend both knees up and bring them to the chest. Grab the tops of the shins and round the lower back. Take the knees in small circles to massage the muscles around the sacrum.

Benefits: This pose releases lower back tension and calms the nervous system.
Contraindications: Avoid with lumbar herniation or during pregnancy after first trimester.
Chakra: sacral

488. Eka Pada Sukha Balasana (one foot happy baby pose)

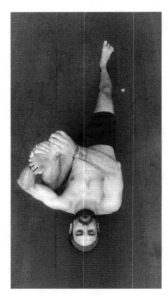

From a supine position, bring one leg toward the chest and take hold of the foot with both hands. One hand holds the heel and the other holds the outside edge of the foot. The straight leg is pressing down into the floor to stabilize the form. Kick up into your hands to engage the hamstrings and then pull the knee down to the floor.

Benefits: This pose releases lower back and hamstring tension. It opens the hip and prepares the body for relaxation.
Modification: Bend the stabilizing leg up to the ceiling, or use a strap to hold the foot.
Chakra: root, sacral

489. Sukha Balasana (happy baby pose)

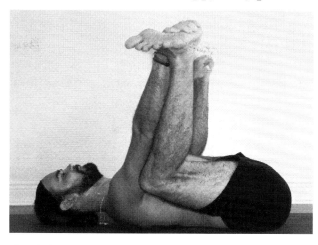

From a supine position, bring both knees up toward the chest and grab the inside or the outside edges of the feet. Flex the feet and push up then pull down to open the hips.

Benefits: This pose releases lower back tension and opens the hips.
Contraindications: Avoid with lumbar herniation or during pregnancy after first trimester.
Chakra: sacral

490. Supta Parvritta Garudasana (twisting reclined eagle pose)

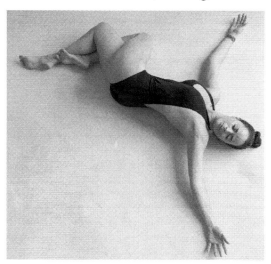

From a supine position, wrap the legs into eagle position and twist to the opposite side of the leg that is wrapped on top. Hold the knees down with one hand, and reach the other arm out to the side to stretch the upper body.

Benefits: This pose stretches the abductors and relieves lower back tension. It opens the chest and expands the lungs. It stimulates the abdominal organs and pancreas.
Contraindications: Avoid with lumbar herniation or pregnancy.
Modification: Use one hand to pull the knee across to the floor. The expanding hand can rest on the rib cage if the shoulder is tight.
Chakra: sacral, solar plexus

491. Jathara Parivartanasana (firmly rooted pose I, simple supine twist)

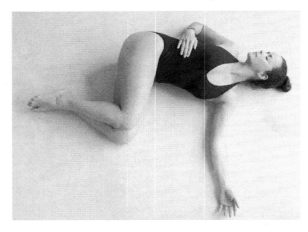

From a supine position, twist both knees over to one side. One hand can pull the top knee down if it hovers. Rest the other hand on the ribcage to release the shoulder or extend it out to the side to stretch the chest.

Benefits: This pose relieves lower back tension. It opens the chest and expands the lungs. It stimulates the abdominal organs and pancreas.
Contraindications: Avoid with lumbar herniation or pregnancy after first trimester.
Modification: Place a blanket between the knees if the piriformis is strained.
Chakra: sacral, solar plexus

492. Jathara Parivartanasana II (firmly rooted pose II)

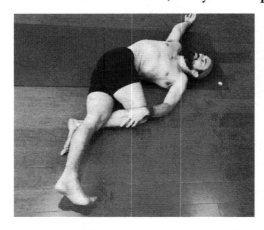

From a figure four supine leg position, twist and take the legs over to the side of the top leg. The bottom leg extends out to the side and hovers off the floor with the support of the ankle underneath. Hold the knee down with one hand and reach the opposite arm out to the side.

Benefits: This pose relieves lower back tension. It stretches the chest and shoulder muscles. It stimulates the abdominal organs and pancreas.
Contraindications: Avoid with lumbar herniation or pregnancy after first trimester.
Chakra: sacral, solar plexus

493. Jathara Parivartanasana III (firmly rooted pose III)

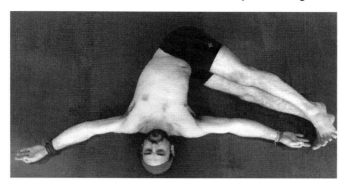

From a supine position, extend both legs straight up and reach the arms out to the sides. Slowly twist over in one direction bringing the feet toward one hand. Keep the opposite arm and shoulder pressing down into the floor. Outer rotate the hip of the top leg.

Benefits: This pose relieves lower back tension. It stretches the chest and shoulder muscles. It stimulates the abdominal organs and pancreas.

Contraindications: Avoid with lumbar herniation or pregnancy after first trimester.

Chakra: sacral, solar plexus

494. Shavasana (corpse pose)

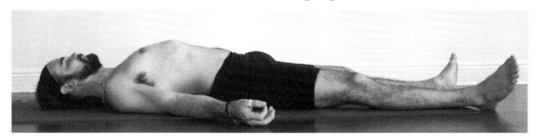

Lie flat on the back with the feet mat width apart. Bring the shoulder blades toward the spine with the arms extended out to the side. The outer three knuckles of the hands should be in contact with the floor and the index knuckles hovers off the floor. The head is neutral with the top and bottom eyelids level. The feet are pointing to the sides at 45-degree angles.

Benefits: This pose releases all tension in the body and mind. It alleviates headaches, fatigue, and insomnia. It relieves mild depression and hyperactivity. It decreases heart and respiratory rates. It reduces blood pressure and increases happiness.

Contraindications: Avoid lying flat during pregnancy after first trimester.

Modification: The body can be supported in many ways with props. For pregnancy, a blanket is under the sitting bones and a bolster under the spine. Blankets are used as a pillow under the head. To relieve lower back tension, place a bolster or blankets under the knees. To relieve shoulder tension, place a small blanket roll under the bottom tips of the shoulder blades. If the feet drop lower than 45 degrees, then support them with blocks.

Chakra: root, sacral, solar plexus, heart, throat, brow, crown

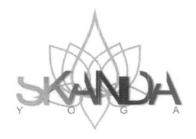

CHAPTER 16

Synchronizing With Natural Cycles of Time

Early in my teaching career, I primarily taught Hatha Yoga and the Ashtanga Yoga system. I then began to study and teach Anusara® Yoga, a modern form of Hatha Yoga derived from the Iyengar style of yoga. This system emphasized anatomical alignment, and classes were structured around a teaching or theme. Lina Vallejo suggested that instead of using themes, I synchronize my classes with a conscious alignment to natural cycles and patterns of time. She believed that this would put us in tune to the ebb and flow of universal energy. I followed her suggestion and began to base my classes on the energies and characteristics of the days, as described in both ancient and modern time-keeping systems. These systems followed the cyclical and ever-repeating astronomical patterns that the ancient peoples believed encoded certain possibilities that affected all life in the cosmos. These patterns were so consistently predictable that ancient astronomers and calendar keepers were able to establish an oracle for each day. By following the calendar, one would come into alignment with natural, cyclical patterns and develop a harmonious relationship with time and all of creation. When I began to base my classes on the living oracle of repeating patterns of time, our community began to experience more magic, grace and synchronicity. Skanda Yoga classes use a natural-time calendar system that was adapted from the ancient calendar systems of the Maya. The energies found within this system complement the attributes of Indian mythological characters and are utilized for personal growth and the development of spiritual qualities of being.

Ancient Mesoamerican Calendar Systems

Mesoamerican societies evolved around mythology, religion, astronomy and political organizations. Their genius in these areas produced vital civilizations, complex hieroglyphic writing, and calendar systems. The Olmecs were the first organized culture in the region, taking root in the swampy Gulf Coast area of Mexico around 1800 B.C. Olmec astronomers were adept sky-watchers. They left ample evidence that they were aware of precession[27] and tracking its resulting shift in the rise times of stars. Their keen observations revealed how precessional movement changed the Earth's relationship to the heavens and how these changes exerted dramatic effects on evolving humanity.

As the first Millennium was coming to a close, the Olmec had faded away, leaving a 260-day calendar system called the Tzolkin and a cultural style that would come to define the Maya. The early Maya were obsessed with time and endeavored to find a holistic model of it that embodied evolution and human nature. They used two different time-keeping systems, one accounting for short counts and the other for long counts.

Short counts were defined by the 260-day Tzolkin calendar. The 365-day solar-year calendar was called the Haab and, when combined with the Tzolkin, it produced the 52-year Calendar Round.

The Long Count was based on nested cycles of days multiplied at each level by the key number 20. From the time of its chosen base date in 3114 B.C., this system tracked perpetually repeating sequences of 5,125 days. These were "world ages" and they were one-fifth of the 26,000-year precessional cycle. The Maya did not conceive of the Long Count calendar on its base date in August 11, 3114 B.C. The date was chosen to begin a precessional cycle that the Maya believed would end with the winter solstice on December 21, 2012. On the following day, a new world age and precessional cycle began, bringing with it new possibilities for spiritual and cultural evaluation.

The creation of the Long Count calendar is attributed to the site of Izapa in Chiapas, Mexico and it flourished from 250 B.C.E to 50 C.E. From this ritual center came the creation story of the Maya, the *Popol Vuh*, and sophisticated cosmological ideas that would help humanity recognize its place in the great chain of creation.

The Tzolkin consists of 20-day signs combined with the numbers one to 13. Thirteen refers to the 13 full moons within a solar year, and the day signs were certain animals, things and concepts that by their name and nature conveyed a particular energy, possibility or characteristic. This timing frequency of 13:20 was a natural, rhythmic constant. In this base cycle, every day could be described and understood, making the Tzolkin a system of divination and prophecy. It guided the Maya through the classic period.

Today, in tiny village towns in the highlands of Guatemala, Quiche Maya Ajk'ijaab (calendar keepers and spiritual guides) keep a continuity of tradition that survived the collapse of their once-great civilization and the ravages of the Conquest. Through their ceremonies and rituals, the short count of days has remained unbroken for all these thousands of years. The Long Count of days faded into the past along with the great Maya kings, astronomers, and shamans.

---

27 Axial precession is the slow and continuous change in the orientation of an astronomical body as it rotates around its axis. Like a wobbling top, the earth's axis traces out two cone patterns in the sky as it moves through a full rotational cycle over a period of approximately 26,000 years.

The Dreamspell Calendar

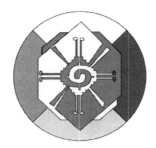

In 1987 the 13-moon natural-time calendar called the Dreamspell was popularized by Jose Arguelles, in conjunction with a Yucatec Maya elder named Humbatz Men. The Dreamspell combines a 365-day lunar-solar year with the 260-day cycles of the Tzolkin. The result is a harmonic constant that entrains the mind to repetitions, patterns, and synchronicity.

1	21	41	61	81	101	121	141	161	181	201	221	241
2	22	42	62	82	102	122	142	162	182	202	222	242
3	23	43	63	83	103	123	143	163	183	203	223	243
4	24	44	64	84	104	124	144	164	184	204	224	244
5	25	45	65	85	105	125	145	165	185	205	225	245
6	26	46	66	86	106	126	146	166	186	206	226	246
7	27	47	67	87	107	127	147	167	187	207	227	247
8	28	48	68	88	108	128	148	168	188	208	228	248
9	29	49	69	89	109	129	149	169	189	209	229	249
10	30	50	70	90	110	130	150	170	190	210	230	250
11	31	51	71	91	111	131	151	171	191	211	231	251
12	32	52	72	92	112	132	152	172	192	212	232	252
13	33	53	73	93	113	133	153	173	193	213	233	253
14	34	54	74	94	114	134	154	174	194	214	234	254
15	35	55	75	95	115	135	155	175	195	215	235	255
16	36	56	76	96	116	136	156	176	196	216	236	256
17	37	57	77	97	117	137	157	177	197	217	237	257
18	38	58	78	98	118	138	158	178	198	218	238	258
19	39	59	79	99	119	139	159	179	199	219	239	259
20	40	60	80	100	120	140	160	180	200	220	240	260

The Dreamspell is based upon the timing frequency of 13:20. Thirteen lunar cycles combine with 20-day signs (solar seals) to produce a 260-day count calendar. Arguelles wrote in *The Mayan Factor* that the number 20 comes from 20 different pulsations from the galactic center that are amplified by the sun as a lens, and directed towards Earth. We experience these pulsations as different energies each day. The combination of the lunar tones and solar seals creates a natural system that provides a daily oracle or prophecy.

Modern civilization has created an artificial timing mechanism based on a 12-month year and a 60-minute hour. A year begins at one point and ends at another, establishing time as a linear progression. This 12:60 timing frequency is artificial; it is disconnected from the astronomical cycles and energies that influence everything in the natural world. This model of linear time presents a concept of time always ending, and this leads to the sensation that there is never enough time. Current economic systems link earnings with finite time; this tie creates the concept that time is money.

The ancient calendar keepers believed that by orienting human activities and initiatives to these natural, cyclical patterns, a life would be lived in harmony with the higher energies of creation and achieve its fullest potential. The higher energies of creation can be known and described mathematically. One of the most intriguing examples of harmony and synchronicity with the mathematical patterns of time can be found in the life and death of K'inich Janaab' Pakal – a late-classic-period ruler of the Maya city of Palenque. Pakal understood that all natural systems and phenomena could be described mathematically and that the language of mathematics transcended the subjectivity of human experience and language. He anticipated the rise and fall of an artificial construction of time. The timing of his death and burial, and the discovery of his tomb, bears out an incredible synchronicity of time and numbers. He died in 683 C.E., his tomb was completed nine years later in 692 C.E., and it was discovered in 1952. Subtract 692 from 1952, and you are left with 1,260 years. 12:60 is the frequency of our artificial and linear construct of time. The Long Count calendar ended and began a new cycle in the year 2012. Subtract 692 from that number, and you get 1,320. This is the frequency or pattern of natural, cyclical time.

The Dreamspell was intended to provide an accessible alternative to artificial time cycles and to reacquaint users with the energies, opportunities and challenges present in each day. While we can't ignore the Gregorian calendar altogether, we can avail ourselves to the spiritual guidance offered by the Dreamspell and to conceive of time as an energetic possibility. Arguelles proposed that the "law of time" (Time/Energy=Art) would result in a refinement of being – the convergence of energetic intent with natural cycles produces art.

Many people around the world support replacing the 12-month calendar system with the 13-month lunar calendar, believing that attunement with natural cycles would result in alignment, cooperation, peace and harmony. In 1939, the global calendar was to be reformed by the League of Nations in favor of the more simplified 13-month system. The Vatican argued that changing the calendar would throw the world into chaos and war, and blocked its adoption. Since then, chaos, war and violence continue to increase with atrocities that would have been unimaginable in 1939. Perhaps alignment with natural time would indeed produce a more peaceful planet.

Dreamspell in Skanda Yoga

When teaching or practicing a Skanda Yoga sequence, the Dreamspell calendar is used for the development of spiritual qualities and the *asana* routine. The oracle reminds us of the quality of the day's energy. The 20 solar seals and 13 lunar tones activate energies of our psyche and neural DNA and, when applied in physical actions, create a union between physical and spiritual energies. This is the essence of Skanda.

In a Skanda Yoga class, there are six energies that direct and structure the sequencing of the practice. Three ascending energies (solar seals) are consciously encoded through *manas shakti* (mental energy) and three descending energies (lunar tones) are embodied through *Prana shakti* (force of life energy). The energy of the day sign is used to structure the sequencing of the practice. The lunar tone is used for the number of repetitions of specific actions or the amount of time held in a pose. The use of the tone in the sequencing automatically makes some days easier and others harder.

These ascending/solar and descending/lunar energies are illustrated by the image of interlocking triangles pointing in opposite directions. The downward-pointing triangle symbolizes manifesting, coagulating feminine energy and the upward-pointing triangle represent ascending, aspiring masculine energy. This six-pointed star is an ancient sacred symbol and the geometric symbol or *"yantra"* of Skanda. Skanda's spiritual powers or *shaktis* are manifested in an ascending-descending/male-female paradigm where there is a spiritual and physical union. This aligns with the lunar tone and solar seal of the Dreamspell calendar.

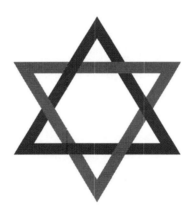

The Dreamspell calendar embodies the three primary *shaktis* or supreme energies of creation: will power/intention (*iccha*), action/knowledge (*jnana*), and essence/cleansing action (*kriya*). The application of power, action, and essence from the solar seals defines the attitude or energy of the day. The lunar tone represents the quality of actions that are physically embodied. Through the confluence of seal and tone, a spiritual cleansing or manifestation arises. This combination of three components of right view with three components of right knowledge leads to a positive outcome.

The 13 Lunar Tones

The 13 lunar tones are the downward-manifesting feminine energies that are embodied physically. Each tone has unique energy qualities. These qualities prescribe certain actions that can be embodied on or off the mat.

	Name	Power	Action	Essence
1	Magnetic	Unify	Attract	Purpose
2	Lunar	Polarize	Stabilize	Challenge
3	Electric	Activate	Bond	Service
4	Self-existing	Define	Measure	Form
5	Overtone	Empower	Command	Radiance
6	Rhythmic	Organize	Balance	Equality
7	Resonant	Channel	Inspire	Attunement
8	Galactic	Harmonize	Model	Integrity
9	Solar	Pulse	Realize	Intention
10	Planetary	Perfect	Produce	Manifestation
11	Spectral	Dissolve	Release	Liberation
12	Crystal	Dedicate	Universalize	Cooperation
13	Cosmic	Endure	Transcend	Presence

1. Magnetic: Initiate a new creation in tune with a higher purpose. Build energy to achieve your purpose and mission in this world. In *asana*, magnetically attract and repel energies in sync with the breath. Inhalations are contracting and resisting, exhalations expanding and deepening.

2. Lunar: Honestly recognize your limitations in order to embrace and overcome them. Challenge yourself in all ways of being in the world. In *asana*, polarize energies through rooting and rising, while seeking stability in postures.

3. Electric: Serve your heart's desires. Be open to all possibilities. Be part of the solution. In *asana*, activate muscle energy in concentric and eccentric actions.

4. Self-Existing: Form a plan of action. Define boundaries. Create a blueprint of success. Be definitive in your actions, while striving towards good form and alignment. In *asana*, measure your level of commitment between self-effort and surrender.

5. Overtone: Gather resources for empowerment. In *asana*, create expansion of the inner body and lengthen the sides of the body. Shine bright with radiance.

6. Rhythmic: Organize resources with efficiency. In *asana*, balance actions with the breath - resisting on inhalation and expanding on exhalation. Seek equality in action. Equality leads to unity.

7. Resonant: Align with the source of Spirit. Channel your inspiration. In *asana*, seek attunement with breath, energy, and nature. Channel energy from the periphery into the core.

8. Galactic: Represent the greatest expression of your Self. Integrity is gained through embracing that which you hold true or close to your heart. Gain solidarity by embodying your level of integrity. In *asana*, inform the form by harmonizing with breath and energy.

9. Solar: Cultivate passionate action. In *asana*, embody *spanda* (pulsation) in action, while staying in remembrance of the intentions for practice.

10. Planetary: Manifest the highest to bring completion to projects. Make every action perfect by giving it your best effort. In *asana*, produce life force through linking actions with the breath.

11. Spectral: Relax, surrender and smile. Let go of anything holding you back, and celebrate freedom in the moment. In *asana*, dissolve and release tension with the breath. Let go of self-effort and striving.

12. Crystal: Discover and share your experiences with love. In *asana*, dedicate actions for your higher purpose. Focus on connecting to back-body strength, which represents the universal and leads to a greater expression of the self. Use the energy cultivated to enhance cooperation in all aspects of your life.

13. Cosmic: Overcome any negative inertia and remember the presence of spirit. This is the peak of the cycle and it embodies all preceding energies. The practice should be the strongest to create more endurance to transcend limitations with more presence to what matters most.

Each tone is represented as a dot for numbers 1-4 and a straight line for the number 5. The 20 day signs (solar seals) repeat a color sequence associated with the four cardinal directions: red-east, white-north, blue-west, and yellow-south. Red days initiate, white days refine, blue days transform, and yellow days manifest. The color for each day has an influence on the practice sequence. Red days have more backbends to fire up the practice to initiate a new energy. White days have more forward bends and twists for introspection. Blue days have more arm balances and inversions for self-empowerment, and yellow days are a strong mix of the three previous energies to build strength to manifest your intentions.

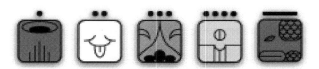

20 Day Signs (Solar Seals)

Seal Name	Timecell	Power	Action	Essence
Red Dragon	Input	Birth	Nurture	Being
White Wind	Input	Spirit	Communicate	Breath
Blue Night	Input	Abundance	Dream	Intuition
Yellow Seed	Input	Flowering	Target	Awareness
Red Serpent	Store	Life Force	Survive	Instincts
White Worldbridger	Store	Death	Equalize	Opportunity
Blue Hand	Store	Accomplishment	Know	Healing
Yellow Star	Store	Elegance	Beautify	Art
Red Moon	Process	Water	Purify	Flow
White Dog	Process	Heart	Love	Loyalty
Blue Monkey	Process	Magic	Play	Illusion
Yellow Human	Process	Free Will	Influence	Wisdom
Red Skywalker	Output	Space	Explore	Wakefullness
White Wizard	Output	Timelessness	Enchant	Receptivity
Blue Eagle	Output	Vision	Create	Mind
Yellow Warrior	Output	Fearlessness	Question	Intelligence
Red Earth	Matrix	Navigation	Evolve	Synchronicity
White Mirror	Matrix	Endlessness	Reflect	Order
Blue Storm	Matrix	Self-generation	Catalyze	Energy
Yellow Sun	Matrix	Universal Fire	Enlighten	Life

Each day also has a guiding power that can influence the sequencing. When you know the guiding power, then you can bring key poses from that class sequence into the sequence of the day of the solar seal. The guiding power of each day will be one of the other four powers of the input, store, process, output, or matrix groups. If the tone is one, six, or eleven, then the guiding power is double the energy of the solar seal for the day. For example, Red Rhythmic Dragon is guided by the power of Birth. Consult the Dreamspell calendar each day to find the guiding power or use the table below. With the guiding power, you can complete the affirmation to seal the energy at the end of the practice. The formula for the daily or personal affirmation is as follows:

I **Tone** *Power* in order to **Tribe** *Action,*

Tone *Action* ing **Tribe** *Essence,*

I seal the **Timecell** of **Tribe** *Power,*

with the **Tone's** *Name* tone of **Tone** *Essence.*

I am guided by the power of the *Guiding **Tribe** *Power.*

Example Affirmations:

Blue Spectral Eagle seal 115

"I Dissolve in order to Create,
Releasing Mind,
I seal the output of Vision,
with the Spectral tone of Liberation.
I am guided by my own power doubled."

Yellow Crystal Warrior seal 116

"I Dedicate in order to Question,
Universalizing Fearlessness,
I seal the output of Intelligence,
with the Crystal tone of Cooperation.
I am guided by the power of Elegance."

Key for finding the guiding power for each day:

Solar Seals with Tones:	Guide Power Energy
1, 6, or 11:	The guiding power is the solar seal of the day.
2, 7, or 12:	12 seals ahead or 8 seals back of solar seal of the day.
3, 8, or 13:	4 seals ahead or 16 seals back of solar seal of the day.
4 or 9:	4 seals back or 16 seals ahead of solar seal of the day.
5 or 10:	8 seals ahead or 12 seals back of solar seal of the day.

Dreamspell Oracle

Red Dragon (nurtures-birth-being): Initiates a new beginning and a new cycle of energy. The Red Dragon represents the beginning of all life and the essence of motherly love. It is an invitation to nurture on all levels of our being, and accept healing from the universe. Allow your Self to be supported by life. Dragons were often used in the image of the Uroborus by the alchemical and mystery schools to represent the 'eternal return'. The Dragon turning back on itself to bite its own tail represents the process of birth, death, and rebirth. The practice is always beginning again and this day opens us to the possibility of starting a new creation.

In the *asana* sequence, there is focus on the upper back and cervical spine while performing backbends. Backbends represent the unknown potential because we can't see where we are going. They build trust and confidence to go into the unseen territory of our being. There is also a focus on hip-openers to activate the root chakra and to balance the energies of *prana* and *apana*.

White Wind (communicate-breath-spirit): Breath is synonymous with wind and spirit. Our bodies communicate to us through the breath. When you enter into an uncomfortable space or the body is strained, then the breath will become constricted. It is a sign that you should not be there. The breath will guide you deeper into the posture. If you can release tension on exhale, then stay in the pose. If the tension does not release, then do not force the opening.

This day encourages us to focus on the conscious breath. When you are present with the breath, you are present with the moment. The mind can go into the past or future, but the breath is always present. The conscious breath in *asana* activates the five *Prana vayus*, the winds of the life force. This class focuses on *vinyasa* transitions to build power in the breath. It incorporates forward bends, hip-openers, twists, and arm balances to bring awareness to the *Prana vayus*.

Blue Night (dreams-abundance-intuition): Utilize your dreams to develop more awareness of what your aspirations are in life. Trust in your intuition and stay in gratitude to attract more abundance into your life. The more thankful you are for what you have in life, the more you will attract more blessings for personal growth and development. If you constantly tell yourself that there isn't enough and that you are lacking and in need, that is what you get from life - nothing. Abundance is not measured in material wealth but in the spiritual wisdom cultivated through practice.

Blue Night energy builds conscious energy to reach the super-conscious state of lucid awareness while awake and asleep. In *asana* practice, use the hands to stabilize awareness in the moment. The hands are the most powerful tools for dreamers because they can always be found in the dream, as they are attached to the dream body. The hands are the foundation for *asana* and dreaming practices. When you visualize your hands, repeat internally, "I'm dreaming, this is a dream." The more this is repeated as a mantra, the more likely the thought will occur when you actually are dreaming. If you never tell yourself that you are dreaming when you are awake, you will never gain enough awareness to perceive through the illusion of the dream to gain lucidity. When we are lucid in a dream, we are unbound by limitations, but when we awake, we may feel separate from others or from God. The goal of the dreaming practice is to attain the super-conscious state of inherent unity through dreaming and then apply it while awake to create a totality or unification of the self.

This *asana* practice is a flow of variations, arm balance transitions and inversions to stay in remembrance of the dream space.

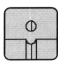

Yellow Seed (targets-flowering-awareness): This energy reminds us that we are gardeners of awareness and that we must target what we want to flourish in our life. Plant a seed in your heart as an intention of what you would like to manifest. Nourish it with breath and energy. We prepare the ground for growth through *asana* practice. The *vinyasa* prepares the body to dig deep. The standing poses and inversions break down the outer shell of the seed, which must fall away and decay if the inner fruit is to flower. We must drop attachment to our limitations and obstacles if we are to grow. The backbends and shoulder openers create an expansion of heart-space, allowing the seed of intentions to flourish.

Red Serpent (survives-life force-instincts): This energy is synonymous with the *kundalini shakti*, the dormant spiritual energy that dwells at the base of the pelvic floor. In the hatha yoga tradition, it is said that the serpent must be decapitated so that its body will uncurl to awaken the upper *chakras*. The *kundalini* is powerful energy that, if raised too quickly, can lead to extreme emotional states or hallucinations. This occurs through long practices of *pranayama* or Kundalini Yoga. To slowly raise the energy, we use *asana* to safely unravel the *granthis* (psychic knots), which constrict its upward flow to the crown chakra. Deep lunges and hip-openers performed with the bandhas slowly release the *kundalini shakti*.

Red Serpent energy reminds us that our bodies are our temples. They are vehicles for exploration and heightened states of spiritual attainment. The body has an intelligence, which we experience as instincts. Our body knows what it needs and through *asana* practice, we become more aware of instincts and honor them as an embodiment of divine energy. By honoring our body's temple through *asana* and doing the internal work through meditation, the life force is strengthened along with the will to survive.

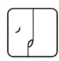

White Worldbridger (equalizes-death-opportunity): Release everything in your life that no longer serves you. There is great freedom in surrender. By letting go of what is unnecessary, we free up energy, and make space for new things to come into our life. By overcoming our obstacles in life, and letting go of our desire to control, we bridge the gap between our former self and the person we are capable of becoming. Worldbridger energy brings death to energies that hinder us, but it is also humbling by reminding us of our own impermanence. By staying in remembrance of our own death, we live more fully in the moment. Death is not the end but is a new beginning. In death, you must surrender to be successful; paradoxically, in life, you must surrender to opportunities to be successful.

Worldbridger energy is neutralizing, nullifying, and equalizing. The yoga *asana* practice embodies forward bends, twists, and backbends to equalize the body and take the mind back to *sesha* (the 0 point) or nothingness. We enter *shavasana* as a symbolic death to the ego and are thus reborn to pursue a new accomplishment (Blue Hand).

Blue Hand (knows-accomplishment-healing): Hands are instruments of personal power. They have the power to heal, mend, lend, and support. Hands engage us in our activities, which bring the sensation of accomplishment. Embrace your activities and practice as a master craftsman and artist of light. The process of actualizing an accomplishment requires patience and personal healing. It cannot be forced with self-effort. When activities are done in the spirit of *isvara-pranidhana* (dedication to God), then every act becomes an instrument of personal healing. When we heal ourselves, we become more sensitive to the healing process of others. Socrates said, "Be kind, for everyone you meet is fighting a great battle." The battle for personal freedom requires the healing support from others. Nobody can do it alone. Accept healing from the universe so you can become an instrument of healing for others.

The Blue Hand practice focuses on empowering our hands to stay in remembrance of their connection to our inner being. The hands are used in all the alternate positions throughout the sequence. It is encouraged that when the arm balances become easy with hands flat, they are then performed on ridgetop, fists, or fingertips. The variations in *asana* build power in the hands, which correlates to strengthening our personal power.

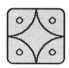

Yellow Star (beautifies-elegance-art): Inner beauty is achieved through self-acceptance and kindness towards others. Yoga teaches us to be humble and to surrender to a power greater than ourselves. In humility there is great power. Yellow Star energy reminds us of our inner power and beauty but reminds us that it is not created by us but through us. When we give up asserting ourselves over others in a show of dominance for the empowerment of our false self, and start uplifting others by the power of our inner radiance, then that is art. The artist refines and beautifies nature. Whenever we generate art from within, either through yoga or by witnessing art, then there is a suspension of consciousness and an uprising of energy. The experience of art and acts of beauty creates more *sattva*, balanced energy, and a desire to experience elegance or a refinement of consciousness in all experiences. The experience of *sattva* is the balance between the two extremes of *rajas* (excessive) and *tamas* (deficiency). Yoga teaches us to find the midline between the extremes to manifest more beauty, art, and elegance.

The Yellow Star practice is all-encompassing with powerful poses to create inner strength and humility.

Red Moon (purifies-universal water-flow): The energy of the Red Moon purifies the senses to bring us back into remembrance of our essence as divine beings. Through yoga, we purify our minds and bodies, so we don't fall into forgetfulness. We purify by embodying the attributes of Universal Water; fluidity and resiliency. We flow in *asana* to gain the strength to yield when necessary. To 'go with the flow' is not always what is in one's best interests; sometimes it is best to yield and observe the flow before merging. Yoga develops the inner confidence and awareness of when you need to yield and when it is time to flow.

The Red Moon practice focuses on backbends to initiate remembrance of the universal, twists to purify, and hip-openers to activate *sacral chakra* (water element).

White Dog (loves-loyalty-heart): The energy of White Dog honors the heart as a medium of spirit. It asserts that the essence of our being is love, and the all-curing medicine is compassion. It invites us to cultivate our relationships and to draw power from our spiritual family. By generating love in yoga, we are able to extend the energy to others. When we are clear, there shouldn't be anything that obstructs the energy of love and acceptance. Yoga removes all obstructions so the heart energy can develop fully. By strengthening the connection to the heart-space, we develop more loyalty and trust in the Supreme.

The White Dog practice is playful with standing poses and twists to cultivate puppy love energy. The practice develops mad dog energy through arm balances and backbends. White dog day balances puppy love with mad dog energy, so that we are compassionate and receptive, yet strong and determined in our actions.

Blue Monkey (plays-magic-illusion): The energy of Blue Monkey reminds us that we are children of the universe. It develops a playful spirit, so we can bring spontaneity and fun into our life. If we identify with the struggles in life, then we become trapped in *maya*, the illusion. When we embrace the spirit of playfulness, we are more aligned with the *lila*, the sport of God. In Hindu mythology, the blue monkey is Hanuman, the devotional servant of Lord Rama. Hanuman is often described as the monkey god of war, but his main quest is to re-unite the god and goddess, Ram and Sita.

In the epic of the Ramayana, Ram was set to marry Sita, but she was kidnapped by the evil demon king Ravana, who stole her away to Sri Lanka. Ram had no army and was overcome with grief. He asked Hanuman to locate Sita, deliver his ring, and help build his army. Hanuman was filled with self-doubt, but then he turned within and connected to his heart. He realized his only desire was to re-unite Ram and Sita. He was filled with love for them and realized that love for the god and goddess dwelled within him and not outside. Upon this recognition, he gained all eight *siddhis*, supernatural powers. He became very large, and made one symbolic leap from India to Sri Lanka. He located Sita and delivered the ring. He assisted Ram in defeating the demons, and saving Sita. The story is symbolic of our own process in yoga, where the goal is to reunite the god/goddess (solar/lunar) energies of the human body. Ravana symbolizes the Lower Self, or the ego, and creates a state of dualism within, where the god/goddess energies are separate. Hanuman represents the Higher Self, and the state of remembrance. The Higher Self triumphs over the Lower Self, and succeeds in re-creating a state of unity when we connect to the Truth and the hearts desire.

The Blue Monkey practice is playful with variations, arm balances, and inversions. It also prepares the hamstrings for *Hanumansana* to represent the symbolic leap from India to Sri Lanka, and our own path to unite the god and goddess energies.

Yellow Human (influence-free will-wisdom): Yellow Human energy reminds us that our individuality contributes to the diversity of humanity. Our experiences bring wisdom that influences those around us. We are all microcosmic reflections of the macrocosm, and through yoga, we learn to transcend our identification with the finite and connect to the power of the infinite. The Yellow Human practice is dedicated to the sages, gurus, and teachers who have transcended the finite and manifested the infinite.

This is a list of the sage poses incorporated in the sequencing and their historical significance:

Vasistha: famous for living in a cave and training three wish-fulfilling cows. He taught proper worship for Skanda by abstaining from meat on Fridays and repeating the mantra "Om Saravanabhava Namaha."

Vishvamitra: famous for his conquest for worldly power, but was defeated by Vasistha's super empowered cows. He thus surrendered to Vasistha and became his devotee. He then shifted his focus toward attaining spiritual power.

Koundinya: a sage of Vasistha's family who founded the Koundinya Gotra (lineage). The goddess Parvati for the purpose of making intoxicating drinks created him.

Galava: a student of Vishvamitra.

Gheranda: the author of the Gheranda Samhita, one of the three classical texts on hatha yoga. The other two main texts are the Hatha Yoga Pradipika and the Shiva Samhita. The Gherandha Samhita is the most detailed on the practice. It categorizes seven limbs of yoga compared to the eight-fold path of Patanjali's ashtanga yoga. The seven limbs of the Gheerandha Samhita are:

1: Shatkarma: purification
2: Asana: posture for strengthening
3: Mudra: for steadying energy flow
4: Pratyahara: for sense withdrawal and calming
5: Pranayama: for breath control and lightness of being
6: Dhyana: for focus and perception
7: Samadhi: for the experience of bliss in aloneness

Marichi: son of the creator Brahma given the task of finishing the creation process. He is married to Kala and fathers Kasyapa.

Kasyapa: son of Marichi who was seducced by Maya while meditating. He fathered three children with her who grew up to be the three demons defeated by Skanda's lance: Surapadma, Simhamukha, and Taraka.

Matsyendranath: the first teacher of hatha yoga. He overheard a conversation between Shiva and Parvati on the techniques to manifest divine awareness and was granted a human form due to his success in the practice.

Goraknath: the first student of Matsyendranath and founder of the Nath sect of yoga. There is a myth that his mother was barren and asked a wandering sage for a blessing so she may be with child. He instead gave her some seeds that he instructed her to drink. She instead threw them in the field behind her due to her disbelief. When the sage returned nine months later, he asked where her child was. She told him what she had done and he went into the field and located a pile of cow dung where the seeds had fallen. He repeated some mantras and a child grew out of the cow dung. This child was Goraknath.

Red Skywalker (explore-space-wakefulness): Red Skywalker energy invites us to transcend old paradigms, conditionings, and limitations. It awakens new levels of awareness and alternate states of consciousness. No one can transcend without the support of a partner or teacher. The two descending lines of the Red Skywalker glyph represent the grounding into the earth with the teachings, and then using them to uplift toward the heavens. In yoga we root and ground ourselves physically and energetically, so that our spirits can soar with the awareness of the Higher Self. This practice can be done in isolation, but Skywalker energy encourages us to seek the support of another for elevation. It is only when we surround ourselves with positive people that we gain the courage to step into unknown territory.

The Red Skywalker practice incorporates backbends and inversion variations that are challenging and playful.

White Wizard (enchant-timelessness-receptivity): White Wizard energy reminds us that we are all magicians of our lives when we are present in the moment. We lose our power to cultivate magic when our mind drifts into regrets of the past or fears of the future. In the present moment, anything is possible. We create magic through our thoughts, words, and actions. Develop your own personal myth and honor your own legend. The present moment is the wizard's playing field.

The White Wizard practice is built upon twisting. When we spiral the body, it brings us into the depths of our being and the uprising sensations of the moment.

Blue Eagle (create-vision-mind): The energy of the Blue Eagle is transformative. In order to transform, we must establish a clear vision of where we are directing our energy. Focusing on the horizon attains the goal. Ignore the minor details that may deter your flight path. Establish "eagle vision" in your life and stay focused on the big picture. All eagles reach a point in their life where their talons overgrow and they are no longer able to capture prey. At this time they must fly to the peak of a mountain and bash their talons against the rocks to break them off. If they do not endure this painful process, they face certain death. There comes a time for humans also to endure the pains of the transformative process. We have to stay focused on the horizon to overcome all discomfort. This can only be accomplished through mindfulness and contemplation.

The Blue Eagle practice incorporates variations of the eagle pose to stay in remembrance of the vision of spirit, and to build strength for transformation on all levels of being.

Yellow Warrior (question-intelligence-fearlessness): Yellow Warrior encourages you to question your limitations and fears with an intelligent attitude, so that you can pursue your path with a fearless attitude. To follow your path of spiritual development, it requires that you follow your heart and its convictions. The heart commands truth regardless of where it takes you. Follow your heart and you will achieve success on the path. The spiritual warrior overcomes the fear to fight for what is just, right, and honorable. Yoga develops the inner strength to fight for what you believe in and also for the rights of others.

The practice of the Yellow Warrior is strong and challenging to develop the attitude of the spiritual warrior. The energy of Skanda is embodied throughout the practice by building positivity to overcome the energies of negativity, fear, and ignorance.

Red Earth (evolve-navigate-synchronicity): Red Earth energy recognizes the mother earth as a conscious living being. When you align with nature's cyclical patterns, you experience more synchronicity in your life. When you witness synchronicity, you must recognize that it occurs because you are aligned with the universal energy. If you dismiss it as pure chance, then your energetic vibration is diminished. When it is acknowledged as Grace, your vibration increases, and the process accelerates.

In mythology, Skanda's brother Ganesha represents the earth element. Elephants embody the heaviness and grounding of the earth element. The elephant has no natural predator and is the remover of obstacles, as nothing stands in the path of an elephant. When the energy of Ganesha is embodied, it clears the path for the uprising energy from the root *chakra*, and the experience of synchronicity.

Ganesha's elephant head symbolically represents the practice of yoga. The large ears are for listening to the quality of the breath. The long nostrils are for deepening the breath. The small mouth represents less talk and more action. The whole idea of having an elephant head on a human body is somewhat ridiculous, so it reminds us not to take anything too seriously. Elephants have no predator in nature, but they are scared of marsupials, and thus Ganesha's vehicle is a rat. This shows that the practice of yoga has the power to control one's natural fears.

The practice of the Red Earth contains backbends to awaken the life force energy and hip-openers to activate the lower *chakras* and the earth element. Releasing tension in the hips synergistically releases mental holding patterns and creates a natural uprising of energy. By freeing physical tension, we release mental tension, which allows us to be more present in the moment. Evolution occurs after involution. By going within ourselves and removing self-imposed obstacles, we can navigate our path towards our optimal state of wellbeing.

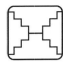

White Mirror (reflect-endlessness-order): The mirror is the mind that reflects our inner reality and projects it externally as our reality. Yoga clears the mirror of the mind so that we reflect the truth of our divine nature. White Mirror energy reminds us that all perspectives are relative to their point of view. Honor the viewpoints of others by recognizing they are all subjectively true, even if not based in reality. Use all experiences as a self-reflective meditation to see how we are co-creators of our reality, and to witness how others are creating theirs.

The White Mirror sequence incorporates forward bends, twists, and hip-openers to develop more introspective and reflective awareness. The path is endless. By reflecting upon how far you've come on your journey, you honor the process, which results in patience with yourself and others. Nobody can awaken overnight. It is a practice that requires you to set up life in order so progress can be achieved.

Blue Storm (catalyze-self-generation-energy): Blue Storm energy reminds us not to identify with the chaos in our lives. It invites us to cultivate "the eye of the storm," where we are peaceful and tranquil. Cultivate strength in the center of your being and then you will have a greater capacity to influence others with positivity. The stronger we are in our center, the less likely we are to lose ourselves when the storm of life hits.

The Blue Storm sequence focuses on midline techniques to develop more awareness of the center.

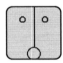

Yellow Sun (enlighten-universal fire-life): Yellow Sun is the peak of the cycle, and carries the highest energy. It reminds you to celebrate life fully and to walk the path of enlightenment. Developing more *tapas*, inner heat blazes the path, to burn off all impurities so the divine light of your being can shine bright. Enlightenment can be thought of as a noun, as some place you finally reach or something that is attained. Or enlightenment can be thought of as a verb, where you are being enlightened or are enlightening yourself by actions or activities. According to Descartes, enlightenment could be defined by what it is not. If you accept what you are told without question from religious authorities, government agencies, or any other position of power, this is not an enlightened state of mind. An enlightened being is able to think for itself without being influenced by outside forces. Use the awareness and strength gained through the practice to trust in your Self, and don't be concerned with the thoughts of others.

The Yellow Sun sequence builds inner heat through powerful poses. It is designed to be a fun and challenging practice that inspires you to celebrate your life. It incorporates arm balances and inversions for self-empowerment.

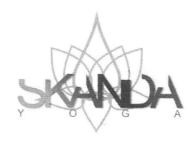

CHAPTER 17: Dreamspell Class Sequences

The following sequences are structured for classes or for personal practice. The level 0 initiation classes (red, white, blue, yellow) develop the opening and technique necessary for levels I-III. The initiation sequences can also be practiced as hot yoga sequences by removing *vinyasa* after the strength recruiting section. They should be performed between 60-75 minutes and between 78-87 degrees, or 88-98 degrees for hot yoga. There are three levels for each day of the 20-day sequence of solar seals from the Dreamspell calendar. They are designed for 90-minute classes, but can be done in 75 minutes by dropping the challenging section. The room temperature should be between 82-87 degrees. The level 1 sequences can be rendered level 0 by eliminating arm balances and the challenging section. The levels are for Skanda Yoga classes only and are not meant as a comparison with other schools. For example, a level 1 Skanda Yoga class might be a level 2 or 3 class in a different system.

The sequences are open to slight modifications and variations. If wall space is unavailable, or teaching is mixed-level, then skip the challenge section and place a shortened version of it after the deepening section. All of the poses should be held for five breaths in the warm-up and strength recruiting section. Poses can be held longer in the challenging, opening, and deepening sections. The poses listed in the warm-up should be incorporated into the opening Sun Salutations. *Vinyasas* should be added in between the poses, or blocks of poses in the strength recruiting and opening sections. They should be performed in the challenging section when working arm balances. There are no *vinyasas* in the deepening or restorative section of the practice (except on yellow days). All poses should be performed evenly on both sides with *vinyasa* between the right and left side. When there is a group of poses like "triangle, half moon, sugarcane, standing split," they should performed all on one side with a *vinyasa* after, and then enter the second side. When (x2) appears in the sequence, then the pose is repeated twice. When you see "xTone" in the sequence, that indicates that the pose should be performed in repetitions of 1-13 as indicated by the tone number of each day on the Dreamspell. If it is tone 1, 6, or 11, then the number can be doubled. Practice the sequence on the appropriate day of the Dreamspell calendar. You can go to **www.skandayoga.com** to see the energy of the day.

All of the sequences are balanced for the body. However, the color of the day will determine the focus for the body. For example, Red days will incorporate more backbends. White days will focus on forward bends, twists, and hip-openers. Blue days will prepare the body for inversions and arm balances. Yellow days are a combination of the three preceding energies and are strong practices to represent the completion of a cycle. The sequences should be practiced at one's own level. If a pose is not available, then work as close as you can, or skip to the next pose. Progression will be noticed as one repeats the same sequences every twenty days. When practicing, it is important to listen to your body first; if something doesn't feel right, then don't do it. It is not possible to practice hard every single day, so mix in some easy days with the hard practices. It is also good to take rest days with massages periodically. Do not be concerned with trying to acquire poses, but instead use the poses as tools to enhance meditation and introspection. It is not about what we can do externally that matters, but it is the inner state of being that matters most. Celebrate life and live fully. Enjoy the practice.

*Please note that for the sake of brevity "Utthita" has been left out in front of poses such as Parsvakonasana, Trikonasana, and Ardha Chandrasana. Also, in some cases, the common name is used in English instead of a direct translation.

*Also note that drop-backs, Natarajasana, and Viparita Chakrasana are all optional at the end of sequences.

INITIATION SEQUENCES

Level O: Red

Intention: Initiate a new pattern of existence.
Focus in asana: stability in form
Mudra: *jnana* (knowledge seal)
Pranayama: *viloma* (ladder breath on inhalation)
Direction: East
Element: Earth

Introduction: (5-10 min)
Meditation, Mudra, and Pranayama
Chant

Warm-Up: (10 min)
Sun Salutation A [0] (x2)
Bound hand locust [311]
Elixir of the moon pose I [17]
Side angle pose [49]

Strength Recruiting: (10 min)
Warrior I [34]
Triangle [59]
Sage Vasistha prep [214]
Upward facing Kali pose [106], sage Shankara's pose [107]
Extended wide leg forward bend I [88]

Child's pose [388]

Opening: (15 min)
Locust pose I-III [307-309]
One arm auspicious pose [326]
Half frog [261], child's pose [388]
Pigeon pose [400]
Fire log pose [405]
Half fish pose [374]
Extended legs wide pose [88]
Bound angle pose [410]

Deepening: (10 min)
Leg lifts (xTone) [350 & 351]
Bridge [295]
Upward bow [300]

Restorative: (10-20 min)
Shoulder stand [164]
Eye of the needle [486]
Single leg stretch I, II, III [474, 476, 477]
Happy baby [489]
Corpse pose [494]

Level O: White

Intention: Refine existence through breath and spirit.
Focus in asana: victorious breath
Mudra: *Vishnu* (savior seal)
Pranayama: *nadi shodhana* (alternate nostril breathing)
Direction: North
Element: Wind

Introduction: (5-10 min)
Meditation, Mudra, and Pranayama
Chant

Warm-Up: (10 min)
Sun Salutation A [0] (x2)
Side angle pose [49], elixir of the moon IV [20]
Action pose [8], mountain pose [1]

Strength Recruiting: (10 min)
Warrior I [34], revolved side angle [57]
Wind vinyasa [345] (xTone)
Bound hands warrior [41], humble warrior [47]
Triangle [59], intense side stretch [87]

Half moon [70], revolved half moon, standing split [69]
Child's pose [388]

Opening: (15 min)
Twisting thigh stretch [288]
Pigeon prep pose [400]
Forehead to knee pose [366], revolved forehead to knee pose [369]
Sage Marichi pose I & III [424, 426]
Extended leg wide pose [381], revolved seated wide angle pose [382]
Two arm hero [332], yogi's staff pose prep [443]

Deepening: (5min)
Windshield wipers (xTone)
Bridge pose
Upward bow pose

Restorative: (10)
Shoulder stand, plow pose
Single leg stretch I, II, III
Happy baby
Corpse pose

Level 0: Blue

Intention: Seek a transformation on all levels of being.
Focus in asana: Moving from the inside out
Mudra: *jnana* (wisdom seal)
Pranayam*a*: *viloma* (ladder breath on exhalation)
Direction: East
Element: Water

Introduction: (5-10 min)
Meditation, Mudra, and Pranayama
Chant

Warm-Up: (10 min)
Sun Salutation A [0] (x3)
Monkey lunge I pose [14]
Side angle pose [49]

Strength Recruiting: (10 min)
Warrior I [34]
Sage Vasistha prep [214]
Warrior I [34], warrior II [43], side warrior [45]
Triangle [59], half moon [70], standing split [86], eagle pose I [104], standing split [86]
Half garland pose [101], extended wide leg stretch [88]

Monkey frog [434]
Child's pose [388]

Opening: (10-15 min)
One arm auspicious pose [326], bow pose [265]
Pigeon prep [400]
Camel [275], supine hero pose [468]
Half fish prep [374], one foot cow face forward bend [365]
Seated wide angle [381], revolved seated wide angle [382]
West side stretch [357]

Deepening: (5-10 min)
Eagle crunches [349] (xTone)
Bridge pose [295]
Upward bow pose [300]

Restorative: (10-20 min)
Shoulder stand [164], plow pose [171]
Single leg stretch I-III [477]
Supine auspicious pose [481]
Supine twist III [491]
Corpse pose [492]

Level O: Yellow

Intention: Manifest a greater possibility in life.
Focus in asana: muscle energy (intention in action)
Mudra: *Rudra* (ruler of the solar plexus)
Pranayama: *bhastrika* (breath of fire)
Direction: West
Element: Fire

Introduction: (5-10 min)
Meditation, Mudra, and Pranayama
Chant

Warm-Up: (10 min)
Sun Salutation A [0] (x3)
Side angle pose [50]
Sun Salutation B [00] (x2)

Strength Recruiting: (10 min)
Extended bound hands warrior [42]
Bound hands warrior I [41], humble warrior [47]
Triangle [59], half moon [70], standing split [86]
Extended legs wide forward bend I-IV [81-84]
Child's pose [388]

Opening: (15 min)
Twisting thigh stretch [288], Hanuman prep [436],
Subramanya's pose [22]
One foot pigeon prep [400]
Camel [275]
Half fish [375], cow face pose [395]
Seated wide angle pose [381], revolved seated wide angle [382]
Baby cradle [441], half bound west side stretch [363]

Deepening: (10min)
Boat pose & half-boat [346, 347] (x3)
Bridge pose [295]
Upward bow [300] (x2)

Restorative: (15-20 min)
Shoulder stand [164], plow pose [171]
Fish pose [319], intense foot pose [321]
Single leg stretch I, II, III [474, 476, 477]
One foot happy baby [488], happy baby [489]
Supine twist I & II [491, 492]
Corpse pose [494]

1) Red Dragon: NURTURE – BEING – BIRTH

The energy of the Red Dragon initiates a new beginning, a new cycle of energy, and a pattern of existence. It represents the abundance of potential energy, and the source of all, to which all return. Red Dragon is the beginning and end of the transformative cycle. Start anew again like you are doing the practice for the first time. The aim for today is to take the re-birth or renewing energy off the mat and into the world, so everything feels fresh and alive. Take the time to nurture yourself with the energy of 'mother love'. The Red Dragon harnesses life force (*Prana*) to initiate the refining, transformative, and manifesting processes. The class focuses on backbends to move into the unknown, while targeting the upper back and cervical spine to awaken new energies of awareness.

"The Truth is your birthright. No one can take it from you." – Sri Svami Purna

Intention: Accept healing from the universe.
Allow yourself to be supported by life.
Focus in asana: *mula bandha*
Digit: right index finger

Chakra: throat
Mudra: *shunya* (heaven energy seal)
Pranayama: *viloma* (ladder breath on inhalation), *moorcha* (swooning breath)

Level I

Introduction: (5-10 min)
Meditation, Mudra, and Pranayama,
Chant

Warm-Up: (5-10 min)
Sun Salutation A [0] (x2)
Bound hand locust [311], Crocodile pose [306]
Elixir of the moon pose I [17]
Side angle pose variation [50] (one hand behind head)

Strength Recruiting: (15 min)
Warrior I [34, 35] (x2)
Warrior I [36] (two hands behind the head), Warrior III [46], standing split [86]
Bound side angle [55]
Upward facing Kali pose [106], sage Shankara's pose [107]
Extended wide leg forward bend I-III [88-90]
Crane pose [185], child's pose [388]

Challenging: (10 min)
Handstand prep technique at wall [147]
Handstand scorpion prep [160]
-or-
Locust pose I-IV [307-310]

Opening: (15 min)
One arm auspicious pose [326]
One foot bow pose [269], bow pose [265], child's pose [388]
One foot king pigeon prep [400]
Fire log pose I, II [405, 406]
Seated wide angle pose [381], revolved seated wide angle [382]
Two arm hero [332], east side stretch [294]
Supported baby cradle [442], yogi's staff pose prep [443]

Deepening: (10 min)
Leg lifts [350 & 351] (xTone)
Bridge pose [295]
Upward bow pose [300] (x2)

Restorative: (10-20 min)
Shoulder stand [164], plow pose [171]
Fish pose [319], intense foot pose [321]
Single leg stretch I, II, III [474, 476, 477]
Happy baby [489], supine twist [491]
Corpse pose [494]

Level II

Introduction: (5-10 min)
Meditation, Mudra, and Pranayama
Chant

Warm-Up: (5-10 min)
Sun Salutation A (x3) [0]
Bound hand locust [311], Crocodile pose [306]
Elixir of the moon pose I-III [17-19]
Side angle pose variation (one hand behind head) [50]

Strength Recruiting (10 min):
Warrior I [34, 35] (x2)
Sage Vasistha's pose [215], wild thing [219]
Warrior I (with two hands behind head) [36], Warrior III (both hands behind head) [46], Standing split [86], handstand [146]
Triangle [59], half-moon [70], sugarcane [77], standing split [86], handstand [146]
Upward facing Kali pose [106], sage Shankara's pose [107], extended legs wide forward bend pose IV-V [91, 92]
Crane pose [185], child's pose [388], dragon pose [260]

Challenging: (10-15 min)
Handstand prep technique at wall [147]
Handstand one leg scorpion prep [160]
Scorpion [162]
-or-
Locust poses I-IV [307-310]
One arm auspicious pose [326]

Bound one leg bow pose [270], bound bow pose [266], bow pose [265], child's pose [388]

Opening: (10-15 min)
Half frog [261], sage Gherandhasana prep [272], child's pose [388]
One foot king pigeon [285]
Fire log pose I-III [405-407]
Half fish [374], cow face [396]
Seated wide angle pose [381], revolved seated wide angle pose [382]
Two arm hero [332], east side stretch [294]
Yogi's staff pose prep [443]

Deepening: (10 min)
Dragon flags [353] (xTone)
Bridge pose [295]
Upward bow [300] (x2)
Lord of the dance pose [115] (x2)

Restorative: (10-20 min)
Shoulder stand [164], plow pose [171]
Fish pose [319], intense foot pose [321]
Eye of the needle [486], Supine upward foot diamond pose prep [478]
Happy Baby [489], sleeping yogi's pose [463]
Supine twist I & II [491, 492]
Corpse pose [494]

Level III

Introduction: (5-10min)
Meditation, Mudra, and Pranayama
Chant

Warm-Up: (10min)
Surya Namaskar A [0] (x5)
Baddha Hasta Shalabhasana [311], Makarasana [306]
Soma Chandrasana I-III [17-19]

Parsvakonasana [50]

Strength Recruiting: (10-15 min)
Virabhadrasana I [34]
Virabhadrasana I [35]
Virabhadrasana I [36], Virabhadrasana III [46], Urdhva Prasarita Ekapadasana [86], Adho Mukha Vrksasana [146]
Trikonasana (one hand behind head) [63], Ardha

Chandrasana [70], Ardha Chandra Chapasana [77], Parivrtta Ardha Chandrasana [71], Nindra Eka Pada Dhanurasana [78], Urdhva Prasarita Ekapadasana [86], Adho Mukha Vrksasana [146]

Baddha Parsvakonasana [55], Eka Pada Koundinyasana II [199], Ghanda Bherundasana [316]

Purna Vasisthasana [218], Camatkarasana [219]

Urdhva Kaliasana [106], Shankarasana [107]

Prasarita Padattonasana IV, V [91, 92]

Bakasana [185], Balasana [388], Araniasana [260]

Challenging: (10 min)
Adho Mukha Vrsksasana [146], Eka Pada Vrischikasana [161]
Vrischikasana II [162]
Pincha Mayurasana [133]
Vrischikasana I [139]
Mandalasana [304]

Opening: (15 min)
Agnistambha Eka Bhuja Swastikasana [329]
Purna Eka Pada Dhanurasana (x2) [271], Purna Dhanurasana [268], Balasana [388]

Eka Pada Rajakapotasana [285]

Agnistambhasana I-III [405-407]

Baddha Ardha Matsyendrasana [376], Gomukhasana [397]

Upavishta Konasana [381], Parivrtta Upavishta Konasana [382]

Dwi Bhuja Virasana [332], Purvottanasana [294]

Yoga Dandasana (444)

Maksikanagasana I-IV (242-245), Valgulasana [247]

Deepening: (10 min)
Pincha Araniasana [353] (xTone)
Setu Bandha Sarvangasana [295]
Urdhva Dhanurasana [300] (x2)
Natarajasana [115], Baddha Natarajasana [116]
Drop-backs [322] (xTone)

Restorative: (10-20 min)
Sarvangasana [164], Halasana [171], Karnapidasana [173]
Sucirandrasana [486], Supta Urdhva Padma Vajrasana [172], Eka Pada Sirsa Shayanasana [464]
Yoga Nidrasana [463]
Jathara Parivartanasana I & III [491, 493]
Shavasana [494]

2) White Wind: COMMUNICATE – BREATH – SPIRIT

The energy of White Wind enhances the conscious breath to build spirit, so we can communicate our truth. The breath is the most important aspect of yoga and life. By consciously bringing structure to the breath, we can learn how to tame the mind. By liberating the breath, we enhance the flow of the *prana vayus*, the vital winds, which enhances the bodies health and vitality. The breath and the wind come and go with complete freedom, with no attachment, and they both can be playful, strengthening, or resisting. Ultimately, when we connect to the conscious breath, we connect to the spirit of the higher self. This class focuses on *vinyasa* transitions, forward bends, hip-openers, and twists.

"Life itself is the vehicle given to you that you may learn the mysteries of life." – Sri Svami Purna

Intention: Let the breath guide and support you.
Focus in asana: *ujjayi* breath and *spanda*
Digit: right middle finger
Chakra: heart

Mudra: *vayu* (wind seal)
Pranayama: *sheetali* (cooling breath with *jalandhara bandha*)

Level I

Introduction: (5-10 min)
Centering Meditation, Mudra, and Pranayama
Chant

Warm-Up: (10 min)
Sun Salutation A [0] (x2)
Side angle pose [49], elixir of the moon IV [20]
Fierce pose [10], revolved fierce pose [12], half fierce pose [11]

Strength Recruiting: (10-15 min)
Warrior I [34], revolved side angle [57]
Wind Vinyasa [345] (xTone)
Bound hands warrior [41], humble warrior [47]
Triangle pose [59], half moon [70], revolved half moon [71], intense side stretch [87], standing split [86]
Extended wide leg stance [88], revolved extended legs wide [94], monkey frog pose [434], child's pose [388]
Crane pose [185], child's pose [388], puppy pose [257]

Challenging: (10-15 min)
Sage Marichi's pose I [424], one arm pressure pose [182]

Sage Marichi's pose III [426], side crane pose [191]

Opening: (10-15 min)
Revolved one foot king pigeon prep II [288]
Camel [275], supine hero [467]
Sage Marichi's pose V [428], Sage Marichi's pose VI [429]
Seated wide angle [381], revolved seated wide angle [382]
East side stretch [294]
West side stretch I-III [357-359]

Deepening: (10 min)
Windshield wipers [354] (xTone)
Bridge pose [295]
Upward bow pose [300] (x2)

Restorative: (10-20 min)
Shoulder stand [164], plow [171]
Single leg stretch I, II, III [474, 476, 477]
One foot happy baby [488], happy baby [489]
Supine Twist [491]
Corpse pose [494]

Level II

Introduction: (5-10 min)
Meditation, Mudra, and Pranayama
Chant

Warm-Up: (10 min)
Sun Salutation A (x4) [0]
Side angle pose [49], elixir of the moon IV [20]
Action pose [8], revolved action pose [9]

Strength Recruiting: (10 min)
Warrior I [34], revolved side angle [57]
Wind Vinyasa [345] (xTone)
Bound hands warrior [41], humble warrior [47], sage Koundinya II [199]
Triangle [59], intense side stretch [87], revolved

triangle [65], standing split [86], handstand [146]
Half moon [70], revolved half-moon [71], standing split [86], handstand [146]
Half garland pose [101], extended legs wide I & V [88, 92], monkey frog [434], child's pose [388]

Challenging: (5 min)
Standing wind pose [109], standing wind forehead to knee [110]
Crane pose [185], headstand II [118], crane pose [185]

Opening: (20-25 min)
Sage Marichi's pose I & III [424, 426], one arm pressure pose [182] or sage Ashtavakra's pose [183]

Sage Marichi's pose II [425], half lotus insect pose [213]

Sage Marichi's pose V & VI [428, 429] into side crane pose [191] or uneven side crane [193]

Seated wide angle [381], revolved seated wide angle [382]

Bound angle I & II [410, 411]

Two arm double diamond [338], west side stretch I-III [357-359], revolved west side stretch [361], west side stretch IV [360]

Deepening: (10min)

Level III

Introduction: (5-10 min)
Meditation, Mudra, and Pranayama
Chant

Warm-Up: (10 min)
Surya Namaskar A [0] (x5)
Parsvakonasana [49], Somachandrasana IV [20]
Karmasana [8], Parivrtta Karmasana [9]

Strength Recruiting: (10-15 min)
Virabhadrasana I [34]
Vayu vinyasa (xTone) [345], Eka Pada Koundinyasana I [198]
Baddha Hasta Virabhadrasana [41], Veerastambhasana [47], Eka Pada Koundinyasana II [199]
Baddha Parsvakonasana [55], Baddha Trikonasana [66], Baddha Eka Pada Uttanasana [68], Svarga Dvijasana [75], Baddha Ardha Chandrasana [73], Urdhva Prasarita Ekapadasana [86], Adho Mukha Vrksasana [146]
Parivrtta Prasarita Padottanasana [94], Prasarita Padottanasana IV-V [91, 92], Thavaliasana [434], Balasana [388]

Challenging: (10 min)
Nindra Vayu Muktyasana [109], Nindra Vayu Mukttonasana [110], Eka Pada Bakasana I [189], Adho Mukha Vrksasana [146]
Bakasana [185], sirsasana II [118] or Adho Mukha

Windshield wipers [354] or Krishna crunches [352] (xTone)
Bridge pose [295]
Upward bow [300] (x3)

Restorative: (10-20 min)
Shoulder stand [164], plow [171], ear pressure [173]
Fish pose [319], intense foot pose [321]
Single leg stretch I, II, III [474, 476, 477]
Happy baby [489], sleeping yogi pose [463]
Supine twist [492]
Corpse pose [494]

Vrksasana [146]
Sirsasana II [118], Parsva Bakasana [191]

Opening: (20 min)
Marichiasana I & III [424, 426], Ashtavakrasana [183]
Marichiasana II & IV [425, 427], Ardha Padma Tittibhasana [213]
Marichiasana V & VI [428, 429], Visama Parsva Bakasana [193]
Marichiasana VII & VIII [430, 431], Yoga Dandasana II [239]
Marichiasana IX & X [432, 433]
Upavishta Konasana [381], Parivrtta Upavishta Konasana [382]

Deepening: (10 min)
Navasana [346], Parsva Navasana [348] (xTone)
Urdhva Dhanurasana [300] (x3)
Hanumanasana [438] (x2)

Restorative: (15-20 min)
Sarvangasana [164], Halasana [171], Karnapidasana [173], Parsva Karnapidasana [174]
Matsyasana [319], Uttana Padasana [321]
Supta Bhairavasana [460]
Yoga Nidrasana [463]
Jathara Parivartanasana I [491]
Shavasana [494]

3) Blue Night: Dream – Intuition – Abundance

The energy of the Blue Night merges the awareness of the Dreamer and the Dreamed Being to cultivate lucidity through all experiences. To accomplish anything in life, it must first be dreamed or imagined. When we go to sleep, we become the creators of our own world, and when we are awake, the energy from our dreams can influence our waking reality. Blue Night energy merges the two energies of the dreamed and dreamer, so we become co-creators of the world we experience. We must honor our dreams and visions, and pursue them with the desire to shake them until they become true. This class embodies arm balances and inversions to create the strength to transform our lives by actualizing our dreams.

"Inner Peace is not to be achieved. It is already a part of you. It is your Source. The basis of your Being."
– Sri Svami Purna

Intention: Enter the sanctuary of the Self, and experience the mystery that dwells within you. Unite stillness with your intuition. Become lucidly aware of the dream like nature of life to perceive through the illusion.
Focus in asana: *pratyahara*, turning the senses within
Digit: Right ring finger
Chakra: Solar plexus

Mudra: *Rudra* (ruler of solar plexus), *Vishnu* (Savior seal)
Pranayama: *surya bheda* visualization for women and *chandra bheda* for men (Men block right nostril and inhale green energy up left side, and then exhale blue energy down right side. Females block left side and inhale green energy up right, and then exhale blue energy down left side.)

Level I

Introduction: (5-10 min)
Meditation, Mudra, and Pranayama
Chant

Warm-Up: (10 min)
Sun Salutation A [0] (x3)
Monkey lunge I pose [14]
Side angle pose [50], half warrior side angle pose [51]

Strength Recruiting: (10 min)
Warrior I [34]
Sage Vasistha [215]
Warrior I [34], warrior II [43], side warrior [45], bound side angle pose [55]
Triangle [59], half-moon [70], standing split [86], eagle pose I & II [104, 105], standing split [86]
Half garland pose [101], extended wide leg stretch [88],

Challenging: (10 min)
Crane pose [185], sirsasana II [118], crane pose [185], child's pose [388]
Twisting thigh stretch [288], one foot sage Vasistha II pose [217]
Extended hand to big toe pose I-IV [81-84]
Handstand prep at wall [147]

Opening: (10 min)
One arm auspicious pose [326]
Bow pose [265], child's pose [388]
Camel [275], supine hero pose [468]
Half fish prep [374], one foot cow face forward bend [365]
Seated wide angle [381], revolved seated wide angle [382]
Two arm hero pose [332]

Deepening: (10 min)
Eagle crunches [349] (xTone)

Bridge pose [295]
Upward bow pose [300] (x2)

Restorative: (10-20 min)
Shoulder stand [164], plow pose [171]
Fish pose [319], intense foot pose [321]

Infinity pose [479], single leg stretch III [477]
One foot happy baby [488], happy baby pose [489]
Supine twist [491]
Corpse pose [492]

Level II

Introduction: (5-10 min)
Meditation, Mudra, and Pranayama
Chant

Warm-Up: (10 min)
Sun Salutation A [0] (x4)
Monkey lunge II pose [15]
Side angle [50], half warrior side angle [51]

Strength Recruiting: (10-15 min)
Warrior I [34]
Three limb staff pose [195], sage Vasistha's pose [215]
Warrior I variation [37], side warrior [44], bound side angle [55], sage Koundinya II [199]
Triangle [59], half moon [70], standing split [86], eagle pose [104], standing split [86], handstand [146]
Half garland [101], wide leg forward bend I, IV, V [88, 91, 92]
Crane pose [185], child's pose [388]

Challenging: (10-15 min)
Handstand [146] (timed at wall 3min), child's pose [388] (1 min)
Forearm stand [133] (timed at wall 2min), child's pose [388] (1 min)
Headstand [117] (timed at wall 3min), supported child's pose [389] (1 min)
-or-

Extended hand to big toe pose I-IV [81-84]
Skanda squats [85] (xTone)

Opening: (15 min)
One arm auspicious pose [326]
Locust pose IV [310], child's pose [388]
One foot king pigeon [285]
Camel [275], bound supine hero pose [470]
Peacock pose [229], swan pose [228]
Half fish prep [374], one foot cow face forward bend [365], cow face pose [395]
Seated wide angle sitting [381], revolved seated wide angle [382]
Two arm hero [332], pendant pose [205]

Deepening: (10 min)
Eagle crunches [349] (xTone)
Bridge [295]
Upward bow [300] (x3)

Restorative: (10-20 min)
Shoulder Stand [164], plow pose [171], ear pressure [173]
Fish pose [319], intense foot pose [321]
Infinity pose [479], single leg stretch III [477]
Happy baby pose [489], sleeping yogi pose [463]
Supine twist [491]
Corpse pose [494]

Level III

Introduction: (5-10 min)
Meditation, Mudra, and Pranayama
Chant

Warm-Up: (5 min)
Surya Namaskar A [0] (x5)
Vanarasana II [15]

Parsvakonasana [50], Ardha Vira Parsvakonasana [51]

Strength Recruiting: (10-15 min)
Virabhadrasana I [34] (x2)
Trianga Dandasana [195], Purna Vasisthasana [218]
Virabhadrasana [37], Parsva Virabhadrasana [44],
Baddha Parsvakonasana [55], Eka Pada Koundinyasana
II [199], Ghanda Bherundasana [316]
Baddha Eka Pada Uttanasana [68], Svarga Dvijasana
[75], Tittibhasana II, I [96, 212]
Bakasana [185], Sirsasana II [118] or Adho Mukha
Vrksasana [146]
Balasana [388], Uttana Shishosana [257]

Challenging: (12-18 min)
Adho Mukha Vrksasana [146] (timed at wall 3-5min),
Balasana [388] (1min)
Pincha Mayurasana [133] (timed at wall 3-5min),
Balasana [388] (1min)
Sirsasana [117] (timed at wall 3-5min), Salamba
Balasana [389] (1min)
-or-
Utthita Hasta Padangusthasana I-IV [81-84]
Vira Utthita Hasta Padangusthasana [85] (xTone)

Opening: (15 min)
Eka Bhuja Swastikasana [326]
Shalabhasana IV [310], Viparitta Shalabhasana [312],
Balasana [388]

Eka Pada Rajakapotasana I [285]
Ushtrasana [275], Laghuvajrasana [278], Baddha Supta
Virasana [470]
Mayurasana [229], Hamsasana [228]
Baddha Ardha Matsyendrasana [376], Gomukhasana II
[397]
Upavishta Konasana [381], Parivrtta Upavishta
Konasana [382], Kurmasana [386], Supta Kurmasana
[387]
Baddha Konasana I, II [410, 411], Dwi Bhuja Virasana
[332], Lolasana [205]

Deepening: (10 min)
Garuda vinyasa [349] (xTone)
Setu Bandha Sarvangasana [295]
Urdhva Dhanurasana [300] (x3)
Drop-backs [322] (xTone)

Restorative: (10-20 min)
Sarvangasana [164], Eka Hasta Parsva Sarvangasana
[169], Halasana [171]
Matsyasana [319], Uttana Padasana [321]
Supta Padangusthasana I [475], Anantasana [479]
Supta Eka Bhuja Vira Padangusthasana [336]
Yoga Nidrasana [463]
Jathara Parivartanasana [491]
Shavasana [494]

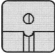

4) Yellow Seed: TARGET – AWARENESS – FLOWERING

The energy of the Yellow Seed strengthens our intentions and our determination to manifest our heart's desires. We plant an intention as a seed within the heart and target it with breath and awareness during the practice so it will flourish into fruition off the mat. It is important to have goals in life to keep us focused and motivated. The spiritual path is one of growth, not of stagnation. Establish *sankalpa mudra* and form a strong intention. Seal the vision within your heart. This class focuses on shoulder openers and backbends to open the heart space.

"The seed has always been there but the ground has to be prepared. All the elements have to be in right order. Then creation starts, and you can see the explosion of energy and life." – Sri Svami Purna

Intention: Break down the outer shell of the seed (intention), so the inner fruit can grow to fruition (manifestation).
Focus in asana: muscle energy (intention in action)

Digit: right pinky finger
Chakra: root
Mudra: *sankalpa* (intention energy seal)
Pranayama: *ujjayi* (victorious breath), *bahya*

kumbhaka (exhale retention with *maha bandha*)

Level I

Introduction: (5-10 min)
Meditation, Mudra, and Pranayama
Chant

Warm-Up: (10 min)
Sun Salutation A [0] (x3)
Side angle pose [50], warrior side angle [52]
Sun Salutation B [00] (x2)

Strength Recruiting: (10 min)
Extended bound hands warrior [42]
Bound hands warrior I [41], humble warrior [47]
Triangle [59], half moon [70], sugarcane [77], standing split [86]
Bound side angle [55]
Extended legs wide forward bend I-IV [81-84]
Crane pose [185], child's pose [388], heart opening pose I [258]

Challenging: (5-10 min)
Handstand [150] (leg raises at wall)
Handstand [158] (legs wide at wall)
Forearm stand prep [132]
-or-
Sage Vasistha's pose [214], wild thing [219], crane pose [185]
Twisting thigh stretch [288], one foot sage Koundinya II [199]

Opening: (15 min)
One arm heart sugarcane [337]
One foot locust pose [314], child's pose [388]
One foot pigeon prep [400], mermaid pose I [283]
One foot pigeon prep II [287]
Half fish [375]
Seated wide angle pose [381], revolved seated wide angle [382]
Bound angle pose [410], wheel of Skanda [324], two arm hero pose [332]

Deepening: (10 min)
Boat pose & half-boat [346, 347] (x3)
Bridge pose [295]
Upward bow [300] (x2)
Drop-back prep [322] (at wall or with spotter)

Restorative: (10-20 min)
Shoulder stand [164], plow pose [171]
Fish pose [319], intense foot pose [321]
Single leg stretch I, II, III [474, 476, 477]
One foot happy baby [488], happy baby [489]
Supine twist [491]
Corpse pose [494]

Level II

Introduction: (5-10 min)
Meditation, Mudra, and Pranayama
Chant

Warm-Up: (10 min)
Sun Salutation A [0] (x4)
Side angle [50], warrior side angle pose [52]
Sun Salutation B [00] (x2)

Strength Recruiting: (10 min)
Bound hands warrior I [41], humble warrior [47],
one foot sage Koundinya II [199]
Triangle [59], half moon [70], sugarcane [77], standing split [86], handstand [146]
Extended legs wide forward fold I-V [88-92]
Crane pose [185], headstand II [118], crane pose [185]
Child's pose [388], heart opening pose I, II [258, 259]

Challenging: (10-15 min)

Handstand [150] (leg raises at wall)
Handstand [158] (legs wide at wall)
Forearm stand [133]
Scorpion [139]
-or-
Full sage Vasistha's pose [218], wild thing [219], crane pose [185]
Sage Vishvamitra's pose [223], one foot sage Koundinya II [199]

Opening: (15 min)
One foot king pigeon prep II [287], Subramanya pose prep [22]
King pigeon [282]
Half fish [375]
Half fish II [378], half bound lotus west side stretch [363]
Seated wide angle pose [381], revolved seated wide

angle pose [382]
Bound angle pose [410], wheel of Skanda [324], two arm hero pose [332]

Deepening: (10 min)
Boat pose & half-boat [346, 347] (x3)
Bridge pose [295]
Upward bow [300] (x3)
Drop-backs [322] (xTone)

Restorative: (15-20 min)
Shoulder stand [164], plow pose [171], ear pressure [173]
Fish pose [319], intense foot pose [321]
Single leg stretch I, II, III [474, 476, 477]
Happy baby [489], sleeping yogi pose [463]
Supine twist [491]
Corpse pose [494]

Level III

Introduction: (5-10 min)
Meditation, Mudra, and Pranayama
Chant

Warm-Up: (10 min)
Surya Namaskar A [0] (x5)
Parsvakonasana [50], Vira Parsvakonasana [52]
Surya Namaskar B [00] (x2)

Strength Recruiting: (15 min)
Baddha Hasta Virabhadrasana [41],
Veerastambhasana [47], Eka Pada Koundinyasana II [199], Ghanda Bherundasana [316]
Baddha Parsvakonasana [55], Baddha Trikonasana [66], Baddha Eka Pada Uttanasana [68], Svarga Dvijasana [75], Baddha Ardha Chandrasana [73], Urdhva Prasarita Ekapadasana [86], Adho Mukha Vrksasana [146]
Parivrtta Baddha Parsvakonasana [58], Eka Pada Koundinyasana I & II [199, 198]
Prasarita Padottanasana I-V [88-92]
Bakasana [185], Sirsasana II [118] or Adho Mukha Vrksasana [146], Bakasana [185]

Balasana [388], Nirakunjasana I-II [258, 259]

Challenging: (10-15 min)
Adho Mukha Vrksasana (leg raises at wall) [150]
Susiravat Prasarita Adho Mukha Vrksasana (legs wide hollow back) [158]
Pincha Mayurasana (133), Susiravat Vrischikasana (140)
-or-
Purna Vasisthasana (218), Camatkarasana (219)
Vishvamitrasana (223), Eka Pada Koundinyasana II (199), Ghanda Bherundasana (316)

Opening: (15 min)
Eka Bhuja Swastikasana [326]
Eka Bhuja Anahata Chapasana [337], Balasana [388]
Eka Pada Rajakapotasana I [285]
Eka Pada Rajakapotasana II [290]
Eka Pada Rajakapotasana III [291]
Eka Pada Rajakapotasana V [293]
Baddha Ardha Matsyendrasana [376]
Ardha Matsyendrasana II [378], Ardha Baddha Padma Paschimottanasana [363], Marichiasana II [425], Ardha Matsyendrasana III [379]

Upavishta Konasana [381], Parivrtta Upavishta Konasana [382]
Baddha Konasana I, II [410, 411], Skanda Chakrasana [324], Dwi Bhuja Virasana [332]

Deepening: (15 min)
Navasana [346] & Ardha Navasana [347] (x3)
Urdhva Dhanurasana [300] (x2)
Dwi Pada Viparita Dandasana [301], Eka Pada Viparita Chakrasana [305]

Hanumanasana [438] (x2-3), Eka Pada Rajakapotasana IV [292]

Restorative: (15 min)
Bharadvajasana II [372], Padmasana [446], Simhasana [317], Goraknathasana [448], Urdhva Kukkutasana [226]
Padmasana [446] (3-5min meditation)
Jathara Parivartanasana I & II [491, 492]
Shavasana [494]

5) Red Serpent: SURVIVE – INSTINCTS – LIFE FORCE

Red Serpent energy is synonymous with the primal life force energy called the *kundalini shakti*. It is the base energy of the root chakra that we draw up the body through the practice to awaken the higher spiritual centers. When we are sensitive to the influence of our own life force energy, it brings us into attunement with our instincts. Throughout the practice, hold *mula bandha, uddiyana,* and *kechari mudra* to increase the flow of life force and assist the natural uprising of energy. This class embodies shoulder openers, hip-openers, and backbends that target the lower back to activate the lower chakras.

"In the pursuit of your Self, you are responsible. You alone are responsible for your own growth, for your own understanding, and for your own achievement." – Sri Svami Purna

Intention: Trust in your instincts. Refine your physical temple. Express your passion, vitality, and sensuality fully.
Focus in asana: Channel *kundalini* by utilizing breath and *bandhas.* Unlock the energy by releasing the *granthis*, the psychic knots of the pelvic floor, through deep lunges, and hip openers.
Digit: Right big toe
Chakra: Crown
Mudra: *Chin mudra* (psychic gesture of consciousness)
Pranayama: *sheetkari* (hissing breath), *antara kumbhaka* (retention after inhalation)

Level I

Introduction: (5-10 min)
Meditation, Mudra, and Pranayama
Chant

Warm-Up: (10 min)
Surya Namaskar A [0] (x3)
Bound hand locust [311]
Elixir of the moon pose I [17]

Strength Recruiting: (10-15 min)
Warrior I (x2) [34]
Sage Vasistha's pose [215]
Warrior I (hands in reverse prayer) [40], Intense side stretch [87]
Triangle [59], half moon [70], standing split [86]
Upward Kali pose [106], sage Shankara's pose [107], extended wide leg pose I & IV [88, 91]

Crane pose [185], child's pose [388], puppy pose [257]

Challenging: (5-10 min)
Full Vasisthasana [218]
Chathaka bird pose prep [221], wild thing [219]
Crane pose [185]
-or-
Handstand (scorpion prep at wall) [160]
Forearm stand (prep at wall) [132]

Opening: (15-20 min)
One arm auspicious pose [326]
One arm lotus pose [330], one arm auspicious pose
II [327], one leg extended wide cobra pose [254]
Two feet extended wide cobra pose [253], child's
pose [388]
Half fish pose [375]
Cow face pose I [396]

Level II

Introduction: (5-10 min)
Meditation, Mudra, and Pranayama
Chant

Warm-Up: (5-10 min)
Sun Salutation A [0] (x3)
Bound hand locust [311]
Elixir of the moon II or III [18 or 19]
Side angle pose [50]

Strength Recruiting: (10-15 min)
Warrior I [34] (x2)
Sage Vasistha's pose [215], one foot sage Vasistha's pose
[216]
Warrior I (hands in reverse prayer) [40], Warrior III [46],
Standing split [86], handstand [146]
Triangle [59], half moon [70], sugarcane [77], standing
splits [86], handstand [146]
Bound side angle [55], one foot sage Koundinya II [199]
Upward Kali pose [106], Shankara's pose [107], extended
wide leg pose I, IV, V [88, 91, 92]
Monkey frog pose [434], child's pose [388]

Challenging: (10 min)

Seated wide angle pose [381], revolved seated wide
angle pose [382]
Two arm hero pose [332], two arm double diamond
[338], west side stretch I & II [357-358]

Deepening: (10 min)
Dragon flags [353] (xTone)
Bridge pose [295]
Upward bow pose [300] (x2)

Restorative: (10-20 min)
Shoulderstand [164], plow [171]
Eye of the needle [486], Supine upward foot
diamond pose prep [478]
Supine Ganesha's pose [483]
Supine twist [491, 492]
Corpse pose [494]

Crane pose [185], headstand II [118], crane pose [185]
Full Vasistha pose [218]
Chathaka bird pose prep [221], wild thing [219], crane
pose [185]
-or-
Handstand scorpion [160]
Forearm stand scorpion [139]
Headstand [117], unsupported headstand [125]

Opening: (15-20 min)
Half frog [261], upward half frog [262], frog pose [264]
One arm auspicious pose [326]
One arm lotus pose [330], one arm auspicious pose II
[327], one leg extended wide cobra pose [254]
Two feet extended wide cobra pose [253], child's pose
[388]
Half fish [375]
Camel [275], one arm auspicious supine hero pose [328],
supine hero [468]
Seated wide angle pose [381], revolved seated wide angle
pose [382]
Two arm hero pose I & II [332, 333], two arm double
diamond [338], west side stretch I-III [357-359]

Celibacy pose [203]

Deepening: (10 min)
Dragon flags [353] or Kali crunches [355] (xTone)
Bridge [295]
Upward bow [300] (x2)
Drop-back [322]

Level III

Introduction: (5-10 min)
Meditation, Mudra, and Pranayama
Chant

Warm-Up: (10 min)
Surya Namaskar A [0] (x4)
Baddha Hasta Shalabhasana [311]
Soma Chandrasana II or III [18, 19]

Strength Recruiting: (15min)
Virabhadrasana I [34]
Purna Vasisthasana [218], Camatkarasana [219]
Atmanjali Virabhadrasana [40], Parsvottanasana
[87], Virabhadrasana III [46], Urdhva Prasarita
Ekapadasana [86], Adho Mukha Vrksasana [146]
Baddha Parsvakonasana [55], Eka Pada
Koundinyasana II [199], Ghanda Bherundasana
[316]
Kapinjalasana [221]
Urdhva Kaliasana [106], Shankarasana [107],
Prasarita Padattonasana IV & V [91, 92]
Bakasana [185], Sirsasana II [118], Bakasana [185],
Balasana [388]
Araniasana [260]

Challenging: (10-15 min)
Drop-backs [322] (x6-13)
Hanumanasana I [438] (x4-6)

Opening: (15 min)
Ardha Bhekasana [261], Urdhva Ardha Bhekasana
[262], Urdhva Uttana Ardha Bhekasana [263]
Bhekasana [264]
Eka Bhuja Swastikasana [326]

Restorative: (15-20 min)
Shoulder stand [164], plow pose [171], supine angle pose
[465]
Eye of the needle [486], Supine upward foot diamond
pose prep [478],
Supine Ganesha's pose [483]
Supine twist I & II [491, 492]
Corpse pose [494]

Eka Bhuja Padmasana [330], Eka Bhuja Swastikasana
II [327], Eka Pada Prasarita Bhujangasana [254]
Dwi Pada Prasarita Bhujangasana [253], Balasana
[388]
Eka Pada Rajakapotasana I [285]
Agnistambhasana I-III [405-407]
Upavishta Konasana [381], Parivrtta Upavishta
Konasana [382]
Baddha Konasana I-III [410-412], Mulabandhasana
I & II [414, 415]
Dwi Bhuja Virasana I & II [332-333], Dwi Bhuja
Visvajrasana [338], Paschimottanasana I-IV [357-
360]
Brahmacharyasana [203], Urdhva Navasana [201]

Deepening: (10 min)
Pincha Araniasana [353] (xTone)
Setu Bandha Sarvangasana [295]
Urdhva Dhanurasana [300] (x2)
Natarajasana [115] (x2)

Restorative: (15 min)
Sarvangasana [164], Halasana [171], Karnapidasana
[173], Supta Baddha Konasana [466]
Sucirandrasana [486], Supta Urdhva Padma
Vajrasana [172], Eka Pada Sirsa Shayanasana [464]
Yoganidrasana [463]
Jathara Parivartanasana I & II [491, 492]
Shavasana [494]

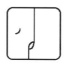

6) White Worldbridger: EQUALIZE – OPPORTUNITY – DEATH

The energy of the Worldbridger bridges the gap between our instincts (Red Serpent) and our accomplishments (Blue Hand). To bridge the gap, we must let go of the past and things that no longer serve our best interests, in order to make room for the New. In *asana*, we let go of self-imposed limitations, and we open up to a greater possibility. We are all capable of more than we can conceive, and the Worldbridger is about finding the limitless potential of our being. This class focuses on forward bends, twists, and backbends that inspire a greater opening of being.

"Utilize every moment in your life. Opportunities do not come again in the same spirit." – Sri Svami Purna

Intention: Surrender your desire to control every situation, and accept that you are part of a larger plan. Let go of the past and that which no longer serves you. Open to a greater possibility.
Focus in asana: Let go of self-effort, and open to grace.
Digit: Right index toe

Chakra: Throat
Mudra: *Vishnu* (seal of Vishnu)
Pranayama: *nadi shodhana* (Alternate nostril breathing. Hold the breath in for a count of 11 or repeat *"om namo Shivaya"* at the pause between breaths.)

Level I

Introduction: (5-10 min)
Meditation, Mudra, and Pranayama
Chant

Warm-Up: (10 min)
Sun Salutation A [0] (x3)
Action pose [8], mountain pose [1]
Intense pose [10], revolved intense pose [12], half intense pose [11]
Side angle [49], elixir of the moon IV [20]

Strength Recruiting: (10 -15 min)
Warrior I [34], revolved side angle [57]
Wind vinyasa [345] (xTone)
Bound hands warrior [41], humble warrior [47]
Triangle [59], intense side stretch [87], standing split [146]
Extended wide leg forward bend [88], revolved wide leg standing forward bend [94], Extended wide legs forward bend IV [91] Garland pose [100]

Challenging: (10 min)
Crane pose [185], child's pose [388], headstand II [118]
Noose pose [99], side crane [191]
Twisting thigh stretch [288], one foot sage Koundinya II pose [199]

Opening: (15 min)
One arm auspicious pose [326], bow pose [265], side bow [267], child's pose [388]
One foot king pigeon prep [400], forehead to knee pose I [366], revolved forehead to knee pose [369]
Camel pose [275], supine hero pose [468]
Wizard's pose [175]
Half lotus west side stretch [363], Sage Marichi pose II [425]
Seated wide angle [381], revolved seated wide angle [382]

Deepening: (10 min)
Windshield wipers [354] or Krishna crunches [352]
(x11)
Bridge [295]
Upward bow [300] (x2)

Restorative: (10-20 min)
Shoulder stand [164], plow pose [171]
Fish pose [319], intense foot pose [321]
Supine single leg stretch I, II, III [474, 476, 477]
One foot happy baby [488], happy baby [489]
Supine twist [491]
Corpse pose [494]

Level II

Introduction: (5-10 min)
Meditation, Mudra, and Pranayama
Chant

Warm-Up: (10 min)
Sun Salutation A [0] (x3)
Action pose [8], mountain pose [1]
Intense pose [10], revolved intense pose [12], half
intense pose [11]
Side angle pose [49], elixir of the moon IV [20]
Down dog twist [29], turbo dog [33]

Strength Recruiting: (15 min)
Warrior I [34]
Warrior I [34], revolved side angle [57]
Wind vinyasa [345] (xTone)
Bound hands warrior [41], humble warrior [47], one
foot sage Koundinya II pose [199]
Triangle [59], intense side stretch [87], revolved triangle
[65], standing split [86], handstand [146]
Extended wide leg forward bend [88], revolved wide leg
standing forward bend [94], extended wide legs forward
bend IV [91]
Crane pose [185], child's pose [388]

Challenging: (10 min)
Handstand [155] (jumping with legs wide, bent, and
straight together)
Forearm stand [133]
Headstand [117]
-or-
Standing hand to big toe pose I-IV [81-84]

Skanda squats [85]

Opening: (15 min)
One arm auspicious pose [326], bow pose [265], side
bow [267], child's pose [388]
One leg king pigeon [285]
Forehead to knee pose I [366], revolved forehead to
knee pose I & II [369, 370]
Camel [275], vajrasana [391], little thunderbolt pose
[278], supine hero's pose [468]
Bound wizard's pose [176]
Half lotus west side stretch [363], sage Bharadvaja's pose
II & III [372, 373]
Sitting legs wide angle [381], revolved sitting legs wide
angle [382]
Bound angle [410], two arm hero [332]
Yogi staff pose prep [443]

Deepening: (10 min)
Windshield wipers [354] and/or Krishna crunches
[352] (x11)
Bridge [295]
Upward bow [300] (x3)

Restorative: (15-20 min)
Shoulder stand [164], plow [171]
Fish pose [319], intense foot pose [321]
Supine single leg stretch I, II, III [474, 476, 477]
Happy baby [489], sleeping yogi pose [463]
Supine twist [491]
Corpse pose [494]

Level III

Introduction: (5-10 min)
Meditation, Mudra, and Pranayama
Chant

Warm-Up: (10 min)
Surya Namaskar A [0] (x5)
Karmasana [8], Tadasana [1]
Utkatasana [10], Parivrtta Utkatasana II [13], Ardha
Utkatasana [11]
Parivrtta Adho Mukha Svanasana [29], Vira Adho
Mukha Svanasana [33]
Adho Mukha Vrksasana [146]

Strength Recruiting: (15 min)
Virabhadrasana I [34]
Prasarita Pada Adho Mukha Vrksasana (jump with
legs wide apart) [155]
Vayu Vinyasa [345] (xTone)
Virabhadrasana I [34], Parivrtta Parsvakonasana [57]
Tarakasana [161]
Baddha Hasta Virabhadrasana [41],
Veerastambhasana [47], Eka Pada Koundinyasana II
[199]
Baddha Parsvakonasana [55], Baddha Trikonasana
[66], Baddha Eka Pada Uttanasana [68], Svarga
Dvijasana [75], Baddha Ardha Chandrasana [73],
Urdhva Prasarita Ekapadasana [86], Adho Mukha
Vrksasana [146]
Vira Adho Mukha Svanasana [33], Bakasana [185],
Balasana [388] Uttana Shishosana [257]

Challenging: (5-10 min)
Utthita Hasta Padangusthasana I-IV [81-84]
Vira Utthita Hasta Padangusthasana [85] (x13)
Nindra Ardha Bhekasana [111]
-or-
Adho Mukha Vrksasana [146] into Ghanda
Bherundasana [316]
Vrischikasana II [162] into Pincha Mayurasana [133]
Sirsasana I [117] into Dwi Pada Viparita Dandasana [301]

Opening: (15 min)
Eka Pada Rajakapotasana I [285], Parivrtta Eka Pada
Rajakapotasana [401]
Ushtrasana [275], Laghuvajrasana [278], Supta
Uttana Virasana [469]
Janu Sirsasana I [366], Parivrtta Janu Sirsasana I, II
[369, 370]
Ardha Baddha Padma Paschimottanasana [363],
Marichiasana II [425], Bharadvajasana II & III [372,
373]
Upavishta Konasana [381], Parivrtta Upavishta
Konasana [382]
Dwi Bhuja Virasana I [332]
Yoga Dandasana [444], Baddha Yoga Dandasana
[445]
Purvottanasana [294]

Deepening: (10 min)
Supta Vayu Vinyasa [354] (x11)
Setu Bandha Sarvangasana [295]
Urdhva Dhanurasana [300] (x3)
Drop-backs [322] (xTone)

Restorative: (15-20 min)
Sarvangasana [164], Halasana [171], Karnapidasana
[173]
Matsyasana [319], Uttana Padasana [321]
Supta Padangusthasana I-III [475, 476, 477]
Yoga Nidrasana [463]
Jathara Parivartanasana [491]
Shavasana [494]

7) Blue Hand: KNOW – HEALING – ACCOMPLISHMENT

The energy of Blue Hand puts our knowledge into action to enhance creativity or to promote healing. Our intentions plus right knowledge initiate the path of transformation, and give us the power to accomplish what we set our minds to. The placement of our hands in hatha yoga is foundational and reflects the strength of our intention to connect with something greater. The Blue Hand energy reminds us to draw upon our past accomplishments to achieve new and greater things. This class focuses on arm balances and inversions that increase hand strength and presence in the moment.

"You are the Creator. You can create your happiness, your own world, your own world of beauty and bliss."
– Sri Svami Purna

Intention: Gain strength from past accomplishments, while bringing completion to the past.
Trust in knowledge received on the path.
Focus in asana: index knuckle rooted
Digit: right middle toe

Chakra: heart
Mudra: *jnana* (knowledge seal) or *Skanda* (spiritual warrior seal)
Pranayama: *viloma* (ladder breath on exhalation)

Level I

Introduction: (5-10 min)
Meditation, Mudra, and Pranayama
Chant

Warm-Up: (10 min)
Sun Salutation A [0] (x5 with hands flat and alternate hand positions: ridgetops, fists, open fists, and fingertips)
Monkey lunge I [14]
Side angle [49], half warrior side angle [51]

Strength Recruiting: (10 min)
Warrior I (x2 with block between the hands) [34]
Sage Vasistha's pose [215]
Triangle [59], half moon [70], standing split [86]
Bound side angle [55]
Extended legs wide forward bend [88], half garland [101]
Crane [185], child's pose [388]

Challenging: (5-10 min)
Handstand [150] (leg raises at wall)
One hand handstand prep [159] (walk feet up wall, extend legs wide, and lift one hand)
Forearm stand prep [132]

Headstand I-III [117-119]

Opening: (15 min)
One foot pigeon prep pose [400]
Camel pose [275], thumb breaker [340], supine hero [468]
Peacock pose [229]
Half fish prep [374], one foot cow west side stretch [365]
Seated wide angle [381], revolved seated wide angle [382]
Bound angle pose I & II [410, 411]
Two arm hero [332]

Deepening: (10 min)
Eagle crunches [349] or Supine arm raises [339] (squeezing block between hands)
Bridge pose [295]
Upward bow pose [300] (x2)

Restorative: (10-20 min)
Shoulder stand [164], plow pose [171]
Single leg stretch I, II, III [474, 476, 477]
One foot happy baby [488], happy baby [489]
Supine twist [492]
Shavasana [494]

Level II

Introduction: (5-10 min)
Meditation, Mudra, and Pranayama
Chant

Warm-Up: (10 min)
Sun Salutation A [0] (x5 with hands flat (grip or claw) and alternate hand positions: ridgetops, fists, open-fists, and fingertips)
Monkey lunge II [15]
Side angle [49], half warrior side angle [51]

Strength Recruiting: (15 min)
Warrior I (with block between the hands) [34]
Extended bound hands warrior [42]
3-limbed staff pose [195], sage Vasistha's pose [215]
Side warrior [44], bound side angle [55], one foot sage Koundinya pose II [199]
Triangle [59], half moon [70], sugarcane [77], standing split [86], handstand [146]
Extended legs wide forward bend [88], half garland pose [101]
Crane pose [185, 186, 187] (x2-3 with hands flat, ridgetop or fist position)

Challenging: (10-15 min)
Handstand prep technique [147] (at wall)
One hand handstand [159] (kick up with a block under one hand)
Forearm stand [133] (at wall)

Uneven forearm stand [142] (at wall)
Headstand series [117-123]

Opening: (15-20 min)
Wrist openers [341-343]
One foot king pigeon prep pose [400]
Camel [275], thumb breaker [340]
Peacock pose [229], one hand peacock [234]
Sage Marichi pose III [426], one foot cow west side stretch [365]
Cow face pose II [397]
Seated wide angle [381], revolved seated wide angle [382], intense angle [204]

Deepening: (10 min)
Eagle crunches [349] (xTone)
Supine double diamond pose [480]
Bridge pose [295]
Upward bow [300] (x2)
Drop-backs [322] (at wall or with spotter if needed)

Restorative: (15-20 min)
Shoulder stand [164], one hand side shoulder stand [169], plow [171]
Fish pose [319], intense foot pose [321]
Single leg stretch I, II, III [474, 476, 477]
Supine formidable pose [460], sleeping yogi's pose [463]
Supine twist [491]
Corpse pose [494]

Level III

Introduction: (5-10 min)
Meditation, Mudra, and Pranayama
Chant

Warm-Up: (10 min)
Surya Namaskar A [0] (x5: hasta bandha, utthita hasta, musti, amusti, raja hasta)
Vanarasana II [15]
Parsvakonasana [49], Ardha Vira Parsvakonasana [51]
Hasta Padangusthasana [6], Padahastasana [7], Tadasana [1]

Strength Recruiting (15 min)
Virabhadrasana I [34]
Utthita Baddha Hasta Virabhadrasana [42]
Trianga Dandasana [195], Purna Vasisthasana [218], Camatkarasana [219]
Parsva Virabhadrasana [44], Baddha Parsvakonasana [55], Eka Pada Koundinyasana II [199], Ghanda Bherundasana [316]
Ardha Vira Trikonasana [60], Ardha Chandrasana [70], Ardha Chandra Chapasana [77], Urdhva Prasarita

415

Ekapadasana [86], Adho Mukha Vrksasana [146]
Baddha Ardha Malasana [102], Prasarita Padattonasana I, III, V [88, 90, 92]
Bakasana [185 & 186], Musti Bakasana [187]
Balasana [388], Uttana Shishosana [257]

Challenging: (10 min)
Adho Mukha Vrksasana [146, 153] (work alternate hand positions)
Eka Hasta Adho Mukha Vrksasana [159]
Pincha Mayurasana [133], Visama Pincha Mayurasana [142]
Pincha Mayurasana [134] (*tamasic hasta*), Shayanasana [138]
Sirsasana [117-125]

Opening: (15 min)
Parivrtta Eka Hastasana I & II [341 & 342], Parivrtta Baddha Hastasana [343]
Eka Pada Rajakapotasana [287], Ardha Matsyendrasana [375]
Ushtrasana [275], thumb-breaker [340]
Mayurasana [229], Eka Hasta Mayurasana [234]
Baddha Ardha Matsyendrasana [376]
Eka Pada Gomukha Paschimottanasana [365],

Gomukhasana [396]
Upavishta Konasana [381], Parivrtta Upavishta Konasana [382]
Dwi Bhuja Virasana I, II, III [332-334]

Deepening: (10 min)
Navasana & Ardha Navasana [346-347] (with block between hands)
Setu Bandha Sarvangasana [295]
Urdhva Dhanurasana [300] (x3: on ridge-tops, fingertips, or fists)
Drop-backs [322] (xTone)

Restorative: (15-20 min)
Sarvangasana [164], Eka Hasta Parsva Padma Sarvangasana [169], Halasana [171]
Matsyasana [319], Uttana Padasana [321]
Supta Padangusthasana I, II, III [475-477]
Yoganidrasana [463]
Jathara Parivartanasana [491]
Shavasana [494]

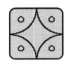

8) Yellow Star: Beauty – Art – Elegance

The energy of the Yellow Star cultivates more beauty, art, and elegance. In Sanskrit this is known as *Sri*, and it is a high spiritual energy in the material world. When we chant Om, we invoke blessings from the spirit world, and when we embody *Sri*, we bring the spiritual into the physical. Yellow Star energy lets our inner strength and beauty shine from the inside out. All of the molecules and atoms in our body are 93% stardust. It can truly be said that we come from the stars, and one day we will return to the stars. The class sequence includes arm balances, inversions, hip-openers, and backbends.

"A diamond lost in the dust will never lose its value, unrecognized and taken for a common stone, it still remains a diamond." – Sri Svami Purna

Intention: Co-create with nature and extend harmony. View life as a work of art.
Focus in asana: *spanda* (pulsation)
Digit: right ring toe

Chakra: solar plexus
Mudra: *rudra* (ruler of the solar plexus)
Pranayama: *kapalabhati* (skull shining), *bahya kumbhaka* (exhale retention with *maha bandha*)

Level I

Introduction: (5-10 min)
Meditation, Mudra, and Pranayama
Chant

Warm-Up: (10 min)
Sun Salutation A [0] (x3)
Side angle [49], warrior side angle [52]
Sun Salutation B [00] (x2)

Strength Recruiting: (10 min)
Warrior I [34], Warrior III [46], standing split [86]
Triangle [59], half moon [70], standing splits [86]
Bound side angle [55], one foot Koundinya II pose [199]
Revolved side angle [57], one foot Koundinya I pose [198]
Warrior splits [93], extended legs wide forward bend [88]
Crane [185], child's pose [388], heart opening pose [258]

Challenging: (10 min)
Handstand [147, 151,] (x2)
Forearm stand [132] (at wall)
Headstand [117] (at wall)
-or-
Crane pose [185], headstand II [118], crane pose [185]
Twisting thigh stretch [288], one foot Vasistha II [217]

Opening: (10 min)
One foot king pigeon prep [400]
Camel [275], supine hero [468]
Marichi's pose I, III [424, 426]
Marichi's pose V, VI [428, 429]
Heron pose [421], revolved heron pose [423], one arm pressure pose [182]
Seated wide angle pose [381], revolved seated wide angle [382]
Bound angle pose [410], star pose [416], revolved star pose [417]

Deepening: (10 min)
Boat pose [346] & half boat pose [347] (x3)
Bridge pose [295]
Upward bow pose [300] (x2)

Restorative: (15-20 min)
Shoulder stand [164], plow pose [171]
Fish pose [319], intense foot pose [321]
Supine single leg stretch I, II, III [474, 476, 477]
One foot happy baby [488], happy baby [489]
Supine twist [491]
Corpse pose [494]

Level II

Introduction: (5-10 min)
Meditation, Mudra, and Pranayama
Chant

Warm-Up: (10 min)
Sun Salutation A [0] (x4)
Side angle [49], warrior side angle [52]
Sun Salutation B [00] (x2)

Strength Recruiting: (15 min)
Warrior I [34], warrior III [46], standing splits [86], handstand [146]
Triangle [59], half moon [70], standing splits [86], kick to handstand [146]

Bound side angle [55], one foot Koundinya pose II [199]
Revolved bound side angle [58], one foot Koundinya I pose [198]
Subramanya pose [22], Vishvamitra's pose [223]

Challenging: (10 min)
Handstand (practice jumping with legs straight and bent) [146, 155]
Forearm stand (balancing away from wall) [133]
Headstand [117], lotus headstand [126-129]
-or-
Crane pose [388], headstand II [118], side crane pose [191], headstand II [118], two foot Koundinya pose [197], headstand II [118]

Opening: (15 min)
One foot king pigeon pose [280]
Camel pose [275], supine hero pose [468]
Marichi pose V, VI [428, 429]
Heron pose II [422], sundial pose [420], sage Ashtavakra's pose [183], sage Koundinya II [199]
Seated wide angle pose [381], revolved seated wide angle pose [382]
Bound angle pose [410], star pose [416], revolved star pose [417]

Level III

Introduction: (5-10 min)
Meditation, Mudra, and Pranayama
Chant

Warm-Up: (10 min)
Surya Namaskar A [0] (x5)
Parsvakonasana [49], Vira Parsvakonasana [52]
Surya Namaskar B [00] (x3)

Strength Recruiting: (15 min)
Purna Vasisthasana [218], Camatkarasana [219]
Virabhadrasana I [34], Virabhadrasana III [46], Urdhva Prasarita Ekapadasana [86], Adho Mukha Vrksasana [146]
Baddha Parsvakonasana [55], Baddha Trikonasana [66], Baddha Eka Pada Uttanasana [68], Svarga Dvijasana [75], Baddha Ardha Chandrasana [73], Urdhva Prasarita Padattonasana [86], Adho Mukha Vrksasana [146]
Parivrtta Baddha Parsvakonasana [58], Eka Pada Koundinyasana I [199]
Subramanya [22], Sri Subramanyasana [246], Vishvamitrasana [243], Eka Pada Koundinyasana II [199], Ghanda Bherundasana [316], Balasana [388], Nirakunjasana II [259]

Challenging: (10 min)
Adho Mukha Vrksasana [146], Prasarita Pada Adho Mukha Vrksasana [155]
Padma Adho Mukha Vrksasana [157]
Pincha Mayurasana [133], Susiravat Vrischikasana [140]
Sirsasana [117], Padma Sirsasana [127], Sirsasana II [118], Urdhva Kukkutasana [226], Sirsasana II [118], Parsva Kukkutasana [227]

Deepening: (10 min)
Boat pose & half boat with twisting [346, 347] (xTone)
Bridge pose [295]
Upward bow pose [300] (x2)
Drop-backs [322] (xTone)

Restorative: (15-20 min)
Hanuman's pose (x2) [437]
Sage Bhardvaja's pose II [372], lotus pose [446], lion pose [317], revolved lion [318]
Happy baby [489], sleeping yogi's pose [463]
Supine twist [491]
Corpse pose [494]

Opening: (15 min)
Parivrtta Eka Pada Rajakapotasana II [288 or 289], Eka Pada Bakasana I & II [189, 190]
Eka Pada Rajakapotasana I [285]
Ushtrasana [275], Supta Virasana [468], Kapotasana [279]
Krounchasana [422], Parivrtta Krounchasana [423], Eka Pada Sirsasana II [456], Ashtavakrasana [183], Eka Pada Koundinyasana II [199] or Adho Mukha Vrksasana [146]
Upavishta Konasana [381], Parivrtta Upavishta Konasana [382]
Baddha Konasana [410], Tarasana [416], Parivrtta Tarasana [417], Parivrtta Baddha Tarasana [418]
Eka Pada Sirsasana [455], Skandasana [457], Chakorasana [236], Yoga Dandasana II [239]
Purvottanasana [294]

Deepening: (10 min)
Navasana & Ardha Navasana [346, 347] (x3)
Setu Bandha Sarvangasana [295]
Urdhva Dhanurasana [300] (x2)
Drop-backs [322] (xTone)
Viparita Chakrasana [323] (xTone)

Restorative: (15-20 min)
Hanumanasana I-III [438- 440]
Bharadvajasana II [372], Padmasana [446], Simhasana [317], Goraknathasana [448], Musti Padma Mayurasana [232]
Supta Bhairavasana [460], Yoga Nidrasana [463]
Jathara Parivartanasana I & II [491, 492]
Shavasana [494]

9. Red Moon: PURIFY – FLOW – UNIVERSAL WATER

Red Moon is the cosmic seed of self-remembrance and the meta-pattern, which unites all beings. It encourages us to enter a "flow" to purify mind, body, and spirit. Essentially Red Moon energy is dedicating your Self to a spiritual discipline until it over rides all existing patterns of attachments and habits. It nullifies *karma*, and sustains *dharma*. This class focuses on hip-openers, twists, and backbends.

"Sooner or later, you will have to realize. There is no return. You cannot go back now. You are caught. Do not even think of going back. It is only ahead, further. You give up your own identity in Total Merger. You become part of the Whole." – Sri Svami Purna

Intention: Purify the instruments of perception to flow in life in a state of remembrance.
Focus in asana: undulate and flow with breath.
Digit: right pinky toe

Chakra: root
Mudra: *Varuna* (water seal) or *Vishnu* (seal of Vishnu)
Pranayama: *nadi shodhana* (alternate nostril), *moorcha* (swooning breath)

Level I

Introduction: (5-10 min)
Meditation, Mudra, and Pranayama
Chant

Warm-Up: (10 min)
Sun Salutation A [0] (x3)
Bound hand locust [311]
Elixir of the moon I [17]

Strength Recruiting: (15 min)
Warrior I [34]
Warrior I [34], revolved side angle [57]
Tree pose [25], side tree [26], warrior II [43], side angle [49], triangle [59], half moon [70], triangle [59], side angle [49], warrior II [43], Tree pose [25], bent tree pose [27]
Bound side angle pose [55]
Upward Kali pose [106], sage Shankara's pose [107], extended wide leg pose I & IV [88, 91]
Garland pose [100], crane pose [185], child's pose [388], heart opening pose [258]

Challenging: (10 min)
Handstand [150] (leg raises at wall)
Handstand [149] (balancing technique)
Headstand [117] (leg raises xTone), supported child's pose [389] -or-
Locust pose I-III [307-310]
One foot locust [314] (push-ups xTone)

Opening: (15 min)
Half frog [261]
One arm heart opening sugarcane pose [337]
Bow pose [265]
One foot king pigeon pose [400], revolved one foot pigeon [401]
Camel [295], supine hero [468]
Half fish pose [375]
Seated wide angle (PNF technique) [381], revolved seated wide angle [382]
Bound angle pose [410]
Half fish II [378], half lotus forward bend [363], sage Marichi pose II [425], lotus pose [446]

Deepening: (10 min)
Leg lifts [350, 351] (x13 with single leg and then both)
Bridge pose [295]
Upward bow pose [300] (x2)

Restorative: (15-20 min)
Shoulder stand [164], plow [171], fish pose [319], intense foot pose [321]

Level II

Introduction: (5-10 min)
Meditation, Mudra, and Pranayama
Chant

Warm-up: (10 min)
Sun Salutation [0] (x4)
Bound hand locust [311]
Elixir of the moon pose [17]

Strength Recruiting: (15 min)
Warrior I [34]
Warrior I [34], revolved side angle [57]
Tree pose [25], side tree [26], warrior II [43], side angle [49], triangle [59], half moon [70], sugarcane [77], revolved half moon [71], one foot standing bow [78], standing split [86], tree pose [25], bent tree pose [27]
Bound side angle [55], one foot sage Koundinya's pose II [199], formidable face pose [316]
Upward Kali pose [106], sage Shankara's pose [107], extended wide leg pose I & IV [88, 91]
Garland pose [100], Crane pose [185], child's pose [388], heart opening pose I [258]

Challenging: (10 min)
Handstand [150] (leg raises at wall)
Handstand [149] (balancing technique)
Forearm stand, Scorpion pose
Headstand [117] (leg raises xTone), supported child's pose [389]
-or-
Locust pose I, II [307, 308]
One foot locust pose [314 or 315] (push-ups xTone or bound one foot locust pose)
Locust pose IV [310], child's pose [388]

Opening: (15 min)
Half frog [261], upward half frog pose [262]
One arm heart opening sugarcane pose [337]
Sage Gheranda's pose prep [272], child's pose [388]
One foot king pigeon [285]
Camel [275], little thunderbolt [278] (with "pigeon droppings" xTone), supine hero [468]
Bound half fish pose [376]
Seated wide angle pose [381] (PNF technique), revolved seated wide angle [382]
Bound angle pose I, II [410, 411] (PNF technique)
Half fish II [378], half lotus forward bend [363], sage Marichi pose II [425], lotus pose [446], scale pose [224]

Deepening: (10-15 min)
Dragon flags [353] (xTone)
Bridge [295]
Upward bow [300] (x2)
Drop-back [322] (at wall or with spotter)

Restorative: (10-20 min)
Shoulder stand [164], plow [171], fish pose [319], intense foot pose [321]
Supine baby cradle [484]
Eye of the needle [486], Supine upward foot diamond pose prep [478]
Happy baby [488], sleeping yogi pose [463]
Supine twist I & II [491, 492]
Corpse pose [494]

Supine baby cradle [484]
Eye of the needle [486], supine upward foot diamond pose prep [478]
One foot happy baby [488], happy baby [489]
Supine twist I & II [491, 492]
Corpse pose [494]

Level III

Introduction: (5-10 min)
Meditation, Mudra, and Pranayama
Chant

Warm-up: (10 min)
Surya Namaskar A [0] (x5)
Baddha Hasta Shalabhasana [311]
Somachandrasana III [19]
Somachandrasana V [21]

Strength Recruiting: (15 min)
Virabhadrasana I (x2) [34]
Vrksasana [25], Parsva Vrksasana [26], Baddha
Parsvakonasana [55], Baddha Trikonasana [66], Baddha
Ardha Chandrasana [73], Vira Ardha Chandrasana
[72], Urdhva Prasarita Eka Padasana [86], Vrksasana
[25], Vakra Vrksasana [27], Tadasana [1]
Adho Mukha Vrksasana [146]
Trianga Dandasana [195], Eka Pada Koundinyasana II
[199], Ghanda Bherundasana [316]
Urdhva Kaliasana [106] Shankarasana [107], Prasarita
Padottanasana [88, 92]
Malasana [100], Bakasana [185], Adho Mukha
Vrksasana [146] or Sirsasana II [118], Bakasana [185]
Balasana [388], Araniasana [260]

Challenging: (10 min)
Adho Mukha Vrksasana [146], Vrischikasana II [162],
Bakasana [185]
Pincha Mayurasana [133], Padma Pincha Mayurasana
[135], Karandavasana [136]
Sirsasana II [118], Urdhva Kukkutasana [226]
Balasana [388]

Opening: (15-20 min)
Ardha Bhekasana[261], Urdhva Adha Bhekasana [262],
Urdhva Uttana Ardha Bhekasana [263]
Eka Bhuja Anahata Chapasana [337]
Gherandasana I & II [273, 274], Balasana [388]
Baddha Ardha Matsyendrasana [376], Gomukhasana
[396]
Baddha Uttana Ardha Matsyendrasana [377]
Upavishta Konasana [281] (PNF technique), Parivrtta
Upavishta Konasaana [282]
Baddha Konasana I-III [410-412] (PNF technique)
Bhardvajasana II & III [372-373], Padmasana [446],
Tolasana [224]
Eka Pada Sirsasana [455], Ruchikasana [112],
Durvasana [113], Kala Bhairavasana [237],
Somanathasana [238], Dwi Pada Sirsasana [240]

Deepening: (10-15 min)
Pincha Araniasana [353] (x13)
Setu Banda Sarvangasana [295]
Urdhva Dhanurasana [300] (x2)
Drop-Backs [322] (xTone)
Natarajasana [115] (x2)

Restorative: (15-20 min)
Sarvangasana [164], Urdhva Padma Sarvangasana
[167], Pindasana [168]
Padma Matsyasana [320], Uttana Padasana [321]
Supta Hindolasana I [484], Supta Urdhva Pada
Vajrasana [172], Eka Pada Sirsa Shyanasana [464]
Yoganidrasana [463]
Jathara Parivartanasana I & III [491, 493]
Shavasana [494]

10) White Dog: LOVE – HEART – LOYALTY

The energy of the White Dog strengthens the connection to the heart and its qualities of love, trust, and loyalty. In yoga and in life, we must be strong and determined, yet receptive and compassionate. Enter the cave of the heart to find what matters most, then move out from that space. These classes focus on refining actions in upward and down dog, forward bends, and twists.

"Unity cannot come through fear, only through tolerance and Love." – Sri Svami Purna

Intention: Be loyal to your essence and your kin. Bring more heart into your path and trust in the higher power.
Focus in *asana*: merging the *apana* and *prana* in the heart space
Digit: left thumb

Chakra: crown
Mudra: *hridaya* (heart seal)
Pranayama: *bhastrika* (breath of fire), *bahya kumbhaka* (retention after exhalation with *maha bandha*)

Level I

Introduction: (5-10 min)
Meditation, Mudra, and Pranayama
Chant

Warm-Up: (10 min)
Sun Salutation (x3) [0]
Down dog [28], up dog [256] (xTone with arms and legs straight during transitions)
Downward facing monkey lunge [24]
Revolved one hand down dog [29], turbo dog [33], up dog [256]

Strength Recruiting: (15 min)
Warrior I (x2) [34], revolved side angle [57]
Turbo dog [33], up dog [256]
Bound hands warrior [41], humble warrior [47]
Turbo dog [33], up dog [256]
Triangle [59], half moon [70], revolved half moon [71], intense side stretch [87]
Bound side angle [55]
Extended legs wide forward bend [88], revolved extended legs wide forward bend [94]
Crane pose [185], child's pose [185], puppy pose [388]

Challenging: (10 min)
Turbo dog [33] jump into crane pose [185]

Twisting thigh stretch [288], Hanuman's prep pose [436], one foot Vasistha II [217]

Opening: (15 min)
One arm auspicious pose [326]
Bow pose [265], side bow [267], child's pose [388]
One foot pigeon prep [400]
Camel [275], supine hero [468]
Sage Marichi's pose I & III [424, 426]
Seated wide angle pose [381], revolved seated wide angle pose [382]
Bound angle I & II [410, 411], east side stretch [294], west side stretch I & II [357, 358]

Deepening: (5-10 min)
Windshield wipers [354] or Krishna crunches [352] (xTone)
Bridge pose [295]
Upward bow [300] (x2)

Restorative: (10-20 min)
Shoulder stand [164], plow pose [171]
Single leg stretch I, II, III [474, 476, 477]
One foot happy baby [488], happy baby [489]
Supine twist [491]
Corpse pose [494]

Level II

Introduction: (5-10 min)
Meditation, Mudra, and Pranayama
Chant

Warm-Up: (10 min)
Sun Salutation A [0] (x4)
Downward facing monkey lunge [24]
Revolved one hand down dog [29], turbo dog [33], up
dog [256]
Side angle pose [49], elixir of the moon pose IV [20]

Strength Recruiting: (15 min)
Warrior I [34]
Warrior I [34], revolved side angle [57]
Wind vinyasa [345] (xTone)
Turbo dog [33], up dog [256]
Bound hands warrior [41], humble warrior [47]
Turbo dog [33], up dog [256]
Triangle [59], half moon [70], sugarcane [77], revolved
half moon [71], standing one foot bow [78], standing
split [86]
Bound side angle [55], Eka Pada Koundinya II [199]
Bound single leg forward bend [88], bird of paradise [75]
Insect pose II [96], arm pressure pose [211], Insect pose I
[212], crane pose [185]
Child's pose [388], puppy pose [257]

Challenging: (10 min)
Twisting thigh stretch [288], Hanuman's prep pose [436],
one foot Vasistha II [217], one foot crane II pose [190]
Mermaid pose II [283], one foot crane [189]

Opening: (15 min)
One arm auspicious pose [326]
Bound one foot bow pose [270], bow pose [265], child's
pose [388]
One leg king pigeon I [285]
One leg king pigeon II [287, 290]
Wizard's pose [175]
Seated wide angle pose [381], seated wide angle pose
[382]
Bound angle I & II [410, 411]
East side stretch [294], west side stretch pose I-III [357-
359], revolved west side stretch [361]

Deepening: (10 min)
Boat pose [346], half boat [347], side boat [348] (xTone)
Bridge [295]
Upward bow [300] (x2-3)
Drop-back [322] (xTone)

Restorative: (15-20 min)
Shoulder stand [164], plow pose [171], ear pressure
[173], side ear pressure [174]
Single leg stretch I, II, III [474, 476, 477]
Happy baby [488], sleeping yogi pose [463]
Supine twist [491]
Corpse pose [494]

Level III

Introduction: (5-10 min)
Meditation, Mudra, and Pranayama
Chant

Warm-Up: (10 min)
Surya Namaskar A [0] (x5)
Parivrtta Eka Hasta Adho Mukha Svanasana [29]
Vira Adho Mukha Svanasana [33], Urdhva Mukha
Svanasana [256]
Eka Pada Dhanur Adho Mukha Svanasana [32]

Strength Recruiting: (15 min)
Virabhadrasana I [34], Adho Mukha Vrksasana [146]
Virabhadrasana I [34], Parivrtta Baddha Parsvakonasana
[58]
Vayu Vinyasa [345] (xTone)
Baddha Hasta Virabhadrasana [41], Veerastambhasana
[47], Eka Pada Koundinyasana II [199]

Trikonasana [59], Parsvottanasana [87], Parivrtta Trikonasana [65], Urdhva Prasarita Ekapadasana [86], Adho Mukha Vrksasana [146]
Baddha Eka Pada Uttanasana [68], Svarga Dvijasana [75]
Tittibhasana II, III & I [96, 97, 212], Bhujapidasana [211], Bakasana [185]
Balasana [388], Uttana Shishosana [257]

Challenging: (10 min)
Vira Adho Mukha Svanasana [33] into Bakasana [185]
Vira Adho Mukha Svanasana [33] into Sirsasana II, Parsva Bakasana [191]
Adho Mukha Vrksasana [146] into Pincha Mayurasana [133]
-or-
Parivrtta Eka Pada Rajakapotasana II [287], Eka Pada Bakasana I & II [189, 190]
Nasginyasana II, Eka Pada Vasisthasana II [217], Eka Pada Bakasana II [190], Eka Pada Koundinyasana II [199], Ghanda Bherundasana [316]

Opening: (15 min)
Eka Pada Rajakapotasana I [285]
Eka Pada Rajakapotasana II [287]
Ushtrasana [275], Supta Virasana [468], Kapotasana [279]

Baddha Shramanasana [176]
Agnistambhasana I-III [405-407], Parivrtta Agni Stambhasana I, II [408, 409]
Upavishta Konasana [381], Parivrtta Upavishta Konasana [382]
Dwi Bhuja Virasana [332], Purvottansana [294], Paschimottanasana III [359], Parivrtta Paschimottanasana [361]
Yoga Dandasana [444], Baddha Yoga Dandasana [445]

Deepening: (10 min)
Navasana [346], Ardha Navasana [348], Parsva Navasana [348] (xTone)
Urdhva Dhanurasana [300] (x2)
Dwi Pada Viparita Dandasana I & II [301, 302]
Drop-backs [322] (xTone)

Restorative: (15-20 min)
Sharvangasana [164], Halasana [171], Karnapidasana [173], Parsva Karnapidasana [174]
Matsyasana [319], Uttana Padasana [321]
Supta Padangusthasana I, II, III [475, 476, 477]
Yoganidrasana [463]
Jathara Parivartanasana I [491]
Shavasana [494]

11) Blue Monkey : PLAY – ILLUSION – MAGIC

Blue Monkey energy is playful and reminds us not to take anything too seriously, especially ourselves. Perceive through the illusion of separation, and stay in remembrance of the *lila*, the divine play, and sport of God. When we are playful in life and in yoga *asana*, then we are open to the possibility of experiencing magic. This practice embodies the attributes of Hanuman, while focusing on arm balances, inversions, and the hamstrings.

"And let there be Love within you and around you. Let there be Light within you and around you. Let there be peace and reconciliation within you and around you." – Sri Svami Purna

Intention: Celebrate spontaneity and perceive through the illusion of separation.
Focus in asana: Be serious about being playful.
Digit: Left index finger
Chakra: Throat

Mudra: *shunya* (heaven seal), or *chin* (psychic gesture)
Pranayama: *ujjayi* (victorious), *viloma* (ladder breath on exhalation)

Level I

Introduction: (5-10 min)
Meditation, Mudra, and Pranayama
Chant

Warm-Up: (10 min)
Sun Salutation A (x3) [0]
Monkey lunge I [14], Anjaney's pose [23]
Side angle [49], half warrior side angle [51]

Strength Recruiting: (15 min)
Warrior I [34]
3-limb staff pose [195], sage Vasistha's pose [215]
Warrior I [34], warrior III [46], standing split [86]
Triangle [59], Half moon [70], standing split [86],
intense side stretch [87]
Half garland pose [101], extended legs wide forward
bend [88]
Monkey frog [434], child's pose [388]

Challenging: (10 min)
Standing split [86] (at wall) into handstand prep [147]
Handstand [146] (kick up to wall)
Handstand "Superman walk-outs" [163]

-or-
Extended hand to big toe pose I-IV [81-84]
Skanda squats (xTone) [85]
Half bound lotus forward fold [80]

Opening: (15 min)
Twisting thigh stretch [288], Hanuman prep [438]
Camel pose [275], supine hero [468]
Heron pose [421], one arm pressure pose [182]
Seated wide angle [381], revolved seated wide angle [382]
West side stretch I, II [357-358], east side stretch [294]

Deepening: (10-15 min)
Eagle crunches [349] (xTone or 11)
Bridge pose [295]
Upward bow pose [300] (x2)
Hanuman's pose [438] (x2 with PNF technique)

Restorative: (10-15 min)
Shoulder stand [164], plow pose [171]
Supine auspicious pose [481], happy baby [489]
Supine twist [491]
Corpse pose [494]

Level II

Introduction: (5-10 min)
Meditation, Mudra, and Pranayama
Chant

Warm-Up: (10 min)
Sun Salutation A [0] (x4)
Monkey lunge I [14], Anjaney's pose [23]
Side angle [49], half warrior side angle [51]

Strength Recruiting: (15 min)
Warrior I (x2) [34]
3-limb staff pose [195], sage Vasistha's pose [215], wild
thing [219]
Warrior I (reverse prayer) [40], intense side stretch [87],
standing splits [86], handstand [146]
Triangle [59], half moon [70], sugarcane [77], standing

split [86], half garland II pose [103], standing split [86],
handstand [146]
Warrior splits (x2) [93], extended legs wide forward bend
I, IV [88, 91]
Monkey frog [434], child's pose [388]
Crane pose [185], headstand II [118], crane pose [185]

Challenging: (15 min)
Standing splits (press into handstand) [152]
Handstand [146]
Superman walkouts [163]
Forearm stand [133], uneven forearm stand [142]
Sirsasana [117-123] (alternate hand positions)
-or-
Extended hand to big toe pose I-IV [81-84]

Skanda squats [85]
Half bound lotus forward fold [80]
Full Vasistha's pose [218] into Hanuman's pose [438]

Opening: (15 min)
Twisting thigh stretch [289], revolved Hanuman prep [437], one foot Koundinya II [199]
One foot king pigeon [285]
Camel [275], supine hero [468]
Heron pose [421], sage Ashtavakra's pose [183]
Seated wide angle pose [381], revolved seated wide angle [382]
Bound angle pose II [411], two arm hero [332]
West side stretch III [359], east side stretch [294], staff

Level III

Introduction: (5-10 min)
Meditation, Mudra, and Pranayama
Chant

Warm-Up: (10 min)
Surya Namaskar A [0] (x5)
Vanarasana III [16]
Parsvakonasana [49], Ardha Vira Parsvakonasana [51]

Strength Recruiting: (15 min)
Virabhadrasana I (x2) [34]
Trianga Dandasana [195], Purna Vasisthasana [218], Camatkarasana [219]
Atmanjali Virabhadrasana [40], Parsvottonasana [87], Urdhva Prasarita Ekapadasana [86], Ardha Malasana II [103], Urdhva Prasarita Ekapadasana [86], Adho Mukha Vrksasana [146]
Baddha Parsvakonasana [55], Baddha Trikonasana [66], Baddha Eka Pada Uttanasana [68], Svarga Dvijasana [75], Baddha Ardha Chandrasana [73], Urdhva Prasarita Ekapadasana [86], Adho Mukha Vrksasana [146]
Vira Prasarita Padattonasana (x2) [93], Prasarita Padattonasana I & V [88, 92], Rajasamakonasana [384]
Thavaliasana [434], Urdhva Thavaliasana [435], Balasana [388]

Challenging: (15 min)
Adho Mukha Vrksasana [152] (press up from standing split)

pose [356], celibacy pose [203]

Deepening: (10 min)
Eagle crunches [349] (xTone or 11)
Bridge pose [295]
Upward bow pose [300] (x2)
Hanuman's pose [438] (x3 with PNF technique)

Restorative: (15-20 min)
Shoulder stand [164], plow pose [171], ear pressure [173]
Fish pose [319], intense foot pose [321]
Supine auspicious pose I & II [481, 482]
Supine twist [491]
Corpse pose [494]

Adho Mukha Vrksasana [146] (work on touching the wrist with toes)
Adho Mukha Vrksasana [155]
Pincha Mayurasana [133], Visama Pincha Mayurasana [142], Visama Parsva Bakasana [193]
Shayanasana [138]
-or-
Utthita Hasta Padangusthasana I-IV [81-84]
Vira Utthita Hasta Padangusthasana [85] (xTone)
Ardha Baddha Padmottanasana [80]
Purna Vasisthasana [218] into Hanumanasana [438]

Opening: (10-15 min)
Eka Pada Rajakapotasana I [285]
Ushtrasana [275], Supta Virasana [468], Mayurasana [229]
Krounchasana [422], Parivrtta Krounchasana [423], Eka Pada Sirsasana II [456]
Skandasana [457], Chakorasana [236] or Ashtavakrasana [184]
Upavishta Konasana [381], Parivrtta Upavishta Konasana [382], Uttana Konasana [204]
Paschimottanasana IV [360], Brahmacharyasana [203], Uttana Paschimottanasana [362]

Deepening: (15 min)
Supta Visvajrasana [490]
Garuda crunches [349] (x11)
Setu Bandha Sarvangasana [295]

Urdhva Dhanurasana [300] (x2)
Drop-backs (xTone) [322]
Hanumanasana [438-440] (x3 or xTone), Eka Pada
Rajakapotasana IV [292]

Restorative: (15-20 min)
Sarvangasana [164], Halasana [171], Karnapidasana [173]
Matsyasana [319], Uttana Padasana [321]
Supta Swastikasana I & II [481, 482]
Supta Bhairavasana [460], Yoganidrasana [463]
Jathara Parivartanasana I & II [491, 492]
Shavasana [494]

12. Yellow Human: INFLUENCE – WISDOM – FREE WILL

The energy of Yellow Human influences our path with the collective wisdom we have gained from all of our experiences. We use this wisdom as a power, *jnana shakti*, that gives us strength to overcome any habits or addictions. The energy of the Yellow Human invites us to bring the Divine into our human experiences. It invokes the power of the sage, teacher, and guru. Draw inspiration from the wisdom of those who live the Highest Truth and have connected to the power of the infinite. This class focuses on the poses dedicated to the sages and teachers who have influenced the development of yoga. It embodies arm balances, hip-openers, twists, and backbends. Honor the limitations of the human form, but play the edge fully and enjoy being an avatar of the one Self.

"Only when we accept things as they really are, renouncing all our assumed needs, can we become truly free."
– Sri Svami Purna

Intention: Honor your own unique abilities. Enjoy being human. Honor those who have transcended the finite and have connected to the power of the infinite.
Focus in asana: Activate and breathe into the 7 major chakras.
Digit: left middle finger

Chakra: heart
Mudra: *Vishnu* (seal of Vishnu), *jnana* (wisdom gesture), *hakini* (ruler of the third eye)
Pranayama: *nadi shodhana* (alternate nostril), *bahya kumbhaka* (retention after exhalation with *maha bandha*)

Level I

Introduction: (5-10 min)
Meditation, Mudra, and Pranayama
Chant

Warm-Up: (10 min)
Sun Salutation A [0] (x3)
Side angle [49], warrior side angle [52]
Sun Salutation B [00] (x2)

Strength Recruiting: (10 min)
Warrior I [34]
Sage Vasistha prep [214]
Triangle [59], half moon [70], standing split [86]
Bound side angle [55]
Sage Vasistha's pose [215]
Extended legs wide forward bend I-IV [88-91]
Crane pose [185], child's pose [388]

Challenging: (10 min)
Handstand (x2) [147, 148]
Forearm stand [132]
Headstand [117]
-or-
Standing baby cradle [108]
Standing half lotus tree [79], half lotus forward bend [80]

Opening: (15 min)
Twisting thigh stretch [288]
Camel [275]
Sage Marichi's pose I & III [424, 426], one arm pressure pose [182]
Half fish [375], cow face pose [396]
Seated wide angle [381], revolved seated wide angle

[382]
Bound angle pose [410]
Baby cradle [441], Arjuna's pose [454]

Deepening: (10 min)
Boat and half boat [346, 347] (x3)
Bridge [295]
Urdhva Dhanurasana [300] (x2)

Restorative: (10-20 min)
Shoulder stand [164], plow [171]
Single leg stretch I, II, III [474, 476, 477]
One foot happy baby [488], Happy baby pose [489]
Supine twist [491]
Corpse pose [494]

Level II

Introduction: (5-10 min)
Meditation, Mudra, and Pranayama
Chant

Warm-Up: (10 min)
Sun Salutation A [0] (x3)
Side angle [49], warrior side angle [52]
Sun Salutation B [00] (x2)

Strength Recruiting: (10-15 min)
Sage Vasistha's pose [215]
Triangle [59], half moon [70], sugarcane [77], standing split [86]
Full sage Vasistha pose [218], wild thing [219]
Bound angle pose [410], one foot sage Koundinya II [199]
Extended legs wide forward bend I-IV [88-91]
Crane pose [185], child's pose [388], heart opening pose [258]

Challenging: (15 min)
Sage Vishvamitra's pose [223]
Standing baby cradle [108], one foot Galava's pose I [208]
Standing half lotus tree [79], half lotus forward bend

[80], sage Kasyapa's pose [220]

Opening: (15 min)
One foot king pigeon [285]
Marichi I & III [424, 426], one arm pressure pose [182], sage Ashtavakra's pose [183]
Bound half fish [376], cow face pose II [397]
Seated wide angle pose [381], revolved seated wide angle [382]
Bound angle pose [410]
Baby cradle [441], Arjuna's pose [454]
One foot behind head [455]

Deepening: (10 min)
Boat pose, half boat [346, 347] (x3)
Bridge [295]
Upward bow [300] (x2)
Drop-backs [322] (xTone)

Restorative: (10-15 min)
Shoulder stand [164], plow [171]
Single leg stretch I, II, III [474, 476, 477]
Happy baby pose [488], sleeping yogi pose [463]

Supine twist [491]

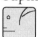

Corpse pose [494]

Level III

Introduction: (5-10 min)
Meditation, Mudra, and Pranayama
Chant

Warm-Up: (10 min)
Surya Namaskar A [0] (x4)
Parsvakonasana [49], Vira Parsvakonasana [52]
Surya Namaskar B [00] (x3)

Strength Recruiting: (15 min)
Purna Vasisthasana [218], Camatkarasana [219]
Virabhadrasana I [36], Virabhadrasana III [46], Adho Mukha Vrksasana [146]
Baddha Parsvakonasana [55], Baddha Trikonasana [66], Baddha Eka Pada Uttanasana [68], Svarga Dvijasana [75], Baddha Ardha Chandrasana [73], Urdhva Prasarita Ekapadasana [86], Adho Mukha Vrksasana [146]
Bakasana [185], Balasana [388]
Parivrtta Baddha Konasana [58], Eka Pada Koundinyasana I [198]
Subramanyasana [22], Vishvamitrasana [223], Eka Pada Koundinyasana II [195], Ghanda Bherundasana [316]
Balasana [388], Nirakunjasana II [259]

Challenging: (15 min)
Nindra Hindolasana [108], Eka Pada Galavasana I & II [208, 209], Ardha Bhujapidasana [210]
Ardha Baddha Padma Vrksasana [79], Ardha Baddha Padmottanasana [80], Kasyapasana [220]

Opening: (15 min)
Eka Bhuja Swastikasana [326]
Gherandasana (x2) [272, 273], Balasana [388]
Eka Pada Rajakapotasana [285]
Marichiasana V & VI [428, 429], Eka Pada Bakasana I & II [189, 190]
Baddha Ardha Matsyendrasana [376]
Upavishta Konasana [381], Parivrtta Upavishta Konasana [382], Uttana Konasana [204]
Baddha Konasana [411], Dwi Bhuja Virasana [332]
Hindolasana [441], Arjunasana [45]
Eka Pada Sirsasana [455], Marichiasana VIII [431], Yoga Dandasana II [239]

Deepening: (10 min)
Navasana & Ardha Navasana [347] (x3)
Setu Bandha Sarvangasana [295]
Urdhva Dhanurasana [300] (x3)
Drop-backs [322] (xTone)
Viparita Chakrasana [323]

Restorative: (15-20 min)
Hanumanasana [438] (x2-3)
Bahardvajasana II, III [372, 373], Padmasana [446], Simhasana [317], Goraknathasana [446], Galavasana [206]
Padmasana [446] (meditation 3-4 minutes)
Jathara Parivartanasana I & II [491, 492]
Shavasana [494]

13) Red Skywalker: Explore – Wakefullness – Space

The Red Skywalker energy initiates the exploration and the adventure of life. It gives us the courage to step outside of our comfort zone to experience the unknown. Red Skywalker elevates consciousness and new levels of awareness. It builds the strength to pursue spiritual and physical motivations, while creating a greater potential of being in the world. The class focuses on inversions and backbends that take us into the unknown.

"Enjoy your health. Enjoy your happiness, freedom and peace. Enjoy all the beauty that life has presented to you. Why not? Why restrict yourself? Keep opening. The sky is the limit. There is no limit to the infinite."
– *Sri Svami Purna*

Intention: Voyage beyond your habitual self and comfort zone. Actively participate in creating a new you.
Focus in asana: Make an energetic connection between heaven and earth, and become a conduit for divine energy.
Digit: left ring finger

Chakra: solar plexus
Mudra: *khechari* (to move the sky), *rudra* (ruler of solar plexus)
Pranyama: *viloma* (ladder breath on inhalation), *moorcha* (swooning breath)

Level I

Introduction: (5-10 min)
Meditation, Mudra, and Pranayama
Chant

Warm-Up: (10 min)
Sun Salutation A [0] (x3)
Bound hand locust [311]
Elixir of the moon I [17]

Strength Recruiting: (15 min)
Warrior I [34]
Warrior I [34], warrior II [43], side warrior [45], side angle pose [49]
Warrior I [36], Warrior III [46], standing split [86]
Side angle [49], triangle [59], half moon [70], standing split [86]
Upward Kali pose [106], sage Shankara pose [107], extended legs wide forward bend I [88]
Child's pose [388]

Challenging: (10 min)
Handstand prep at wall [147]
Handstand (single leg raises into one leg scorpion) [160]

Forearm stand prep at wall [132]
Headstand [117]

Opening: (15 min)
Half frog pose [261]
Bow pose [265], child's pose [388]
Camel pose [275], supine hero pose [468]
Three limb face to knee pose "hurdler stretch" [364]
One foot supine hero single leg stretch [471]

Deepening: (10 min)
Supine leg raises [350, 351] (xTone)
Bridge pose [295]
Upward bow [300] (x2)

Restorative: (10-20 min)
Supine child's pose [487], shoulder stand pose [164], plow pose [171], supine angle pose [465]
Fish pose [319], intense foot pose [321]
Eye of the needle pose [486], supine upward foot diamond pose prep [478]
One foot happy baby [488], happy baby [489]
Supine twist I & II [491, 492]
Corpse pose [494]

Level II

Introduction: (5-10 min)
Meditation, Mudra, and Pranayama
Chant

Warm-Up: (10 min)
Sun Salutation A [0] (x4)
Bound hand locust pose [311]

Elixir of the moon II [18]
Side angle pose variation [50]

Strength Recruiting: (15 min)
Warrior I [34] (x2)
Sage Vasistha's pose [215], wild thing [219]
Warrior I [36], Warrior III [46], standing split [86],

handstand [146]

Triangle [59], half moon [70], sugarcane [77], standing splits [86], handstand [146]

Upward Kali [106], sage Shankara pose [107], extended leg wide forward bend I, IV [88, 92]

Crane [185], child's pose [388]

Challenging: (15 min)

Handstand [152] (one foot on block in standing split and press up)

Handstand wide legs [158, 155]

Forearm stand [133], scorpion [139]

Inverted ear pressure pose [177] or Headstand [117]
-or-
Full Sage Vasistha's pose [218], crane pose [185]

Sage Vishvamitra's pose [223], sage Koundinya pose II [199]

Opening: (15 min)0

Half frog pose [261], upward half frog [262]

One foot king pigeon [285]

Camel [275], supine hero [468],

Level III

Introduction: (5-10 min)

Meditation, Mudra, and Pranayama

Chant

Warm-Up: (10 min)

Surya Namaskar A [0] (x5)

Baddha Hasta Shalabhasana [311]

Somachandrasana II, III [18, 19]

Parsvakonasana [50]

Strength Recruiting: (15 min)

Virabhadrasana I [34], Adho Mukha Vrksasana [146]

Purna Vasisthasana [218], Camatkarasana [219]

Virabhadrasana I [36], Virabhadrasana III [46], Adho Mukha Vrksasana [146]

Raja Baddha Parsvakonasana [56], Eka Pada Koundinyasana II [199], Gandha Bherundasana [316]

Baddha Eka Pada Uttanasana [68], Svarga Dvijasana [75], Tittibhasana II, III, I [96, 97, 212],

Bakasana [185], Balasana [388]

Three limb face to knee pose "hurdler stretch" [364]

One foot supine hero single leg stretch I & II [471, 472], one foot pigeon [280]

Half fish [376]

Seated wide angle [381], revolved seated wide angle [382]

Deepening (10 min)

Dragon flags (x13 or x20) [353]

Upward bow [300]

Two foot upward staff pose [301, 302]

Lord of the dance pose [115] (x2)

Restorative: (15- 20 min)

Shoulder stand pose II [165], plow pose [171], ear pressure pose [173], supine angle pose [465]

Fish pose [319], intense foot pose [321]

Eye of the needle [486], supine upward foot diamond pose prep [478]

Happy baby [489], sleeping yogi's pose [463]

Supine twist I & II [491, 492]

Corpse pose [494]

Challenging: (15 min)

Prasarita Pada Adho Mukha Vrksasana [155]

Padma Adho Mukha Vrksasana [157]

Pincha Mayurasana [132], Vrischikasana [139], Susiravat Vrischikasana [140]

Viparita Karnapida Urdhva Padmasana [181]
-or-
Kapinjalasana [222], Camatkarasana [219], Bakasana [185]

Vishvamitrasana [223], Eka Pada Koundinyasana II [199], Ghanda Bherundasana [316]

Opening: (10-15 min)

Ardha Bhekasana [261], Urdhva Uttana Ardha Bhekasana [263], Bhekasana [264]

Ushtrasana II [275], Supta Virasana [468], Kapotasana [279]

Triangamukhaikapada Paschimottanasana [364], Marichiasana V & VI [428, 429], Eka Pada Supta Virasana I-III [471- 473], Eka Pada Kapotasana I & II [280, 281]

Baddha Ardha Matsyendrasana [376], Gomukhasana [396]

Agnistambhasana I-III [405-407]
Upavishta Konasana [381], Parivrtta Upavishhta Konasana [382]
Baddha Konasana II [411]

Deepening: (15 min)
Pincha Araniasana [353] (x13 or x20)
Urdhva Dhanurasana [300]
Dwi Pada Viparita Dandasana I & II [301, 302], Eka Pada Viparita Chakrasana [305]
Natarajasana [115], Baddha Natarajasana [116]
Drop-backs [322] (xTone)

Viparita Chakrasana [323] (xTone)
Hanumanasana [438, 439] (x2)

Restorative: (15 min)
Sarvangasana [165], Halasana [171], Karnapidasana [173], Supta Baddha Konasana [466]
Supta Hindolasana I [484], Supta Urdhva Pada Vajrasana [172]
Supta Valgulasana [462], Yoganidrasana [463]
Jathara Parivartanasana I & II [491, 492]
Shavasana [494]

14) White Wizard: ENCHANT – RECEPTIVITY – TIMELESSNESS

The energy of the White Wizard brings us into the timeless and eternal present moment. It reminds us that we are all magicians when we cultivate the power of Now. We lose personal power when we go into our past regrets or fears of the future. Throughout the practice, increase receptivity to the breath and energy, while ignoring the thoughts of the lower self. There is nothing that we can't accomplish or overcome when we are present in the moment. This class sequence focuses on twisting to spiral awareness into the moment and forward folds to increase sense withdrawal.

"That inner call, the longing, the burning Fire for Knowledge is unfolding. The Path is Eternal. Knowledge is Perennial. You are the Perennial Being. You are the Eternal Being." – Sri Svami Purna

Intention: To be fully present in the Here and Now.
Focus in asana: releasing tension to increase receptivity
Digit: left pinky finger
Chakra: root

Mudra: *khechari* (to move the sky), *Bahirava/Bhairavi* (gesture of formidable attitude)
Pranayama: *viloma* (ladder breath on exhalation), *bahya kumbhaka* (breath retention after exhalation with *maha bandha*)

Level I

Introduction: (5-10 min)
Meditation, Mudra, and Pranayama
Chant

Warm-Up: (10 min)
Sun Salutation A [0] (x3)
Side angle pose [49], elixir of the moon IV [20]
Fierce pose [10], revolved fierce pose [12], half fierce pose

[11]
Revolved one foot down dog [31], turbo dog [33]
Mountain pose [1]

Strength Recruiting: (15 min)
Warrior I [34], revolved side angle [57]
Wind vinyasa (xTone) [345]
Bound hands warrior I [41], humble warrior [47]
Extended legs wide forward fold [88], revolved extended

legs wide forward fold [94]
Crane pose [185], child's pose [388]

Challenging: (10 min)
Noose pose [99]
Side crane pose [191]
Twisting thigh stretch [288], Hanuman prep pose [436]

Opening: (15-20 min)
One foot king pigeon prep [285], revolved one foot pigeon prep [401], one arm lotus one foot pigeon [402]
Camel [275], supine hero [468]
Wizard's pose [175]
Seated wide angle [381], revolved seated wide angle [382]
Two arm hero pose [332], west side stretch I & II [357, 358], east side stretch [294]

Level II

Introduction: (5-10 min)
Meditation, Mudra, and Pranayama
Chant

Warm-Up: (10 min)
Sun Salutation A [0] (x3)
Side angle pose [49], elixir of the moon IV [20]
Fierce pose [10], revolved fierce pose [12], half fierce pose [11]
Revolved one hand down dog [29], turbo dog [33]
Mountain pose [1]

Strength Recruiting: (15 min)
Warrior I [34]
Warrior I [34], revolved side angle [577]
Wind vinyasa (xTone) [345]
Bound hands warrior I [41], humble warrior [47], one foot sage Koundinya II [199]
Triangle [59], intense side stretch [87], revolved triangle [65], standing split [86], handstand [146]
Extended legs wide forward fold [88], revolved extended legs wide forward fold [94]
Crane pose [185], child's pose [388]

Challenging: (10 min)
Handstand [146] (2 min timed at wall)

Yogi staff pose prep [443]

Deepening: (5 min)
Windshield wipers [354] or Krishna crunches [352] (xTone)
Bridge [295]
Upward Bow pose [300] (x2)

Restorative: (10-20 min)
Shoulder stand [164], plow pose [171], ear pressure pose [173]
Single leg stretch I, II, III [474, 476, 477]
One foot happy baby [488], happy baby [489]
Supine twist [491]
Corpse pose [494]

Forearm stand [133] (3min timed at wall)
Headstand [117] (5min timed at wall)
-or-
Noose pose [99]
Side crane pose [191]
Twisting thigh stretch [288], Hanuman prep pose [436], one foot crow I & II [189, 190]

Opening: (15 min)
One foot king pigeon [285], revolved one foot pigeon [401], one arm lotus one foot pigeon [402]
Camel [275], supine hero [468]
Wizard's pose [175]
Fire log pose II [406], revolved fire log pose [408]
One foot half lotus forward bend [363], sage Marichi II [425]
Seated wide angle [381], revolved seated wide angle [382]
Two arm hero pose [332], west side stretch III [359], revolved west side stretch twist [361]
East side stretch [294]
Yogi staff pose [444]

Deepening: (10 min)
Windshield wipers [354] and/or Krishna crunches [352] (xTone)
Boat pose, half boat, revolved boat [346, 347, 348]

(xTone)
Bridge [295]
Upward bow [300] (x3)

Restorative: (15-20 min)
Shoulder stand [164], plow pose [171] ear pressure [173], side ear pressure [174]

Fish pose [319], intense foot pose [321]
Single leg stretch I, II, III [474, 476, 477]
Happy baby [489], sleeping yogi pose [463]
Supine twist [491]
Corpse pose [494]

Level III

Introduction: (5-10 min)
Meditation, Mudra, and Pranayama
Chant

Warm-Up: (10 min)
Surya Namaskar A [0] (x5)
Parsvakonasana [49], Somachandrasana IV [20]
Parivrtta Eka Hasta Adho Mukha Svanasana [29], Vira Adho Mukha Svanasana [33]
Hasta Padangusthasana [6], Parivrtta Uttanasana [5], Padahastasana [7]
Tadasana [1]

Strength Recruiting: (15 min)
Virabhaasana I [34]
Virabhaasana I [34], Parivrtta Baddha Parsvakonasana [58]
Vayu Vinyasa (xTone) [345], Eka Pada Koundinyasana I [198]
Baddha Hasta Virabhadrasana [41], Veerastambhasana [47], Eka Pada Koundinyasana II [199]
Trikonasana [59], Parsvottanasana [87], Parivrtta Trikonasana [65], Urdhva Prasaritta Ekapadasana [86], Adho Mukha Vrksasana [146]
Prasarita Padattonasana I, IV [88, 91], Parivrtta Prasarita Padattonasana II [95]
Bakasana [185], Sirsasana II [118], Balasana [388]

Challenging: (15 min)
Adho Mukha Vrksasana (5min) [146]
Pincha Mayurasana (3min) [133]
Sirsasana (5min) [117]
-or-
Bakasana [185], Sirsasana II [118], Parsva Bakasana [191], Sirsasana II [118], Dwi Pada Koundinyasana [197], Sirsasana II [118], Eka Pada Galavasana [208],

Sirsasana II [118], Ashtavakrasana [183], Sirsasana III [119], Mayurasana [229]

Opening: (15 min)
Eka Pada Rajakapotasana I [285], Parivrtta Eka Pada Kapotasana [401], Eka Bhuja Padma Eka Pada Kapotasana [402]
Ushtrasana [275], Eka Bhuja Swastika Supta Virasana [328], Supta Virasana [468]
Baddha Shramanasana [176]
Ardha Matsyendrasana II [378], Ardha Baddha Padma Paschimottanasana [363], Marichiasana II [425], Bharadvajasana II [372], Padmasana [446], Tolasana [224], Urdhva Kukkutasana [226], Padma Adho Mukha Vrksasana [157]
Upavishta Konasana [381], Parivrtta Upavishta Konasana [382]
Paschimottanasana III [359], Parivrtta Paschimottanasana [361], Uttana Paschimottanasana [362]

Deepening: (10 min)
Navasana [346], Ardha Navasana [347] & Parsva Navasana [348] (xTone)
Setu Bandha Sarvangasana [295]
Urdhva Dhanurasana [300] (x3)
Drop-backs [322] (xTone)

Restorative: (15-20 min)
Sarvangasana [164], Halasana [171], Karnapidasana [173], Parsva Karnapidasana [174]
Matsyasana [319], Uttana Padasana [321]
Supta Padangusthasana I, II, III [475, 476, 477]
Yoga Nidrasana [463]
Jathara Parivartanasana I [491]
Shavasana [492]

15) Blue Eagle: CREATE – MIND – VISION

The Blue Eagle energy is transformative, but in order to transform, we must first open up to a greater possibility of being in the world. The Blue Eagle initiates the transformation by creating a vision of our life and how we can soar to new heights of greater potential. It represents the clear light of conscious thought. The eagle doesn't focus on little things, but soars to a greater horizon where the unexplored territory can be seen. We all have the power of transforming and stepping into a higher light, and when we do, then we inspire those around us to transform as well. This class focuses on variations of Garuda to stay in remembrance of the spirit's vision, while embodying arm balances, inversions, and core work.

"Sincerity means you are completely true. You have a true heart, an open heart, you are completely sincere. What else do you need? Everything else will come." – Sri Svami Purna

Intention: Let go of small thoughts and ideas that are self-limiting in nature, and open to the greater vision of an expansive self.
Focus in asana: Stay present to what you create with your mind.

Digit: left big toe
Chakra: crown
Mudra: *jnana* (knowledge seal)
Pranayama: *sheetkari* (hissing breath), *jalandhara bandha* (throat lock after inhalation)

Level I

Introduction: (5-10 min)
Meditation, Mudra, and Pranayama
Chant

Warm-Up: (10 min)
Sun Salutation A [0] (x3)
Monkey lunge I [14]
Side angle pose [49], half warrior side angle pose [51]

Strength Recruiting: (10 min)
Warrior I [34]
Eagle warrior [39]
Warrior I [34], warrior III [46], standing splits [86], eagle pose [104], standing splits [86]
Bound side angle [55], one foot Koundinya II [199]
Extended legs wide forward bend [88], half garland [101]
Crane pose [185], puppy pose [257]

Challenging: (15 min)
Handstand prep (at wall) [147]
Handstand [146]
Headstand [117] into eagle forearm stand [141]

-or-
Twisting thigh stretch [288]
Camel [275], supine hero [468]
Peacock pose [229]

Opening: (10 min)
One foot king pigeon prep pose [285]
Half fish [375], cow face pose w/ eagle arms [398]
Seated wide angle [381], revolved seated wide angle [382]
Bound angle [410], two arm hero [332]

Deepening: (10 min)
Eagle crunches [349] (xTone)
Bridge [295]
Upward bow [300] (x2)

Restorative: (10-20 min)
Shoulder stand [164], plow pose [171]
Single leg stretch I, II, III [474, 476, 477]
One foot happy baby [488], happy baby [489]
Supine eagle twist [480]
Corpse pose [494]

Level II

Introduction: (5-10 min)
Meditation, Mudra, and Pranayama
Chant

Warm-Up: (10 min)
Sun Salutation A [0] (x4)
Monkey lunge II [15]
Side angle [49], half warrior side angle [51]

Strength Recruiting: (15 min)
Warrior I [34]
Eagle warrior I [39], revolved side angle [57]
Sage Vasistha's pose [215]
Warrior I [34], warrior III [46], standing split [86],
eagle pose II [105], standing split [86]
Bound side angle [55], one foot sage Koundinya II [199]
Standing wide leg forward bend I & IV [88, 92],
bound half garland [102]
Crane [185], child's pose [385]

Challenging: (10 min)
Wide leg handstand [155]
Eagle handstand [156]

Eagle forearm stand [141]

Opening: (15 min)
One foot king pigeon [285]
Camel [275], supine hero [468]
Peacock pose [229], swan pose [228]
Bound half fish [376], cow face pose w/ eagle arms [398]
Seated wide angle [381], revolved seated wide angle [382]
Bound angle [410], two arm hero [332]

Deepening: (10 min)
Eagle crunches [349] (xTone)
Bridge [295]
Upward Bow [300] (x2)

Restorative: (10-15 min)
Shoulder stand [164], plow pose [171], ear pressure
[173]
Fish pose [319], intense foot pose [321]
Single leg stretch I, II, III [474, 476, 477]
Happy baby [489], sleeping yogi pose [463]
Supine eagle twist [491]
Corpse pose [494]

Level III

Introduction: (5-10 min)
Meditation, Mudra, and Pranayama
Chant

Warm-Up: (10 min)
Sun Salutation [0] (x5)
Vanarasana II [15]
Parsvakonasana [49], Ardha Vira Parsvakonasana [51]

Strength Recruiting: (15 min)
Virabhadrasana 1[34]
Garuda Virabhadrasana I [39], Baddha Parivrtta
Parsvakonasana [58]
Trianga Dandasana [195], Purna Vasisthasana [218,
Camatkarasana [219]
Virabhadrasana I [34], Virabhadrasana III [46], Urdhva

Prasarita Ekapadasana [86], Garudasana II [105], Urdhva
Prasarita Ekapadasana [86], Adho Mukha Vrksasana [146]
Baddha Parsvakonasana [55], Eka Pada Koundinyasana II
[199], Ghanda Bherundasana [316]
Baddha Eka Pada Uttanasana [68], Svarga Dvijasana [75]
Titthibasana II & I [96, 212], Bakasana [185] or Adho
Mukha Vrksasana [146]
Balasana [388], Uttana Shishosana [257]

Challenging: (15 min)
Prasarita Pada Adho Mukha Vrksasana [155]
Garuda Adho Mukha Vrksasana [156]
Pincha Mayurasana [133], Garuda Pincha
Mayurasana [141]
Garuada Sirsasana [124]

Opening: (10-15 min)
Eka Bhuja Swastikasana [326], Dhanurasana [265]
Eka Pada Rajakapotasana I [285]
Ushtrasana [275], Supta Virasana [468]
Mayurasana [229], Viparita Mayurasana [231], Purna
Viparita Mayurasana [231]
Baddha Ardha Matsyendrasana [376], Garuda
Gomukhasana [398]
Upavishta Konasana [381], Parivrtta Upavishta Konasana
[382], Uttana Konasana [204]
Supta Visvajrasana [490]

Deepening: (10 min)
Supta Garudasana [349] (xTone)
Setu Bandha Sarvangasana [295]
Urdhva Dhanurasana [300] (x3)
Drop-backs [322] (xTone)

Restorative: (10-15 min)
Sarvangasana [164], Urdhva Padma Sarvangasana [167],
Pindasana [168]
Padma Matsyasana [320], Uttana Padasana [321]
Supta Padangusthasana I, II, III [475, 476, 477]
Supta Bhairavasana [460], Yoganidrasana [463]
Supta Parivrtta Garudasana [480]
Shavasana [494]

16) Yellow Warrior: Question – Fearlessness – Intelligence

The energy of the Yellow Warrior encourages us to question our reality with intelligence. It is playing the edge in life and in our practice with great skill and fervor. The Warrior is always questioning self-imposed limitations, and confronting them with a fearless attitude to overcome all obstacles. In Indian mythology, Skanda represents the divine warrior. He has six heads to represent the six aspects of the higher self: strength, wisdom, dispassion, prosperity, recognition, and spiritual power. All of these naturally develop when we embrace the practice as the vehicle of transformation. This class focuses on warrior variations, arm balances, inversions, and backbends.

"You do not have to make a statement with the body or with your outer strength. It is the inner strength that matters." – Sri Svami Purna

Intention: Embrace your fears. Gather strength as the spiritual warrior to fight for *dharma* and the convictions of the heart.
Focus in asana: *vira*, enthusiasm for the practice

Digit: left index toe
Chakra: throat
Mudra: *Skanda* (spiritual warrior seal)
Pranayama: *ujjayi* (victorious breath)

Level I

Introduction: (5-10 min)
Meditation, Mudra, and Pranayama
Chant

Warm-Up: (10 min)
Sun Salutation A [0] (x3)
Side angle pose [49], warrior side angle pose [52]
Sun Salutation B [00] (x1)

Strength Recruiting: (15 min)
Extended bound hands warrior pose [42]
Warrior II [43], side warrior variation [45]
Warrior I [34], warrior III [46], standing splits [86],
Triangle [59], half warrior triangle [60]
Extended legs wide forward bend [88], warrior splits (x2) [93]
Crane pose [185], child's pose [388]

Challenging: (10-12 min)
Extended hand to big toe pose I-IV [81-84]
Skanda squats [85] (xTone)
Standing half lotus into a forward fold [79, 80]

Opening: (15 min)
One foot pigeon prep [400]
Camel [275], supine hero pose [468]
Fire log pose I & II [405, 406]
Seated wide angle pose [381], revolved seated wide angle pose [382]
Baby cradle pose [441], Arjuna's pose [454]
Wheel of Skanda [324], two arm hero [332]
West side stretch I & II [357, 358]

Deepening: (10-13 min)
Boat pose & half boat [346, 347] (x3)
Bridge [295]
Upward bow [300] (x2)
Hanuman's pose [438] (x2)

Restorative: (10-15 min)
Sage Bhardva pose I or II [371, 372]
Sweet pose [392] or spiritual power pose [393]
(3-5min meditation)
Supine child's pose [487], supine twist [491]
Corpse [494]

Level II

Introduction: (5-10 min)
Meditation, Mudra, and Pranayama
Chant

Warm-Up: (10 min)
Sun salutation A [0] (x3)
Side angle [49], warrior side angle [52]
Sun salutation B [0] (x2)

Strength Recruiting: (15 min)
Extended bound hands warrior II [42]
Warrior II [43], bound side angle [55], Koundinya II [199]
Warrior I [36], warrior III [46], standing splits [86], kick to handstand [146]
Triangle [59], half warrior triangle [60]
Half moon [70], warrior half moon [72], standing split [86], kick to handstand [146]
Extended legs wide forward bend [88], warrior splits [93] (x2)
Crane pose [185], child's pose [388], heart opening pose I, II [258, 259]

Challenging: (15 min)
Standing hand to big toe pose I-IV [81-84]
Skanda squats [85] (xTone)
Standing half lotus into a forward fold [79, 80]

Opening: (15 min)
One foot king pigeon [285]
Camel [275], supine hero [468]
Half fish [374]
Seated wide angle [381], revolved seated wide angle [382]
West side stretch III [359], archer's pose I & II [452, 453]
Baby cradle pose [441], Arjuna's pose [454]
Skanda's pose [457], sage Ashtavakra's pose [183]
Wheel of Skanda [324], two arm hero [332]

Deepening: (10 min)
Boat pose & half boat [346, 347] (x3)
Bridge [295]
Upward bow [300] (x2)
Hanuman's pose [438] (x2)

Restorative: (10-15 min)
Sage Bhardva pose I or II [371, 372]
Spiritual power pose II [394] or lotus pose [446] (3-5min meditation)
Happy baby pose [489], sleeping yogi pose [463]
Supine twist [491]
Corpse [494]

Level III

Introduction: (5-10 min)
Meditation, Mudra, and Pranayama
Chant

Warm-Up: (10 Min)
Surya Namaskar A [0] (x4)
Parsvakonasana [49], Vira Parsvakonasana [52]
Surya Namaskar B [00] (x2)

Strength Recruiting: (15 min)
Utthita Baddha Hasta Virabhadrasana [42]
Virabhadrasana I [36], Virabhadrasana III [46], Urdhva
Prasarita Ekapadasana [86], Adho Mukha Vrksasana [146]
Baddha Parsvakonasana [55], Baddha Trikonasana [66],
Baddha Eka Pada Uttanasana [68], Svarga Dvijasana
[75], Baddha Ardha Chandrasana [73], Urdhva Prasarita
Ekapadasana [86], Adho Mukha Vrksasana [146]
Parivrtta Baddha Parsvakonasana [58], Eka Pada
Koundinyasana I & II [199, 198]
Vira Prasarita Padattonasana [93], Prasarita Padattonasana
I & V [88, 92]
Bakasana [185], Balasana [388], Uttana Shishosana [257]

Challenging: (15 min)
Utthita Hasta Padangusthasana I-IV [81-84]
Vira Utthita Hasta Padangusthasana [85] (xTone)
Ardha Baddha Padma Vrksasana [79], Ardha Baddha
Padma Uttanasana [80], Kasyapasana [220]

Opening: (15 min)
Eka Pada Rajakapotasana I [285]
Ushtrasana [275], Supta Virasana [468], Kapotasana [279]
Mayurasana [229]
Baddha Ardha Matsyendrasana [376]
Upavishta Konasana [381], Parivrtta Upavishta Konasana [382]
Paschimottanasana III [359], Akarna Dhanurasana I & II
[452, 453]
Eka Pada Sirsasana [455], Skandasana [457], Chakorasana [236]
Marichiasana VIII [431], Yoga Dandasana II [239]

Deepening: (15 min)
Navasana & Ardha Navasana [346, 347] (x3)
Setu Bandha Sarvangasana [295]
Urdhva Dhanurasana [300] (x2)
Dwi Pada Viparita Dandasana [301]
Drop-backs or Viparita Chakrasana [323] (xTone)
Hanumanasana [438] (x2)

Restorative: (10-15 min)
Bharadvajasana II [372], Padmasana [446], Simhasana
[317], Goraknathasana [448], Musti Padma Mayurasana
[232], Viparita Musti Padma Mayurasana [233]
Padmasana [446] (3-5min meditation)
Jathara Parivartanasa I [491]
Shavasana [494]

17) Red Earth: Evolve – Synchronicity – Navigation

The energy of the Red Earth is about navigating our spiritual evolution by synchronizing with the harmonics of time and the earth. In the body, the earth element is found in the pelvic region and the *muladhara chakra*. In Indian mythology, *Ganesha*, the brother of *Skanda* and son of *Shiva*, is the ruler of the root *chakra* and remover of obstacles. When we connect to the power of Ganesha we clear the path for personal growth and development. The practice is designed to open the hips and activate the root *chakra*, while integrating backbends to activate *prana*.

"Yoga is universal. It is a means of research, exploration and expansion on many levels. Life itself is yoga."
– Sri Svami Purna

Intention: Give and receive love from the Mother Earth. Reveal and acknowledge synchronicity. Recognize evolution as an unfolding process.
Focus in asana: *mula bandha*
Digit: left middle toe

Chakra: heart
Mudra: *prithivi* (Earth seal), or *Ganesha* (seal of the remover of obstacles)
Pranayama: *viloma* (ladder breath on inhalation), *ujjayi* (if working *Ganesha mudra*)

Level I

Introduction: (5-10 min)
Meditation, Mudra, and Pranayama
Chant

Warm-Up: (10 min)
Sun Salutation A [0] (x3)
Elixir of the moon [17], monkey lunge III [16]

Strength Recruiting: (15 min)
Warrior I [34]
Side angle pose [49], half bound intense side angle [54]
Triangle pose [59]
Half moon [70], sugarcane [77], standing split [86]
Upward Kali pose [106], sage Shankara [107], extended legs wide forward bend [88]
Crane pose [185], child's pose [388]

Challenging: (10 min)
Standing baby cradle [108], one foot sage Galava's pose [208]
Standing half lotus into a forward fold [79, 80]

Opening: (15 min)
One foot king pigeon prep [400]
Fire log pose [405]
Cow face pose [395]
Forehead to knee pose I, II [366, 367]
Earth saluting pose [380], seated wide angle pose [381], revolved seated wide angle [382]
Bound angle I, II [410, 411]

Deepening: (10 min)
Supine leg raises [350, 351] (xTone)
Bridge [295]
Upward bow [300] (x2)
Lord of the Dance pose (x2) [115]

Restorative: (10-20 min)
Shoulder stand [164], plow pose [171]
Eye of the needle pose [486], supine one foot upward diamond prep [478], supine twist II [492]
Supine auspicious leg pose [481], supine Ganesha's pose [483]
Supine twist I [491]
Corpse pose [494]

Level II

Introduction: (5-10 min)
Meditation, Mudra, and Pranayama
Chant

Warm-Up: (10 min)
Sun Salutation A [0] (x3)
Elixir of the moon II [18], monkey lunge III [16]
Side angle pose [49], intense half bound side angle [54]

Strength Recruiting: (15 min)
Warrior I [34]
Intense warrior I [38]
Triangle [59], intense half bound triangle [62]
Half moon [70], sugarcane pose [77], standing splits [86]
Bound side angle [55], one foot sage Koundinya II [199]
Upward Kali pose [106], sage Shankara's pose [107], extended legs wide forward bend [88, 92]
Crane pose [185], child's pose [388], puppy pose [257]

Challenging: (10 min)
Standing baby cradle [108], one foot sage Galava's pose [208]
Standing half lotus into a forward fold [79, 80]
Standing half frog [111]

Opening: (15 min)
One foot king pigeon [185]
Fire log pose I & II [405, 406]
Forehead to knee pose I, II, [366, 367], half root lock pose [413]
Half lotus forward bend [363], lotus pose [446], scale pose [224]
Earth saluting pose [380], seated wide angle [381], revolved seated wide angle [382]
Bound angle II, III [411, 412]

Deepening: (10 min)
Dragon flags [353] and/or Kali crunches [355] (xTone)
Bridge pose with one foot in half frog [297]
Upward bow [295] (x2)
Two foot inverted staff pose [301]
Lord of the Dance pose [115] (x2)

Restorative: (15-20 min)
Shoulder stand [164], plow pose [171], supine angle pose [465]
Supine baby cradle I [484], supine upward foot thunderbolt pose [172]
Supine Ganesha's pose [483], supine twist II [492]
Sleeping yogi pose [463]
Supine twist [491]
Corpse pose [494]

Level III

Introduction: (5-10 min)
Meditation, Mudra, and Pranayama
Chant

Warm-Up: (10 min)
Surya Namaskar A [0] (x5)
Somachandrasana III [19], Vanarasana III [16]
Parsvakonasana [49], Ardha Baddha Uttana Parsvakonasana [54]

Strength recruiting: (15 min)
Virabhadrasana I [34]
Uttana Virabhadrasana [38]
Trikonasana [59], Utthita Uttana Trikonasana [62]
Ardha Chandrasana [70], Ardha Chandra Chapasana [77],
Parivrtta Ardha Chandrasana [71], Nindra Eka Pada Dhanurasana [78], Urdhva Prasarita Ekapadasana [86],
Adho Mukha Vrksasana [146]
Baddha Parsvakonasana [55], Eka Pada Koundinyasana II [199], Gandha Bherundasana [316]
Urdhva Kaliasana [106], Shankarasana [107], Prasarita Padattonasana V [92], Rajasamakonasana [384]
Bakasana [388]
Ardha Bakasana [188], Balasana [185], Araniasana [260]

Challenging: (10 min)
Eka Pada Galavasana I & II [208, 209], Ardha Bhujapidasana [210]
Koundinyasana variation "Hummingbird" [200]
Nindra Ardha Bhekasana [111]

Opening: (15 min)
Eka Pada Rajakapotasana I [285]
Agnistambhasana [405], Ardha Padma Ushtrasana [277]
Janu Sirsasana II & III [367, 368]
Ardha Baddha Padma Paschimottanasana [363],
Marichiasana II [425], Padmasana [446], Tolasana [224]
Bhunamananasana [380], Upavishta Konasana [381],
Parivrtta Upavishta Konasana [382], Kurmasana [386],
Supta Kurmasana [387]
Baddha Konasana III [412], Mulabandhasana I, II [414, 415]

Deepening: (15 min)
Navasana [346] or Pincha Araniasana [353]
Ardha Bheka Setu Bandha Sarvangasana [297], Bheka Setu Bandha Sarvangasana [298]
Urdhva Dhanurasana [300] (x2)
Natarajasana [115], Baddha Natarajasana [116]

Restorative: (15-20 min)
Supta Balasana [487], Sarvangasana II [165], Halasana

[171], Karnapidasana [173], Supta Baddha Konasana [466] Supta Hindolasana I & II [484, 485] Supta Urdhva Pada Vajrasana [172], Eka Pada Sirsa Shyanasana [464]

Supta Ganeshasana [483], Yoga Nidrasana [463] Jathara Parivartasana I [491], Jathara Parivartasana II [492] Shavasana [494]

18) White Mirror: REFLECT – ORDER – ENDLESSNESS

The energy of White Mirror is reflective and meditative. We use every experience as a meditation to reflect the essence of our Self back to us. Through the outward growth of evolution, we learn to turn the process back within through involution. Our outer reality is a reflection of what we create in our minds. We attract everything that we have in our life and the White Mirror encourages us to become more aware of what we have created and what is still possible to create. Our potential is endless, and if we stay positive, then we will reflect our highest aspirations. This class focuses on forward bends, hip-openers, and twists to increase the experience of *pratyahara*, turning the senses within.

"People become known by the quality of their action, not by their words." – Sri Svami Purna

Intention: Clear the mirror of the mind to reflect the highest state of perfection.
Focus in asana: Watch the breath, not the mind.
Digit: left ring toe
Chakra: Solar-plexus

Mudra: *bhairava/bhairavi* (gesture of formidable attitude)
Pranayama: *kapalabhati* (skull shining), *rechaka kumbhaka* (breath retention after exhalation with *maha bandha*)

Level I

Introduction: (5-10 min)
Meditation, Mudra, and Pranayama
Chant

Warm-Up: (10 min)
Surya Namaskar A [0] (x3)
Intense poses [10], revolved intense pose [11]
Side angle [49], elixir of the moon IV [20]

Strength Recruiting: (10 min)
Warrior I [34], revolved side angle [57]
Bound hands warrior I [41], humble warrior [47]
Triangle [59], half moon [70], revolved half moon [71], standing split [86], intense side stretch [87], revolved triangle [65]
Extended legs wide forward bend [88], revolved

extended legs wide forward bend [94]
Crane [185], child's pose [388]

Challenging: (10 min)
Noose pose [99]
Side crane [191]
Twisting thigh stretch [288], Hanuman prep [436], one foot sage Koundinya II [199]
-or-
Handstand [146[(2 min timed at wall), child's pose [388] (1min)
Forearm stand [133] (1min timed at wall), child's pose [388] (1min)
Headstand [117] (3 min timed at wall), supported child's pose [389] (1min)

Opening: (15 min)
One foot king pigeon prep [400]
Camel [275]
Forehead to knee pose [366], revolved forehead to knee pose I [369]
Seated wide angle pose [381], revolved seated wide angle pose [382]
Bound angle [410]
Baby cradle [441]
Yogi's staff pose prep [443]

Deepening: (10 min)
Krishna crunches [352] (xTone)
Supine double diamond [480]
Bridge pose [295]
Upward bow pose [300] (x2)

Restorative: (10-20 min)
Shoulder stand [164], plow [171], ear pressure [173]
Single leg stretch I, II, III [474, 475, 477]
One foot happy baby [488], happy baby [489]
Supine twist [491]
Corpse pose [494]

Level II

Introduction: (5-10 min)
Meditation, Mudra, and Pranayama
Chant

Warm-Up: (10 min)
Sun Salutation A [0] (x4)
Action pose [8], revolved action pose [9]
Side angle [49], elixir of the moon pose IV [20]

Strength Recruiting: (15 min)
Warrior I [34], revolved side angle [57]
Wind vinyasa [345] (xTone)
Bound hands warrior I [41], humble warrior [47]
Triangle [59], intense side stretch [87], revolved triangle [65], standing splits [86]
Half moon [70], revolved half moon [71], standing splits [86]
Extended legs wide forward bend [88], revolved extended legs wide forward bend [94]
Crane pose [185], child's pose [388], puppy pose [257]

Challenging: (10-15 min)
Noose pose [99]
Side crane [191], two foot sage Koundinya pose [197]
Twisting thigh stretch [289], Hanuman prep [436], one foot crane pose I [189], one foot crane pose II [190]
-or-
Handstand [117] (3 min timed at wall or xTone), child's pose [388] (1min)
Forearm stand [133] (2 min timed at wall), child's pose

[388] (1min)
Headstand [117] (4 min timed at wall), supported child's pose [389] (1min)

Opening: (15 min)
One foot king pigeon [400], revolved one foot king pigeon prep [401]
Forehead to knee [366], revolved forehead to knee I, II [369, 370]
Seated wide angle pose [380], revolved seated wide angle pose [381]
Two arm hero [332], two arm double diamond [338]
West side stretch II [358], revolved west side stretch [361]
East side stretch [294]

Deepening: (10 min)
Windshield wipers [354] (xTone) and Krishna crunches [352] (xTone)
Bridge [295]
Upward wheel [300] (x3)

Restorative: (15-20 min)
Shoulder stand [164], plow [171], ear pressure [173]
Single leg stretch I, II, III [474, 476, 477]
Happy baby [488], sleeping yogi pose [463]
Twist [491]
Corpse pose [494]

Level III

Introduction: (5-10 min)
Meditation, Mudra, and Pranayama
Chant

Warm-Up: (10 min)
Surya Namaskar [0] (x5)
Karmasana [8], Parivrtta Karmasana [9]
Parivrtta Eka Hasta Ado Muka Svanasana [29]
Vira Ado Muka Svanasana [33]
Parsvakonasana [49], Somachandrasana IV [20]

Strength Recruiting: (15 min)
Virabhadrasana I [34], Baddha Parivrtta
Parsvakonasana [57]
Vayu Vinyasa (xTone) [345],
Eka Pada Koundinyasana I [198]
Baddha Hasta Virabhadrasana [41],
Veerastambhasana [47],
Eka Pada Koundinyasana II [199]
Trikonasana [59], Parsvottanasana [87], Parivrtta
Trikonasana [65], Urdhva Prasarita Ekapadasana
[86], Adho Mukha Vrksasana [146]
Baddha Eka Pada Uttanasana [68], Svarga Dvijasana [75]
Tittibhasana II & I [96, 212], Bakasana [185]
Balasana [388], Uttana Shishosana [257]

Challenging: (15 min)
Adho Mukha Vrksasana [146] (3-5 minutes timed or
xTone)
Pincha Mayurasana [133] (2-3 minutes timed)
Sirsasana [117] (5 minutes timed)
-or-
Sirsasana II [118], Parsva Bakasana [191], Sirsasana
II [118], Dwi Pada Koundinyasana [197], Sirsasana
II [118], Eka Pada Galavasana [208], Sirsasana II

[118], Ashtavakrasana [183], Sirsasana II [118],
Urdhva Kukkutasana [226], Sirsasana II [118],
Parsva Kukkutasana [227], Balasana [388]

Opening: (15 min)
Eka Pada Rajakapotasana I [285], Parivrtta Eka Pada
Rajakapotasana [401]
Ushtrasana [275], Vajrasana [391], Supta Uttana
Virasana [469]
Ardha Matsyendrasana II [378], Ardha Baddha
Padma Paschimottanasana [363], Marichiasana II
[425], Marichiasana IV [427], Padmasana [446]
Upavishta Konasana [381], Parivrtta Upavishta
Konasana [382]
Dwi Bhuja Virasana [332], Dwi Bhuja Visvajarasana
[338], Paschimottanasana [357], Parivrtta
Paschimottanasana [361], Purvottanasana [294]
Yoga Danadasana (x2) [444]

Deepening: (10 min)
Navasana [346], Ardha Navasana [347], Parsva
Navasana [348] (xTone)
Visvajrasana [490]
Setu Bandha Sarvangasana [295]
Urdhva Dhanurasana [300] (x3)
Drop-backs [322] (xTone)

Restorative: (15-20 min)
Sarvangasana [164], Halasana [171], Karnapidasana
[173], Parsva Karnapidasana [174]
Matsyasana [319], Uttana Padasana [321]
Supta Padangusthasana I, II, III [475, 476, 477]
Yoga Nidrasana [463]
Jathara Parivartanasana [491]
Shavasana [494]

19) Blue Storm: CATALYZE – ENERGY – SELF-GENERATION

Blue Storm represents all of the drama and craziness in life that causes us to lose our center. When we lose our center, we overreact, and have less ability to influence positive change. On Blue Storm days, we cultivate the "eye of the storm." In the center of a hurricane it is completely peaceful, and that's how we should be when the storm of life hits. We should hold strong to the center and to our peace. This practice focuses on midline technique and adductor strength to build awareness of the center in all poses.

"Be grateful for life's difficulties. They are opportunities for your growth." – Sri Svami Purna

Intention: Hold the eye of the storm.
Focus in asana: Awaken your thunder being, and ride the lightning. Catalyze transformation thru self-generation.
Embodiment: midline technique
Digit: left pinky toe

Chakra: root
Mudra: *chin* (psychic gesture)
Pranayama: *viloma* (ladder breath on exhalation), *moorcha* (swooning breath)

Level I

Introduction: (5-10 min)
Meditation, Mudra, and Pranayama
Chant

Warm-Up: (10 min)
Sun Salutation A [0] (x3 with block between inner thighs)
Monkey lunge I [14]
Side angle pose [49], half warrior side angle pose [51]

Strength Recruiting: (15 min)
Warrior I (x2 with block between hands) [34]
Sage Vasistha prep [214]
Side warrior pose [45], bound side angle [55], one foot sage Koundinya II [199]
Triangle [59], half moon [70], standing split [86]
Warrior splits [93], extended legs wide forward bend [88]
Monkey frog [434], child's pose [388]
Crane pose [185], child's pose [388], puppy pose [257]

Challenging: (15 min)
Handstand balancing technique [149]
Forearm stand (block between hands with palms face up) [134]

Headstand (leg raises with a block between inner thighs) [117]

Opening: (10 min)
One foot king pigeon prep [400]
Camel [275]
Half fish prep [374], one foot cow forward bend [365]
Seated wide angle [381] (with PNF technique)
Bound angle I & II [410, 411] (with PNF technique)
Two arm hero pose [332]

Deepening: (10 min)
Supine arm raises (x13 with block) [339]
Bridge pose (with block between inner thighs) [295]
Upward bow (with block between inner thighs) [300]
Upward bow (with block between inner edges of feet) [300]

Restorative: (10-20 min)
Shoulder stand [164], plow pose [171]
Fish pose [319], intense foot pose [321]
Single leg stretch I, II, III [474, 476, 477]
One foot happy baby [488], happy baby [489]
Supine twist [491]
Corpse pose [494]

Level II

Introduction: (5-10 min)
Meditation, Mudra, and Pranayama
Chant

Warm-Up: (10 min)
Sun Salutation A [0] (x3 w/ block between inner thighs)
Turbo dog (with block between inner thighs) [33]
Monkey lunge II [15]
Side angle [49], half warrior side angle [51]

Strength Recruiting: (15 min)
Warrior I (x2 with block between hands) [34]
Sage Vasistha [215]
Warrior I [37], side warrior pose [44],
bound side angle [55], Koundinya II [199]
Triangle [59], half moon [70], sugarcane [77], standing splits [86], handstand [146]
Warrior splits [93], wide leg forward bend I & V [88, 92]
Monkey frog [434], child's pose [388]
Crane (with block between big toes only) [185],
Headstand II [118]

Challenging: (10-15 min)
Handstand (practice jumping with block between inner thighs) [146]
Handstand (balancing away from wall) [149]
Forearm stand (with block palms face up) [134]
Headstand (leg raises with block x13) [129]
-or-

Twisting thigh stretch [288], Hanuman prep [436],
one foot Vasistha II [217], one foot crow pose II [190],
one foot crow pose I [189]
Pendant pose [205]

Opening: (15 min)
One foot king pigeon [285]
Camel [275], diamond pose [391], little thunderbolt pose [278], Supine hero [468]
Peacock [229]
Half fish [375], cow face [396]
Seated wide angle [381] (with PNF technique)
Bound angle I & II [410, 411] (with PNF technique)
Two arm hero [332]

Deepening: (10-15 min)
Boat pose [346] & half boat pose [347] (x3)
Bridge [295] (with block between inner thighs or feet)
Upward bow [300] (with block between inner thighs x2)
Upward bow [300] (with block between inner edges of the feet)
Hanuman's pose [438] (x2 with PNF technique)

Restorative: (10-20 min)
Shoulder stand [164], plow pose [171], ear pressure [173]
Fish [319], intense foot pose [321]
Supine arm raises (x13 with block) [339]
Supine auspicious pose [481], sleeping yogi's pose [463]
Supine twist I & III [491, 493]
Corpse pose [494]

Level III

Introduction: (5-10 min)
Meditation, Mudra, and Pranayama
Chant

Warm-Up: (10 min)
Surya Namaskar A [0] (x3 with a block between inner thighs)
Vanarasana II [15]
Parsvakonasana [49], Ardha Vira Parsvakonasana [51]

Strength Recruiting: (15 min)
Virabhadrasana (use block between hands x2) [34]
Purna Vasisthasana [218]
Virabhadrasana [37], Parsva Virabhadrasana [44], Baddha Parsvakonasana [55], Eka Pada Koundinyasana II [199],
Ghanda Bherundasana [316]
Baddha Eka Pada Uttanasana [68], Svarga Dvijasana [75],
Tittibhasana II & I [96, 212]

Vira Prasaritta Padattonasana [93], Prasaritta Padattonasana V [92], Urdhva Thavaliasana [435]
Bakasana [185], Sirsasana II [118] or Adho Mukha Vrksasana [146]

Challenging: (15 min)
Adho Mukha Vrksasana [146] (Jumping with block between legs)
Adho Mukha Vrksasana [150] (leg raises- single leg and then both)
Pincha Mayurasana [134] (palms face up with block), Shayanasana [138]
Sirsasana leg raises [129] (work towards x27, x54, x72, or x108)
Sirsasana II [118] (leg raises with twists xTone)

Opening: (15 min)
Baddha Eka Pada Rajakapotasana I [286]
Ushtrasana [275], Supta Virasana [468], Vajrasana [391], Laghuvajrasana (with pigeon droppings xTone) [278], Supta Virasana [468]
Mayurasana [229], Viparitta Mayurasana [230]

Baddha Ardha Matsyendrasana [375], Gomukhasana [396]
Upavishta Konasana [381] (with PNF technique)
Baddha Konasana I-III [410, 411, 412] (with PNF technique)
Dwi Bhuja Virasana [332]

Deepening: (10 min)
Navasana [346] & Ardha Navasana [347] (x3)
Urdhva Dhanurasana [300] (block between inner thighs)
Urdhva Dhanurasana [300] (block between inner edges of feet)
Drop-backs (xTone) [322]
Hanumanasana (x3) [438]

Restorative: (10-15 min)
Salambha Sarvangasana [164], Halasana [171], Karnapidasana [173]
Matsyasana [319], Uttana Padasana [321]
Supta Bhairavasana [460], Yoga Nidrasana [463]
Jathara Parivartanasana I & III [491, 493]
Shavasana [494]

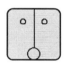

20) Yellow Sun: Enlighten – Life – Universal Fire

Yellow Sun energy is the peak of the energetic cycle and represents the highest attainment. The Sun is a symbol for the invisible Creator and also the divine light of our soul. Honor that light and ignite the practice with Universal Fire to burn off impurities, and to seek an enlightened state of being. This class is strong to develop more inner heat and passion for the practice. It embodies arm balances, inversions, hip-openers, twists, and backbends.

"You have to live in this world, but evolve like a lotus. The lotus flower has a natural wax which, when in water, does not get wet. Live like a lotus flower." – Sri Svami Purna

Focus: Honor the inner divine light and celebrate life.
Embodiment: Inner body bright
Digit: right thumb
Chakra: crown

Mudra: *Vishnu* (seal of Lord Vishnu), *chin* (psychic gesture), *makula* (bud seal is used for final meditation)
Pranayama: *suryabheda* (vitality stimulating), or *bhastrika* with *agni sara* (quintessential fire breath with *chin mudra*)

Level I

Introduction: (5-10 min)
Meditation, Mudra, and Pranayama
Chant

Warm-Up: (10 min)
Sun Salutation A [0] (x3)
Side angle pose [49], warrior side angle pose [52]
Sun Salutation B [00] (x2)

Strength Recruiting: (15 min)
Triangle [59], half moon [70], sugar cane [77],
standing split [86], kick to handstand [146]
Bound side angle
Revolved side angle [57]
Extended legs wide forward bend I-IV [88-91]
Crane pose [185], child's pose [388], heart opening pose [258]

Challenging: (15 min)
Handstand (leg raises xTone) [150]
Handstand (Superman walk-outs x3) [163]
Forearm stand [133]
Headstand I, II, III [117, 118, 119] -or-
Sage Vasistha's pose [215], wild thing [219], crane pose [185]
One arm auspicious pose [326]

Locust pose IV [310], child's pose [388]

Opening: (15 min)
Twisting thigh stretch [288]
Camel [275], supine hero pose [468]
Heron pose [421], sun dial pose [419],
one arm pressure pose [182]
Seated wide angle pose [381],
revolved seated wide angle pose [382]
Bound angle I & II [410, 411]

Deepening: (10 min)
Boat pose [346] and half boat pose [347] (x3)
Bridge pose [295], one foot bridge [296]
Upward bow pose (x2) [300]
Hanuman's pose (x2) [438]

Restorative: (10-20 min)
Sage Bharavaja pose [371], spiritual power pose II [394]
(meditation 2-5 minutes)
One foot happy baby [488], happy baby [489]
Supine twist [491]
Corpse pose [494]

Level II

Introduction: (5-10 min)
Meditation, Mudra, and Pranayama
Chant

Warm-Up: (10 min)
Sun Salutation A [0] (x4)
Side angle pose [49], warrior side angle pose [52]
Sun Salutation B [00] (x2)

Strength Recruiting: (15 min)
Warrior I [34], warrior III [46], standing splits [86],
handstand [146]
Bound side angle [55], bound triangle [66], bound single
leg stretch [68], bird of paradise [75], bound half moon
[73], stand splits [86], handstand [146]
Revolved bound side angle [58], sage Koundinya I [198]
Extended legs wide forward bend I-IV [88-91]
Crow pose [185], headstand II [118], crow pose [185]

Child's pose [388], heart opening pose II [259]

Challenging: (15 min)
Handstand (balance away from wall) [146]
Handstand (Superman walk-outs xTone) [163]
Forearm stand [133], scorpion [139]
Headstand series [117-123] -or-
Subramanya's pose [22], Sage Vishvamitra's pose [223],
sage Koundinya II [199]
Twisting thigh stretch [288], one foot crow pose I & II
[189, 190]

Opening: (15 min)
One foot king pigeon I [285]
Mermaid II [284]
Camel [275], supine hero pose [468], pigeon pose [279]
Heron pose II [422], revolved heron pose [423], sundial
pose II [420], sage Ashtavakra's pose [183]

Seated wide angle [381], revolved seated wide angle [382]
One foot behind the head (x2) [455]
East side stretch [294], west side stretch I-III [357-359]

Deepening: (10 min)
Boat pose [346] and half boat pose [347] (x3)
Bridge pose [295], one foot bridge [296]
Upward bow pose (x3) [300]
Hanuman's pose (x3) [438]

Restorative: (10-20 min)
Sage Bhardvaja pose II, III [372, 373]
Lotus [446], lion [317], rooster pose [225], upward rooster [226]
Lotus [446] or spiritual power pose II [394] (meditation 5-7 minutes)
Supine twist [490]
Corpse pose [492]

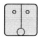

Level III

Introduction: (5-10 min)
Meditation, Mudra, and Pranayama
Chant

Warm-Up: (10 min)
Surya Namaskar A [0] (x5)
Parsvakonasana [49], Vira Parsvakonasana [52]
Surya Namaskar B [00] (x3)

Strength Recruiting: (15 min)
Virabhadrasana I [34], Virabhadrasana III [46], Urdhva Prasarita Ekapadasana [86], Adho Mukha Vrksasana [146]
Baddha Parsvakonasana [55], Baddha Trikonasana [66], Baddha Eka Pada Uttanasana [68], Svarga Dvijasana [75], Baddha Ardha Chandrasana [73], Urdhva Prasarita Ekapadasana [86], Adho Mukha Vrksasana [146]
Parivrtta Baddha Parsvakonasana [58], Parivrtta Baddha Trikonasana [67], Parivrtta Baddha Eka Pada Uttanasana [69], Parivrtta Svarga Dvijasana [76], Parivrtta Baddha Ardha Chandrasana [74], Urdhva Prasarita Ekapadasana [86], Adho Mukha Vrksasana [146]
Tittibhasana II-IV [96-98], Tittibhasana I [212], Bakasana [185], Adho Mukha Vrksasana [146]
Balasana [388], Nirakunjasana II [259]

Challenging: (15 min)
Adho Mukha Vrksasana [146], Vrischikasana II [162], Ghanda Bherundasana [316]
Adho Mukha Vrksasana [146], Eka Pada Koundinyasana II [199]
Adho Mukha Vrksasana, Pincha Mayurasana [133]
Padma Pincha Mayurasana [135], Karandavasana [136]
Sirsasana II [118], Urdhva Kukkutasana [226], Sirsasana II [118], Parsva Kukkutasana [227]

Opening: (15 min)
Eka Pada Rajakapotasana I [285]
Eka Pada Rajakapotasana II [287]
Ushtrasana [275], Eka Pada Bheka Ushtrasana [276], Supta Virasana [468], Kapotasana [279]
Krounchasana II [422], Parivrtta Krounchasana [423], Surya Yantrasana II [420], Eka Pada Sirsasana II [456], Chakorasana [236] or Ashtavakrasana [184]
Upavishta Konasana [381], Parivrtta Upavishta Konasana [382], Uttana Konasana [204]
Raja Kapotasana [282]
Eka Pada Sirsasana I [455], Skandasana [457], Chakorasana [236], Kala Bhairavasana [237], Ruchikasana [112], Durvasana [113], Yoga Dandasana II [239]
Dwi Bhuja Virasana I [332], Purvottanasana [294]

Deepening: (15 min)
Navasana & Ardha Navasana [346, 347] (xTone)
Urdhva Dhanurasana (x2) [300]
Drop-backs (xTone) [322]
Viparita Chakrasana (xTone) [323]
Hanumanasana I-III [438-440]

Restorative: (10-20 min)
Bharadvajasana II & III [372, 373], Padmasana [446], Simhasana [317], Goraknathasana [448]
Yoga Mudrasana I & II [450, 451], Urdhva Kukkutasana [226], Padma Adho Mukha Vrksasana [157]
Parivrtta Padmasana [447], Padmasana [446] (meditation 5-7 minutes)
Jathara Parivartanasa I [491]
Shavasana [494]

CHANTS AND INVOCATIONS

Nataraja mantra:
Nataraja, Nataraja, Nartana Sundara Nataraja
Shiva Raja, Shiva Raja, Shiva Kami Priya Shiva Raja
Chidumbadeshwara Nataraja
Pati Purishwara Nataraja

Lord of the Dance, Soverign of the Dance, Beautiful Dancer
Beloved One, who is Shiva's desire
Auspicious lord, the Lord clothed in consciousness
Sovereign of the Dance, Earthen ruler, Lord of the Universe

Purna mantra:
Om Purnamadah Purnamidam
Purnat Purnamudachyate
Purnasya Purnamadaya
Purnamevavashishyate
Om Shanti, Shanti, Shantihi*

*chanted at the end after 3 repetitions
This is perfect; the perfect evolves out of the perfect. If a part is taken out of the whole then again the original remains complete & perfect. Om, peace, peace, eternal peace.

Gayatri mantra:
Om Bhur Bhuvah Svaha
Tat Savitur Varenyam
Bhargo Devasya Dheemahi
Dhiyo Yo Nah Prachodayat

Let us honor the supremacy of the divine light, the god-head who illumines all, who recreates all, to whom all return, whom we invoke to guide us with divine grace to the highest sacred place.

Saravan mantra:
Om Saravanabhava

I offer salutations to Lord Saravan for protection and prosperity.

Skanda Gayatri mantra:
Om Tha Purushaya Vidhmahe
Maha Senaya Dheemahe
Thanno Skandah Prachodayath

Om, Let me meditate on the great male,
Oh, commander in chief, give me higher intellect,
And let the six faced one illuminate my mind.

Closing Prayer
Lokah Samastah
Sukhino Bhavantu
Om, shanti, shanti, shantihi*

*chanted at the end after 3 repetitions
May All Beings Everywhere Be Happy and Free
Om, peace, peace, eternal peace

Asana Index

Standing Poses

1. Tadasana with anjali mudra (mountain pose with prayer seal)
2. Urdhva Hastasana (upward hand pose)
3. Uttanasana (intense pose)
4. Ardha Uttanasana (extended intense pose)
5. Parivrtta Uttanasana (revolved intense pose)
6. Hasta Padangusthasana (hand to big toe pose)
7. Padahastasana (feet on hands pose)
8. Karmasana (action pose)
9. Parivrtta Karmasana (revolved action pose)
10. Utkatasana (fierce pose)
11. Ardha Utkatasana (half fierce pose)
12. Parivrtta Utkatasana I (revolved fierce pose)
13. Parivrtta Utkatasana II (revolved fierce pose II)
14. Vanarasana I (monkey tail pose I, "monkey lunge" or "lunge position")
15. Vanarasana II (monkey tail pose II)
16. Vanarasana III (monkey tail pose III)
17. Somachandrasana I (elixir of the moon pose I)
18. Somachandrasana II (elixir of the moon pose II)
19. Somachandrasana III (elixir of the moon pose III)
20. Somachandrasana IV (elixir of the moon pose IV)
21. Somachandrasana V (elixir of the moon pose V)
22. Subramanyasana (Subramanya's pose)
23. Anjaneyasana (Anjaney's pose, "monkey lunge")
24. Adho Mukha Anjaneyasana (downward facing Anjaney's pose)
25. Vrksasana (tree pose)
26. Parsva Vrksasana (side tree pose)
27. Vakra Vrksasana (bent tree pose)
28. Adho Mukha Svanasana (downward facing dog pose)
29. Parivrtta Eka Hasta Adho Mukha Svanasana (revolved one hand down dog pose)
30. Parivrtta Eka Hasta Eka Pada Adho Mukha Svanasana (revolved one hand one foot down dog)
31. Parivrtta Eka Pada Adho Mukha Svanasana (revolved one foot down dog)
32. Eka Pada Dhanur Adho Mukha Svanasana (one foot bow down dog pose, "Mad Dog")
33. Vira Adho Mukha Svanasana (powerful downward facing dog, "Turbo Dog")
34. Virabhadrasana I (warrior I pose)
35. Virabhadrasana I (warrior I pose variation, one hand behind head)
36. Virabhadrasana I (warrior I pose variation, two hands behind head)
37. Virabhadrasana I (warrior I pose variation, wrists crossed)
38. Uttana Virabhadrasana I (intense warrior I pose)
39. Garuda Virabhadrasana (Eagle warrior pose)
40. Atmanjali Virabhadrasana (warrior pose with hands in reverse prayer)

41. Baddha Hasta Virabhadrasana (bound hands warrior pose)

42. Utthita Baddha Hasta Virabhadrasana (extended bound hands warrior pose)

43. Virabhadrasana II (warrior II pose)

44. Parsva Virabhadrasana (side warrior pose)

45. Parsva Virabhadrasana (side warrior pose variations)

46. Virabhadrasana III (warrior III pose)

47. Veerastambhasana (warrior Veerastambha's pose, "humble warrior")

48. Salamba Utthita Parsvakonasana (supported side angle with elbow on thigh & hand on block)

49. Utthita Parsvakonasana (extended side angle)

50. Parsvakonasana (side angle pose variation with one hand behind the head)

51. Ardha Vira Parsvakonasana (half warrior side angle)

52. Vira Parsvakonasana (warrior side angle pose)

53. Ardha Baddha Parsvakonasana (half bound side angle pose)

54. Ardha Baddha Uttana Parsvakonasana (half bound intense side angle pose)

55. Baddha Parsvakonasana (bound side angle pose)

56. Raja Baddha Parsvakonasana (kingly bound side angle pose)

57. Parivrtta Parsvakonasana (revolved side angle pose)

58. Parivrtta Baddha Parsvakonasana (revolved bound side angle pose)

59. Utthita Trikonasana (extended triangle pose)

60. Ardha Vira Trikonasana (half warrior triangle pose)

61. Vira Trikonasana (warrior triangle pose)

62. Utthita Uttana Trikonasana (extended intense triangle pose)

63. Trikonasana (triangle pose variation)

64. Trikonasana (triangle pose variation)

65. Utthita Parivrtta Trikonasana (extended revolved triangle pose)

66. Baddha Trikonasana (bound triangle pose)

67. Parivrtta Baddha Trikonasana (revolved bound triangle pose)

68. Baddha Eka Pada Uttanasana (bound one foot intense pose)

69. Parivrtta Baddha Eka Pada Uttanasana (revolved bound one foot intense pose)

70. Utthita Ardha Chandrasana (extended half moon)

71. Utthita Parivrtta Ardha Chandrasana (extended revolved half moon)

72. Vira Ardha Chandrasana (warrior half moon)

73. Baddha Ardha Chandrasana (bound half moon)

74. Parivrtta Baddha Ardha Chandrasana (revolved bound half moon)

75. Svarga Dvijasana (bird of paradise)

76. Parivrtta Svarga Dvijasana (revolved bird of paradise)

77. Ardha Chandra Chapasana (sugarcane pose)

78. Nindra Eka Pada Dhanurasana (standing one foot bow pose)

79. Ardha Baddha Padma Vrksasana (half bound lotus tree pose)

80. Ardha Baddha Padmottanasana (half bound lotus stretched out pose)

81. Utthita Hasta Padangusthasana I (extended hand to big toe pose I)

82. Utthita Hasta Padangusthasana II (extended hand to big toe pose II)

83. Utthita Hasta Padangusthasana III (extended hand to big toe pose III)

84. Utthita Hasta Padangusthasana IV (extended hand to big toe pose IV)

85. Vira Utthita Hasta Padangusthasana (powerful extended hand to foot, "Skanda squat")
86. Urdhva Prasarita Ekapadasana (upward stretched out one foot pose, "standing splits")
87. Parsvottanasana (intense side stretch pose)
88. Prasarita Padottanasana I (extended wide leg pose I)
89. Prasarita Padottanasana II (extended wide leg pose II)
90. Prasarita Padottanasana III (extended wide leg pose III)
91. Prasarita Padottanasana IV (extended wide leg pose IV)
92. Prasarita Padottanasana V (extended wide leg pose V)
93. Vira Prasarita Padottanasana (warrior extended leg pose, "warrior splits")
94. Parivrtta Prasarita Padottanasana I (revolved extended leg pose I)
95. Parivrtta Prasarita Padottanasana II (revolved extended leg pose II)
96. Tittibhasana II (insect pose II)
97. Tittibhasana III (insect pose III)
98. Tittibhasana IV (insect pose IV)
99. Pashasana (noose pose)
100. Malasana (garland pose)
101. Ardha Malasana I (half garland pose I)
102. Baddha Ardha Malasana (bound half garland pose)
103. Ardha Malasana II (half garland pose II)
104. Garudasana I (eagle pose)
105. Garudasana II (eagle pose II)
106. Urdhva Kaliasana (upward facing goddess pose)
107. Shankarasana (sage Shankara's pose, "conqueror of the four corners")
108. Nindra Hindolasana
109. Nindra Vayu Muktyasana (standing wind releasing pose)
110. Nindra Vayu Mukttonasana (standing wind releasing face to knee pose)
111. Nindra Ardha Bhekasana (standing half frog pose)
112. Ruchikasana (sage Ruschika's pose)
113. Durvasana (sage Durvasa's pose)
114. Nindra Baddha Yoga Dandasana (standing bound yogi's staff pose)
115. Natarajasana (lord of the dance pose)
116. Baddha Natarajasana (bound lord of the dance pose)

Inversions

117. Sirsasana I (headstand I)
118. Sirsasana II or Utripada Sirsasana (headstand II or tri-pod headstand)
119. Sirsasana III (headstand III)
120. Salamba Sirsasana I (supported headstand I)
121. Salamba Sirsasana II (supported headstand II)
122. Baddha Sirsasana (bound headstand)
123. Bhujamadya Sirsasana (elbow supported headstand)
124. Garuda Sirsasana (eagle headstand)

167. Urdhva Padma Sarvangasana (upward lotus shoulder stand pose)
168. Pindasana (womb pose)
169. Eka Hasta Parsva Sarvangasana (one hand side shoulder stand pose)
170. Eka Hasta Parsva Padma Sarvangasana (one hand side lotus shoulder stand pose)
171. Halasana (plow pose)
172. Supta Urdhva Pada Vajrasana (supine upward foot diamond pose)
173. Karnapidasana (ear pressure pose)
174. Parsva Karnapidasana (side ear pressure pose)
175. Shramanasana (Ascetic's Pose, "wizard's pose")
176. Baddha Shramanasana (bound ascetic's pose)
177. Viparita Karnapidasana (inverted ear pressure pose)
178. Eka Pada Viparita Karnapidasana (one foot inverted ear pressure pose)
179. Viparita Karnapida Utthita Hasta Padangusthasana (inverted ear pressure extended hand to foot pose)
180. Viparita Karnapida Natarajasana (inverted ear pressure lord of the dance pose)
181. Viparita Karnapida Urdhva Padmasana (inverted ear pressure lotus pose)

Arm Balances

182. Eka Hasta Bhujasana (one hand and arm pose)
183. Ashtavakrasana (sage Ashtavakra's pose)
184. Ashtavakrasana (sage Ashtavakra's pose with elevated hands)
185. Bakasana (crane pose)
186. Bakasana (crane pose with elevated hands)
187. Musti Bakasana (crane pose with fists)
188. Ardha Bakasana (half crane pose)
189. Eka Pada Bakasana I (one foot crane pose I)
190. Eka Pada Bakasana II (elevated one foot crane pose II)
191. Parsva Bakasana (side crane pose)
192. Musti Parsva Bakasana (side crane pose with fists)
193. Visama Parsva Bakasana I (uneven side crane pose I)
194. Visama Parsva Bakasana II (uneven side crane pose II)
195. Trianga Dandasana (three limbed staff pose)
196. Parashuramasana (eternal warrior pose)
197. Dwi Pada Koundinyasana (two foot sage Koundinya pose)
198. Eka Pada Koundinyasana I (one foot sage Koundinya pose I)
199. Eka Pada Koundinyasana II (one foot sage Koundinya pose II)
200. Eka Pada Koundinyasana (one foot sage Koundinya pose variation, "hummingbird")
201. Urdhva Navasana (upward boat pose)
202. Urdhva Ardha Padma Navasana (upward half lotus boat pose)
203. Brahmacharyasana (celibacy pose)
204. Uttana Konasana (intense angle pose)
205. Lolasana (pendant pose)
206. Galavasana (sage Galava's pose)

207. Musti Galavasana (sage Galava's pose with fists)

208. Eka Pada Galavasana I (one foot sage Galava's pose I)

209. Eka Pada Galavasana II (one foot sage Galava's pose II)

210. Ardha Bhujapidasana (half arm pressure pose)

211. Bhujapidasana (arm pressure pose)

212. Tittibhasana I (insect pose I)

213. Ardha Padma Tittibhasana (half lotus insect pose)

214. Vasisthasana (sage Vasistha's prep pose)

215. Vasisthasana (sage Vasistha's pose)

216. Eka Pada Vasisthasana I (one foot sage Vasistha's pose I)

217. Eka Pada Vasisthasana II (one foot sage Vasistha's pose II)

218. Purna Vasisthasana (full sage Vasistha's pose)

219. Camatkarasana (pose of spiritual delight, "wild thing")

220. Kasyapasana (sage Kasyapa's pose)

221. Kapinjalasana (Chathaka bird prep pose)

222. Kapinjalasana (Chathaka bird pose)

223. Vishvamitrasana (sage Vishvamitra's pose)

224. Tolasana (scale pose)

225. Kukkutasana (rooster pose)

226. Urdhva Kukkutasana (upward rooster pose)

227. Parsva Kukkutasana (side rooster pose)

228. Hamsasana (swan pose)

229. Mayurasana (peacock pose)

230. Viparita Mayurasana (inverted peacock pose)

231. Purna Viparita Mayurasana (full inverted peacock pose)

232. Musti Padma Mayurasana (fist lotus peacock pose)

233. Viparita Musti Padma Mayurasana (inverted fist lotus peacock pose)

234. Eka Hasta Mayurasana (one hand peacock) or Pungu Mayurasana (wounded peacock)

235. Eka Hasta Padma Mayurasana (one hand lotus peacock)

236. Chakorasana (moon bird pose)

237. Kala Bhairavasana (destroyer of time pose)

238. Somanathasana (keeper of soma pose)

239. Yoga Dandasana II (yogi's staff pose II)

240. Dwi Pada Sirsasana II (two feet behind head pose II)

241. Viranchyasana II (sage Viranchi's pose II)

242. Maksikanagasana I (dragonfly I)

243. Maksikanagasana II (dragonfly II)

244. Maksikanagasana III (dragonfly III)

245. Maksikanagasana IV (dragonfly IV)

246. Sri Subramanyasana (auspicious Subramanya's pose)

247. Valgulasana (bat pose)

Backbends

248. Sphinx pose
249. Apanavasana (downward corpse pose)
250. Majarasana (cat pose, "all fours position")
251. Bhujangasana (cobra pose preparation)
252. Bhujangasana (cobra pose)
253. Prasarita Bhujangasana (extended wide cobra pose)
254. Eka Pada Prasarita Bhujangasana (one leg stretched wide cobra pose)
255. Utthita Eka Pada Prasarita Bhujangasana (extended one leg stretched wide cobra pose)
256. Urdhva Mukha Svanasana (upward facing dog)
257. Uttana Shishosana (intense birthing pose, "puppy pose")
258. Nirakunjasana I (heart opening pose I)
259. Nirakunjasana II (heart opening pose II)
260. Araniasana (dragon pose)
261. Ardha Bhekasana (half frog pose)
262. Urdhva Ardha Bhekasana (upward half frog pose)
263. Urdhva Uttana Ardha Bhekasana (upward intense half frog pose)
264. Bhekasana (frog pose)
265. Dhanurasana (bow pose)
266. Baddha Dhanurasana (bound bow pose)
267. Parsva Dhanurasana (side bow pose)
268. Purna Dhanurasana (full bow pose)
269. Eka Pada Dhanurasana (one foot bow pose)
270. Baddha Eka Pada Dhanurasana (bound one foot bow pose)
271. Purna Eka Pada Dhanurasana (full one foot bow pose)
272. Gherandasana (sage Gheranda's prep pose)
273. Gherandasana I (sage Gheranda's pose I)
274. Gherandasana II (sage Gheranda's pose II)
275. Ushtrasana (camel pose)
276. Eka Pada Bheka Ushtrasana (one foot frog frog camel pose)
277. Ardha Padma Ushtrasana (half lotus camel pose)
278. Laghuvajrasana (little thunderbolt pose)
279. Kapotasana (pigeon pose)
280. Eka Pada Kapotasana I (one foot pigeon pose I)
281. Eka Pada Kapotasana II (one foot pigeon pose II)
282. Rajakapotasana (king pigeon pose)
283. Nasginyasana I (mermaid I pose)
284. Nasginyasana II (mermaid II pose)
285. Eka Pada Rajakapotasana I (one leg king pigeon I)
286. Baddha Eka Pada Rajakapotasana I (bound one leg king pigeon I)
287. Eka Pada Rajakapotasana II (one foot king pigeon II prep)
288. Parivrtta Eka Pada Rajakapotasana II (revolved one foot king pigeon II prep, "twisting thigh stretch")
289. Parivrtta Eka Pada Rajakapotasana II (revolved one foot king pigeon II prep variation)

290. Eka Pada Rajakapotasana II (one leg king pigeon II)

291. Eka Pada Rajakapotasana III (one leg king pigeon III)

292. Eka Pada Rajakapotasana IV (one leg king pigeon IV)

293. Eka Pada Rajakapotasana V (one leg king pigeon V)

294. Purvottanasana (east side stretch)

295. Setu Bandha Sarvangasana (half bound shoulder stand pose, "bridge pose")

296. Eka Pada Setu Bandha Sarvangasana (half bound shoulder stand pose)

297. Eka Pada Bheka Sarvangasana (one foot frog shoulder stand pose)

298. Bheka Sarvangasana (frog shoulder stand pose)

299. Urdhva Dhanurasana (upward bow prep pose)

300. Urdhva Dhanurasana (upward bow pose)

301. Dwi Pada Viparita Dandasana I (two foot inverted staff pose I)

302. Dwi Pada Viparita Dandasana II (two foot inverted staff pose II)

303. Setu Bandhasana (bound lock pose)

304. Mandalasana (sacred circle pose)

305. Eka Pada Viparita Chakrasana (one foot inverted wheel pose)

306. Makarasana (crocodile pose)

307. Shalabhasana I (locust pose I)

308. Shalabhasana II (locust pose II)

309. Shalabhasana III (locust pose III)

310. Shalabhasana IV (locust pose IV)

311. Baddha Hasta Shalbhasana (bound hand locust pose)

312. Viparita Shalabhasana (inverted locust pose)

313. Purna Viparita Shalabhasana (full inverted locust pose)

314. Eka Pada Shalabhasana (one foot locust pose)

315. Baddha Eka Pada Shalabhasana (bound one foot locust pose)

316. Ghanda Bherundasana (formidable face pose)

317. Simhasana (lion pose)

318. Parivrtta Simhasana (revolved lion)

319. Matsyasana (fish pose)

320. Padma Matsyasana (lotus fish pose)

321. Uttana Padasana (intense foot pose)

322. "Drop-back"

323. Viparita Chakrasana (inverted wheel)

Shoulders, Wrists, and Core

324. Skanda Chakrasana (Skanda's wheel)

325. Uttana Garuda Bhujasana I, II, III (intense eagle arm pose I, II, III)

326. Eka Bhuja Swastikasana I (one arm auspicious pose I)

327. Eka Bhuja Swastikasana II (one arm auspicious pose II)

328. Supta Vira Eka Bhuja Swastikasana (supine hero one arm auspicious pose)

329. Supta Agnistambha Eka Bhuja Swastikasana (supine fire log one arm auspicious pose)

330. Eka Bhuja Padmasana (one arm lotus pose)

331. Eka Bhuja Virasana (one arm hero prep pose)

332. Dwi Bhuja Virasana I (two arm hero pose I)

333. Dwi Bhuja Virasana II (two arm hero pose II)

334. Dwi Bhuja Virasana III (two arm hero pose III)

335. Supta Eka Bhuja Virasana (supine one arm hero pose)

336. Supta Eka Bhuja Vira Padangusthasana (supine one arm hero hand to big toe pose)

337. Eka Bhuja Anahata Chapasana (one arm heart sugarcane pose, "heartbreaker")

338. Dwi Bhuja Visvajarasana (two arm double diamond pose, "blood diamond")

339. Supta Bhuja Vinyasa (arm transitions, "arm raises with block")

340. Adho Baddha Mustiasana (downward bound fists, "thumb breaker")

341. Parivrtta Eka Hastasana I (revolved one hand pose)

342. Parivrtta Eka Hastasana II (revolved one hand pose II)

343. Parivrtta Baddha Hastasana (revolved bound hand pose)

344. Ardha Chaturanga Dandasana (half four limb staff pose)

345. Vayu Vinyasa (wind flow)

346. Navasana (boat pose)

347. Ardha Navasana (half boat pose)

348. Parsva Navasana (side boat pose)

349. Supta Garudasana (supine eagle pose, "eagle crunches")

350. Urdhva Eka Padasana (upward one foot pose)

351. Urdhva Dwi Padasana (upward two foot pose)

352. Supta Krishnasana (supine Krishna pose, "Krishna crunches")

353. Pincha Araniasana (dragon tail pose, "dragon flags")

354. Supta Vayu Vinyasa (supine wind transition, "windshield wipers")

355. Supta Kaliasana (supine Kali pose, "Kali crunches")

Hip Openers, Twists, and Forward Bends

356. Dandasana (staff pose)

357. Paschimottanasana I (west side stretch I, "forward bend")

358. Paschimottanasana II (west side stretch II)

359. Paschimottanasana III (west side stretch III)

360. Paschimottanasana IV (west side stretch IV)

361. Parivrtta Paschimottanasana (revolved forward bend)

362. Uttana Paschimottanasana (intense forward bend)

363. Ardha Baddha Padma Paschimottanasana (half bound lotus west side stretch)

364. Trianga Mukhaikapada Pashimottanasana (three limbs face to one leg west side stretch)

365. Eka Pada Gomukha Paschimottanasana (one foot cow west side stretch)

366. Janu Sirsasana I (head to knee pose I)

367. Janu Sirsasana II (head to knee pose II)

368. Janu Sirsasana III (head to knee pose III)

369. Parivrtta Janu Sirsasana I (revolved head to knee pose I)

370. Parivrtta Janu Sirsasana II (revolved head to knee pose II)

371. Bharadvajasana I (sage Bhardva's pose I)

372. Bharadvajasana II (sage Bhardva's pose II)
373. Bharadvajasana III (sage Bhardva's pose III)
374. Ardha Matsyendrasana (lord of the fish pose prep)
375. Ardha Matsyendrasana I (lord of the fish pose I)
376. Baddha Ardha Matsyendrasana (bound lord of the fish pose)
377. Baddha Uttana Ardha Matsyendrasana (bound intense lord of the fish pose)
378. Ardha Matsyendrasana II (lord of the fish pose II)
379. Ardha Matsyendrasana III (lord of the fish pose III)
380. Bhunamananasana (saluting mother earth pose)
381. Upavishta Konasana (seated wide angle pose)
382. Parivrtta Upavishta Konasana (revolved seated wide angle pose)
383. Samakonasana (even angle pose)
384. Rajasamakonasana (royal even angle pose)
385. Eka Hasta Raja Samakonasana (one hand royal even angle pose)
386. Kurmasana (tortoise pose)
387. Supta Kurmasana (sleeping tortoise pose)
388. Balasana (child's pose)
389. Salamba Balasana (supported child's pose)
390. Virasana (hero's pose)
391. Vajrasana (diamond pose)
392. Sukhasana (sweet pose)
393. Siddhasana (spiritual power pose)
394. Siddhasana II (spiritual power pose II)
395. Gomukhasana (cow face prep pose)
396. Gomukhasana I (cow face pose I)
397. Gomukhasana II (cow face pose II)
398. Garuda Gomukhasana (eagle cow face pose)
399. Swastikasana (auspicious pose)
400. Eka Pada Rajakapotasana (one leg king pigeon prep pose)
401. Parivrtta Eka Pada Kapotasana (revolved one leg pigeon pose)
402. Eka Bhuja Padma Eka Pada Kapotasana (one arm lotus one leg pigeon pose)
403. Vamadevasana I (sage Vamadeva's pose I)
404. Vamadevasana II (sage Vamadeva's pose II)
405. Agnistambhasana I (fire log pose I)
406. Agnistambhasana II (fire log pose II)
407. Agnistambhasana III (fire log pose III)
408. Parivrtta Agnistambhasana I (revolved fire log I pose)
409. Parivrtta Agnistambhasana II (revolved fire log II pose)
410. Baddha Konasana I (bound angle pose I)
411. Baddha Konasana II (bound angle pose II)
412. Baddha Konasana III (bound angle pose III)
413. Ardha Mulabandhasana (half root lock pose)
414. Mulabandhasana I (root lock pose I)

415. Mulabandhasana II (root lock pose II)

416. Tarasana (star pose)

417. Parivrtta Tarasana (revolved star pose, "star gazer")

418. Parivrtta Baddha Tarasana (revolved bound star pose)

419. Surya Yantrasana I (sun dial pose I)

420. Surya Yantrasana II (sun dial pose II)

421. Krounchasana I (heron pose I)

422. Krounchasana II (heron pose II)

423. Parivrtta Krounchasana (revolved heron pose)

424. Marichiasana I (sage Marichi's pose I)

425. Marichiasana II (sage Marichi's pose II)

426. Marichiasana III (sage Marichi's pose III)

427. Marichiasana IV (sage Marichi's pose IV)

428. Marichiasana V (sage Marichi's pose V)

429. Marichiasana VI (sage Marichi's pose VI)

430. Marichiasana VII (sage Marichi's pose VII)

431. Marichiasana VIII (sage Marichi's pose VIII)

432. Marichiasana IX (sage Marichi's pose IX)

433. Marichiasana X (sage Marichi's pose X)

434. Thavaliasana (monkey frog pose)

435. Urdhva Mukha Thavaliasana (upward facing monkey frog pose)

436. Hanumanasana (Hanuman prep pose)

437. Parivrtta Hanumanasana (revolved Hanuman prep pose)

438. Hanumanasana I (Hanuman's pose I)

439. Hanumanasana II (Hanuman's pose II)

440. Hanumanasana III (Hanuman's pose III)

441. Hindolasana (baby cradle)

442. Salamba Hindolasana (supported baby cradle)

443. Yoga Dandasana (yogi's staff pose prep)

444. Yoga Dandasana (yogi's staff pose)

445. Baddha Yoga Dandasana (bound yogi's staff pose)

446. Padmasana (lotus pose)

447. Parivrtta Padmasana (revolved lotus pose)

448. Goraknathasana (sage Goraknath's pose)

449. Garbha Pindasana (baby in the womb pose)

450. Yoga Mudrasana I (yoga seal pose)

451. Yoga Mudrasana II (yoga seal pose II)

452. Akarna Dhanurasana I (archer's pose I)

453. Akarna Dhanurasana II (archer's pose II)

454. Arjunasana (Arjuna's pose)

455. Eka Pada Sirsasana I (one leg over the head pose I)

456. Eka Pada Sirsasana II (one leg over the head pose II)

457. Skandasana (warrior Skanda's pose)

458. Viranchyasana I (sage Viranchya's pose I)

459. Dwi Pada Sirsasana I (two feet behind head pose I)

Supine Poses

460. Supta Bhairavasana I (reclined formidable pose I)

461. Supta Bhairavasana II (reclined formidable pose II)

462. Supta Valgulasana (sleeping bat pose)

463. Yoganidrasana (sleeping yogi's pose)

464. Eka Pada Sirsa Shayanasana (one leg over head resting pose)

465. Supta Konasana (reclined angle pose)

466. Supta Baddha Konasana (supine bound angle pose)

467. Supta Virasana (supine hero's prep pose)

468. Supta Virasana (supine hero's pose)

469. Supta Uttana Virasana (supine intense hero pose)

470. Supta Baddha Virasana (supine bound hero pose)

471. Eka Pada Supta Virasana I (one foot supine hero pose I)

472. Eka Pada Supta Virasana II (one foot supine hero pose II)

473. Eka Pada Supta Virasana III (one foot supine hero pose III)

474. Supta Padangusthasana I (supine single leg stretch prep pose I)

475. Supta Padangusthasana I (supine single leg stretch pose I)

476. Supta Padangusthasana II (supine single leg stretch II)

477. Supta Padangusthasana III (supine single leg stretch III)

478. Supta Urdhva Eka Pada Vajrasana (supine one foot upward diamond pose)

479. Anantasana (infinity pose)

480. Supta Parvritta Garudasana (twisting reclined eagle pose)

481. Supta Swastikasana (supine auspicious pose)

482. Supta Swastikasana II (supine auspicious pose II)

483. Supta Ganeshasana (supine Ganesha's pose)

484. Supta Hindolasana I (supine baby cradle I)

485. Supta Hindolasana II (supine baby cradle II)

486. Sucinrandrasana (eye of the needle pose)

487. Supta Balasana (supine child's pose)

488. Eka Pada Sukha Balasana (one foot happy baby pose)

489. Sukha Balasana (happy baby pose)

490. Supta Visvajrasana (double diamond)

491. Jathara Parivartanasana (firmly rooted pose I, simple supine twist)

492. Jathara Parivartanasana II (firmly rooted pose II, simple supine twist)

493. Jathara Parivartanasana III (firmly rooted pose III, simple supine twist)

494. Shavasana (corpse pose)

GLOSSARY OF TERMS

Sanskrit

A – symbol for Shiva

Abhinivesha – fear of death, cleaning to life

Abhyasa – spiritual practice

Acarya – spiritual master

Adharma – the way of the unjust

Adhikari – dedicated student

Adi-Ananta-Sesha – infinite headed serpent that serves as Vishnu's couch

Adho – downward

Advaita – non-dual, meaning that the Absolute is not separate from the individual souls

Agamas – scriptures of divine origin

Agni – demigod of fire

Aham – "I" principle

Ahamkara – ego or sense of separate self

Ahimsa – non-violence

Aishwarya – divine power

Ajna – third eye chakra

Akarna – up to the ear or from the ear

Akasa – ether

Alamba – supported

Amrit – divine nectar

Anahata – unstruck; heart chakra

Ananda – bliss

Ananta – unlimited

Anga – limb

Anjaney – son of Anjana

Anu – atom

Anusvara – finite space that contains the infinite; 2) the pause between breath

Ananda – bliss

Anjali – prayer

Antara – inhalation

Anugraha – grace

Anuttara – supreme

Apana – downward flowing energy

Apara – other, lesser than

Aparigraha – non-greed, non-coveting

Apauruseya – not the work of man

Arani – dragon

Ardha – half

Arjuna – one of the five Pandava brothers of the Bhagavad Gita

Asana – posture for meditation, exercise, or therapy

Asat – that which is temporary

Ashta – eight

Ashtanga – eight limb

Ashtanga yoga – classical eight-limb yoga of Patanjali; Raja Yoga

Ashtavakra – sage of Hindu scriptures born with eight deformities

Asmita – ego

Asteya – non-stealing

Asura – demon

Atman – individual soul, the true self; sense of I Am

AUM – cosmic sound of Creation; abbreviated as Om

Avatara – incarnation of the Lord who has descended from the spiritual world

Avidya – ignorance

Ayurveda – the science of life; the traditional holistic medicine India

Baddha – bound

Bala – 1) strength; 2) child

Baka – bird, crane

Bandha – lock

Bhakti (apara) – devotional love

Bhakti (para) – the constant feeling of being united

Bhastrika – bellows breath

Bhava – attitude; feeling, sensation; trans migratory existence

Bhairava (apara) – Unity – consciousness of Siddhas

Bhairava (para) – the Highest Reality of Shiva; *bha* indicates maintenance of the world, *ra* withdrawal of the world, *va* projection of the world

Bheda –separating, chasm, dualism

Bheka – frog

Bherunda – formidable, terrible

Bhija mantra – single syllable mantras like Om

Bhoga – enjoyment of sensual pleasure

Bhoodevi – the wife of the five Pandava brothers who was the reincarnation of Sita

Bhuja – arm

Bhujanga – cobra

Bhujamadya – elbow

Bhumika – Role

Bhuvana – Becoming

Bija – seed

Bindu – point; a gathering of potential energy

Brahma – the Creator

Brahma nadi – sushumna, central energy channel

Brahman – 1) spiritual energy; 2) all-pervading impersonal aspect of the Lord; 3) a caste of ascetic priests

Brahmacarya – celibacy, or sexual morality

Buddha – 9th incarnation of Lord Vishnu
Buddhi – enlightened mind, intuitive aspect of awareness

Camatkara – miracle, spectacle, astonishment
Cator – four
Chakora – moon bird pose
Chapa – arc, bow
Chaturanga – four limb
Cit – Absolute; foundational consciousness
Citta – Universal Consciousness manifested in the individual
Citi – power of the Absolute to initiate the world process
Chakra – wheel, energy center
Chakora – celestial moon bird
Chandra – moon deity
Chin – psychic

Danda – staff
Dasa – ten
Deva – demigods
Devayani – first wife of Skanda, daughter of Indra, represents kriya shakti
Devi – goddess
Dhanur – bow
Dharana – concentration
Dharma – duty
Dhrishti – gazing point
Dhyana – meditation
Dosha – biological energies of the body
Dukha – suffering
Durga – the form of Parvati, Shiva's wife, as a warrior goddess
Dvesha – repulsion
Dvi – two
Dvija – twice-born

Eka – one
Ekagrata – one-pointed

Galava – sage from Hindu scriptures that lived during the time of Manu
Gandha – whole side of the face, cheek
Ganesha – a son of Shiva, the remover of obstacles
Ganga – a name for the Ganges river, and the mother energy
Ganges – the sacred river of India
Garbha – womb
Garuda – celestial eagle and vehicle of Vishnu

Gheranda – author of the Gheranda Samhita

Gomukha – cow face

Gopi – cow herder

Goraknath – father of hatha yoga, the founder of the Nath sect

Govinda – a name of Krishna, as one who gives pleasure to the senses

Granthi – psychic knot or entanglement

Guna – qualities of nature (tamas guna, rajas guna, sattva guna)

Guru – spiritual teacher, the remover of darkness

Gustha – big toe

Ha – sun

Hakini – ruler of the third eye

Hala – plow

Hamsa – swan, goose

Hare – the pleasurable potency of the Lord

Hari – Vishnu

Hamsa – the jiva, the soul

Hanuman – lord of the monkeys, son of Anjana and Vayu

Hasta – hand

Hatha – solar (*Ha*)/lunar (*tha*); a force of discipline

Hatha yoga – physical practice of yoga postures; employs physical means to unite the masculine and feminine energies; union with the supreme via discipline

Hari – a name of Krishna

Haribol – a word meaning to chant the name of Krishna

Hindola – cradle, swing

Hridaya – heart

Iccha – will, intention

Ida – lunar energy channel

Indra – the King of Heaven

Indriyam – sense organ

Isvara – God or Creator

Isvara pranidhanam – dedication, self-surrender; worship of God

Ishvari – Divine Mother

Jalandhara – 1) chin lock; 2) flowing like water; 3) a character of Indian mythology that was formed by merging Shiva's third eye with the ocean

Japa – repetition of *mantra*

Jaya – victory, mastery

Jiva – individual soul, the empirical self

Jivanmukta – liberated individual

Jivanmukti – experience of liberation

Jnana – knowledge

Jnana Yoga – Sakta upaya

Kāla – time

Kalā – 1) shakti of consciousness, 2) part, participle, aspect

Kali – demigoddess in wrathful form

Kali yuga – the 4th and final age in the yuga system

Kalpa – a day in the life of Lord Brahma; a cycle of precession

Kama – sensual pleasure

Kamadeva – god of love

Kancuka – coverings of Maya: 1) Kalā; 2) (asuddha) Vidya; 3) Raga; 4) Niyati; 5) Kāla

Kanda – the origin of all nadis and the source from which all *vayus* emanante

Kapa – skull

Kapala – skull

Kapalabhati – skull shining

Kapha – biological energy of earth in the body

Kapila – teacher of Sankhya yoga philosophy

Kapinjala – chataka bird, coming from the francoline partridge

Kapota – pigeon

Karana – cause

Karanda – duck

Karma – effect of past actions

Karna – ear

Karuna – compassion, another name for Lakshmi

Karya – effect; objectivity

Kartikas – 6 river nymphs representing the Pleiades constellation

Keerti – recognition, popularity

Khecharī – to move the mind, or to dwell in the expanse of consciousness

Khecharī Mudrā – tip of the tongue is placed on the soft palate

Klesha – obstruction or obstacle

Kona – angle

Kosha – a sheath, the coverings of atman

Koundinya – sage created by Parvati for the purpose of making intoxicating drinks

Kriya – cleansing technique

Krishna – the 8th avatar of Vishnu who is Arjuna's charioteer in the Bhagavad Gita

Krouncha – heron

Kukkuta – rooster

Kumbhaka – retention of breath

Kundalini – creative power of Shiva, a distinct energy that lies at the base of the root chakra

Kuruksetra – battlefield of the Pandavas and the Kauravas, where Krishna spoke the Bhagavad Gita.

Kurma – 1) life force energy which governs movement of the eyelids; 2) tortoise

Laghu – little

Laya – internalization of consciousness; dissolution

Lila – divine play, sport of God, cosmic dream of Vishnu

Linga – phallic symbol of Shiva

Lola – pendant
Loka – plane of existence
Loma – hair

Madhya – the central I – consciousness; the *susumna*, central energy channel
Madhyama – middle
Maha – great
Mahabharata – the great epic of the Pandavas written by the sage Vyasa
Mahadeva – great god
Mahaprana – great life force energy
Makula – a bud
Mala – necklace, rosary, garland
Man – mind
Mana – imaginary, idea, thought, consideration
Manas – the aspect of the mind that builds impressions from senses
Manipura – solar plexus chakra
Mantra – sacred word or formula that is chanted
Manu – lawgiver of mankind; demigod of Brahma
Marici – son of Brahma and grandfather of Surya
Masikanaga – dragonfly
Matrika – Shakti, or energetic power behind spoken words
Matsyendranath – the sage who taught yoga to Goraknath
Maya tattva – the principle that covers consciousness with a veil
Maya – illusion
Mayur – peacock
Mitra – a solar deity who was later adopted by the Zorastrian religion as Mithra Moha – Delusion
Moksha – Liberation
Mula - root
Mudra – energy seal; *mud* (joy) *rā* (to give)
Mukha – face
Mukti – liberation from bondage
Mula – root
Muladhara – root chakra
Murugan – another name for Skanda meaning the divine child

Naga – life force energy that governs belching; 2) serpent
Nandi – the Bull, Shiva's vehicle
Nasginya – mermaid
Nataraja – lord of the dance
Nauli – turning of the abdominal muscles
Nava – 1) nine; 2) boat
Nirakunja – heart opening
Nindra – standing

Niralamba – unsupported

Nirodha – cessation, restraint

Nirvana – Heaven, bliss

Nivrtti – the path of renunciation to elevate being

Niyamas – yogic disciplines, self-observances

Ojas – vital fluids

Pada – foot, chapter, portion

Padma – lotus

Pancha – five

Para – the Highest, the Absolute

Parama Siva – the Highest Reality

Parapara – unity in diversity

Parinama – transformation

Parivrtta – revolved

Parsva – side

Parvati – wife of Shiva, mother of Skanda

Paschima – western

Pasha – noose

Patanjali – author of the Yoga Sutras

Pida – pressure

Pincha – tail

Pinda – solid, compact, dense, ball

Pingala – solar energy channel

Pitta – biological fire energy in the body

Prakriti – matter

Pralaya – dissolution or manifestation

Prana – 1) generic name for vital energy; universal energy; 2) upward rising energy

Prama – exact knowledge

Pranava – same as omkara

Pranayama – 1) liberation of the breath; 2) specific techniques to awaken energies with breath

Prasara – expansion; universe manifested from Shiva through Shakti

Prasarita – stretched out, spread, extended

Pratha – to expand; unfold; shine; the mode of appearance

Pratyahara – turning the senses within

Pratyabhijña – recognition

Pravrtti – the path of engaging the material world to elevate being

Prema – love for Krishna

Prithivi – the earth *tattva*

Puja – ritual worship

Pundarikam – jaguar

Pungu – wounded, injured

Puranas – Hindu texts of divine stories about the epics of the gods

Purna – fullness, completion

Purva – eastern

Purusha – consciousness

Raga – limitation of desire, passion

Raja – King

Raja Yoga – the eightfold path of yoga

Rajas – the principle of motion and activity

Rasa – an enjoyable taste or feeling

Rechaka – retention, exhalation

Risi – seer

Rudra – an aspect of Shiva, residing in the lowest place of Nivrtti kalā

Sadhana – a specific practice or discipline for attaining realization

Sadhu – a holy man

Sahasrara – crown chakra

Salamba – supported

Samkhya – classical philosophy; analytical understanding of material nature

Samsara – the wheel of existence

Samskara – energetic conditioning

Samadhi – bliss through meditation; mental absorption in Love

Samana – life force energy governing the region of the abdomen

Samasthiti – even awareness and attention

Sankalpa – resolution, intention

Sankoca – contraction, limitation

Sanyasi – one who has renounced the world

Shakti – 1) goddess, auspicious energy; 2) the power of Shiva to manifest

Sara – quintessential

Sarvanga – shoulder

Sat – existence or truth

Satchitananda – reality exists as consciousness and bliss

Satha – seven

Sattva – 1) the principle of being; 2) balanced existence; 3) light and harmony

Satya – truthfulness

Satya yuga – first of the four world ages

Saraswati – daughter of Brahma; goddess of knowledge and the arts

Seetkari – hissing

Setu – bridge

Shaivaites – worshippers of Shiva

Shakti – 1) spiritual energy, power, or potency; 2) active principle of creation; 3) first consort of Shiva

Shaktipat – transmission of divine energy from guru to disciple

Shalabha – locust

Shambhavi – 1) eyebrow center; 2) possibility

Shankara – 1) name for Shiva; 2) 9th century C.E. Hindu philosopher

Shastra – authentic revealed scripture

Shata – six

Sheetali – cooling

Shisho – intense birthing

Shiva – the third aspect of the Hindu trinity; the Destroyer; the Benevolent One

Shramana – was a non-Vedic Indian religious movement parallel but separate from the historical Vedic religion

Shruti – Vedic knowledge received from direct transmission, "that which was heard."

Shukra – 1) brother of Lakshmi, the leader of the *asuras;* 2) the planet Venus

Shunya – void; emptiness

Shayana – resting

Siddha – power

Simha – lion

Simhamukha – demon defeated by Skanda who was transformed into a lion

Sirsa – head

Skanda – son of Shiva, protector of the celestial realm

Skandati – one who is in the flow of Skanda's energy

Skanda Yoga – alignment based power yoga to unite with the supreme

Soma – Divine elixir, entheogen

Somanath – keeper of soma

Smriti – Vedic knowledge, "that is remembered"

Spanda – the ecstatic throb of existence that leads to manifestation and maintenance of creation

Stambha – pillar

Sri – beauty, grace, auspiciousness

Sri Yantra – geometric symbol of the goddess Lakshmi

Subramanya – a name for Skanda that implies he has knowledge of Brahman

Sucinrandrasana – eye of the needle

Sukha – ease; sweetness

Surapadma – asura defeated by Skanda and transformed into the peacock

Susiravat – open space, hollowed out

Susupti – dreamless sleep

Svadhya – self-study

Svami – one who can control his mind and senses

Svana – dog

Svapna – dream, dreaming conditioning

Svarga – any of of the seven planes in Hindu cosmology

Svarupa – essential nature

Shava – corpse

Svatatrya – absolute freedom

Swadhistana – sacral chakra

Tadasana – mountain pose

Tara – star

Tantra – technique, to weave or loom

Tamas – principle of inertia, heaviness, darkness, delusion

Tapas – inner heat

Taraka – demon defeated by Skanda who was transformed into an elephant

Tattva – thatness; principle of reality

Tejas – fire on a vital level

Tittibha – insect

Tola – scale

Tra – to free, or deliver

Tratak – candle gazing

Treta yuga – second of the four world ages

Trianga – three limb

Trimurti – the Hindu trinity

Turiya – the fourth state of consciousness; transcendental self that links consciousness, subconscious, and unconscious

Trika – the system of philosophy of the triad – Nara, Sákti and Śhiva; Icchā, Jnana, Kriya

Udaya – rise, appearance, creation

Uddiyana – flying up; abdominal lock

Udyama – the sudden appearance of Supreme I-consciousness

Udana – life force energy governing the region of the head

Ujjayi – victorious breath, yogic breath

Upanishads – a collection of stories from the Vedas that deal with the Absolute

Urdhva – upward

Ushtra – camel

Uttana – intense

Utthita – extended

Vaha – 1) flow, channel; 2) the collective Prana in the *sushumna*

Vairagya – detachment, dispassion, renunciation

Vaishnava – worshipper of Lord Vishnu

Vajra – 1) diamond, hard; 2) weapon of Indra

Vakra – bent

Valgula – species of night bird, bat

Valli – second wife of Skanda; represents iccha shakti

Vamadeva – a Rishi mentioned in the Rigveda and the Upanishads

Vana – forest of reeds, marsh land

Vanara – monkey tail

Varna – 1) letter; 2) object of concentration

Varuna – god of water

Vasistha – sage from the Mahabharata that trained wish fulfilling cows

Vata – biological energy of air in the body

Vatayana – horse

Vayu – wind

Vedas – sacred scriptures revealed to the seers of the forest

Vedanta – philosophical school based upon the Vedas

Veerastambha – humble warrior

Vedha – knowledge, sacred lore, perception

Vi – against

Vibhuti – sacred ash or spiritual power

Vidya – limited knowledge

Vigraha – individual form or shape of body

Vigrahi – the embodied one

Viloma – against the flow

Vikalpa – differentiation of perception; imagination; thought construct

Vikasa – unfoldment; development; expansion

Vimarsa – self-consciousness

Vinyasa – 1) to place in a special way; 2) to flow, to transition

Viparita – inverted

Virabhadra – warrior created from the wrath of Shiva

Viranchi – a name of Brahma

Vishvamitra – 1) friend of the Universe; 2) a great sage who was a student of Vasistha

Visama – uneven

Vishnu – sustainer of the cosmos

Vishuddi – throat chakra

Visva – The Universe

Virya – hero

Vriscika – scorpion

Vrksa – tree

Yantra – geometric symbol

Yamas – self-restraints, moral discipline

Yantra – geometric symbol used for meditation

Yoga – 1) union; 2) to unite, to join, to merge; 3) communion; 4) cessation of thoughts; 5) skill in action

Yoganga – a branch of yoga

Yogin – a male practitioner of yoga

Yogini – a female practitioner of yoga

Yoni – womb, source

Yantra – a mystical diagram or pattern used in rituals and meditation

BIBLIOGRAPHY

Alter, Michael J. **Science of Flexibility.** United States: Human Kinetics, 1988.

Andiappan, Yogananth. **Yoga From the Heart.** Hong Kong: International Yoga Academy Ltd., 2007.

Arguelles, Jose. **The Mayan Factor: Path Beyond Technology.** Santa Fe: Bear & Company, 1987.

Arguelles, Jose. **Time and the Technosphere.** Rochester: Bear & Company, 2002.

Bowditch, Bruce. **The Yoga Practice Guide 2.** Tucson: Third Eye Press, 2012.

Brennan, Barbara Ann. **Hands of Light.** New York: Bantam Book, 1987.

Chalton, Hilda. **Skanda.** New York: Golden Quest. 1989.

DeRose, Maestro. **Yoga Avanzado.** Argentina: Deva's, 2004.

Iyengar, B.K.S. **Light on Yoga.** New York: Schocken Books, 1979.

Iyengar, B.K.S. **Light on Yoga Sutras.** San Francisco: The Aquarian Press, 1993.

Iyengar, B.K.S. **Light on Pranayama.** New York: Crossroad Publishing Company, 2008.

Hirsch, Gertrude. **Mudras: Yoga in Your Hands.** York Beach, Maine: Weiser Books, 2000.

Jenkins, John Major. **The 2012 Story.** New York: Penguin Group, 2009.

Kabade, Rahul. **Sri Muruga.** Wembly: Sri Muruga Publications, 2012.

Kurz, Thomas. **Stretching Scientifically.** Vermont: Stadion Publishing Company, Inc., 1987.

Menen, Rajendar. **The Healing Power of Mudras.** Delhi, India: Pustak Mahal, 2005

Nagar, Shantilal. **Skanda-Karttikeya.** Delhi: B.R. Publishing Corporation, 2006.

Pattanaik, Devdutt. **Shiva: An Introduction.** Mumbai: Vakils, Feffer, and Simons Ltd., 1997

Pinkham, Mark Amaru. **The Truth Behind the Christ Myth: The Redemption of the Peacock Angel.**
    Kempton: Adventure's Unlimited Press, 2002.

Purna, Svami. **The Truth Will Set You Free.** Delhi: New Age Books, 2008.

Purna, Svami. **So You Shall Know the Truth.** Delhi: New Age Books, 2013.

Purna, Svami. **Balanced Yoga.** Delhi: New Age Books, 1990.

Purna, Svami. **Life: A Mysterious Journey.** Charleston, South Carolina: Purna Elements, 2014.

Rhodes, Darren. **Yoga Resource.** Tucson: Tirtha Studios, 2011

Sivananda, Swami. **Lord Shanmukha and His Worship.** Uttaranchal: The Divine Life Society, 2006.

Swenson, David. **Ashtanga Yoga: The Practice Manual.** Texas: Ashtanga Yoga Productions, 1999.

Tsatsouline, Pavel. **Beyond Stretching: Russian Flexibility Breakthroughs.** St. Paul: Dragon Door Publication, 1997.

For more information on the teachings of Sri Svami Purna please visit

www.adhyatmik.org

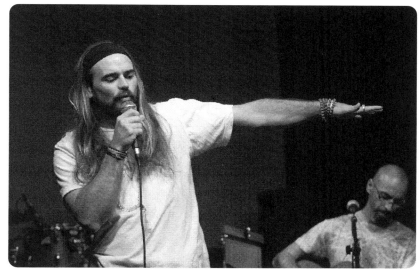

photo by Robert Stolpe

Ken von Roenn III (Yellow Crystal Warrior, ERYT 500) holds a BA in philosophy from the University of Louisville. He is the director of the Skanda Yoga Teacher Training (RYS) at the 200- and 300-hour levels. He lives in Miami, Florida, where he teaches with Lina Vallejo. He is a proud father, lucid dreamer, and a climber.

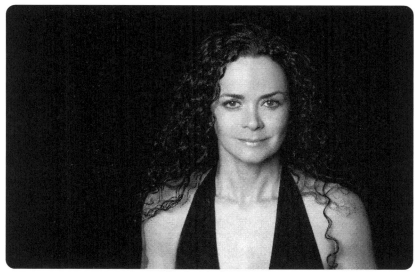

photo by Gabriel Marquez

Lina Vallejo (Blue Spectral Eagle, ERYT) holds a degree in Business from the University of Icesi in Cali, Colombia. She is also a certified AFAA personal trainer. She is the proud mother of two and owner of Skanda Yoga Studio in Miami, Florida. She travels nationally and internationally with Ken, teaching workshops and leading retreats.

Made in the USA
Monee, IL
23 October 2024

68038564R00260